THE COMPLETE
MEDITERRANEAN DIET
COOKBOOK
FOR BEGINNERS

1075
QUICK & EASY MOUTH-WATERING RECIPES THAT ANYONE CAN COOK AT HOME

BY
WILDA BUCKLEY

TABLE OF CONTENTS

Mediterranean
Diet Cookbook
for Beginners

500

Quick and Easy Mouth-watering Recipes that
Busy and Novice Can Cook
2 Weeks Meal Plan Included

By
Wilda Buckley

INTRODUCTION

Mediterranean diet is a specific diet by removing processed foods and/ or high in saturated fats. It's not necessarily about losing weight, but rather a healthy lifestyle choice. It is about ingesting traditional Ingredients consumed by those who live in the Mediterranean basin for a long time. Their diets never changed, so they must be doing something right. This is a diet rich in fruits, vegetables, and fish. Cooking with olive oil is a fundamental ingredient and is an ideal replacement for saturated fats and trans fats. Vegetables and fruits grow well in the heat of the Mediterranean continents, so it's not surprising that the locals devour plenty of them. Studies show that the people who live in these regions live longer and better lives. Changing your own eating habits to one that is proven to be healthy is a good enough reason to begin.

Many studies that have been done on the Mediterranean diet offered promising results.

Heart-healthy diet. Blood pressure tends to drop significantly on the Mediterranean diet; in other words, is a natural way to lower the risk of cardiovascular disease. Researchers have found that the Mediterranean diet can lower your chances of having a stroke and other vascular diseases.

Reduced risk of certain cancers. In general, the Mediterranean diet emphasizes eating plant-based foods and limiting red meat, bad oils, and processed foods. Hence, these eating habits may provide some protection against malignant diseases. People in Mediterranean countries are overall less likely to die from cancer.

Neuroprotective benefits. The Mediterranean diet may improve brain and cogitative functions in older adults (by 15 percent). Clinical trials have shown that those who followed this dietary regimen were less likely to develop Alzheimer's, dementia, or insomnia. A new study has found that antioxidants in the Mediterranean diet plan may protect brain and nerves, cutting the risk of neurological disorders by almost 50 percent.

Weight loss. The Mediterranean diet is the most natural and most delicious way to lose weight and maintain ideal body fat percentage. Low-calorie foods such as fruits, vegetables, yogurt, and fish are widely used in the countries that border the Mediterranean Sea. Natural appetite suppressants include beans, legumes, fat fish, plain dairy products, and high-fiber foods (almost all vegetables, whole grains, apples, avocado, chia seeds). Ginger may control the hunger hormone "ghrelin" too. Consuming a small amount of honey has been shown to reduce appetite. And you will become one step closer to dropping serious pound!

Longevity. Basics of this dietary plan are however vital to longevity and healthy leaving. Other unexpected benefits include reduced risk of developing depression, diabetes management, improved gut health and better mood.

TIPS TO START OFF

Stay Hydrated

Once you've started and are fully immersed in the Mediterranean diet, you might notice that you've started to feel a little bit weak, and a little bit colder, than you're used to. The Mediterranean diet places an emphasis on trying to cut out as much sodium from your diet as possible, which is very healthy for some of us who already have high sodium levels. Sodium, obviously is found in salt, and so we proceed to cut out salt – and then drink enough water to drain every last drop of sodium from our bodies. When it comes to hydration, the biological mechanisms for keeping us saturated and quenched rely on an equal balance of sodium and potassium. Sodium can be found in your interstitial fluid, and potassium can be found inside our cytoplasm – two sides of one wall. When you drink tons of water, sweat a lot at the gym, or both, your sodium leaves your body in your urine and your sweat. Potassium, on the other hand, is only really lost through the urine – and even then, it's rare. This means that our bodies almost constantly need a refill on our sodium levels.

Vitamins and Supplements

Vitamins and minerals can be found in plants and animals, yes, but more often than not fruits and vegetables are much stronger sources. When consume another animal, we are consuming the sum total of all of the energy and nutrition that that animal has also consumed. This might sound like a sweet deal, but the pig you're eating used that energy in his own daily life, and therefore only has a tiny bit left to offer you. Plants, on the other hand, are first-hand sources of things like calcium, vitamin K, and vitamin C, which our bodies require daily doses of.

Meal Preparation and Portion Planning

If you haven't heard of the term "meal prep" before now, it's a beautiful day to learn something that will save you time, stress, and inches on your waistline. Meal prep, short for meal preparation, is a habit that was developed mostly by the body building community in order to accurately track your macronutrients. The basic idea behind meal prep is that each weekend, you manage your free time around cooking and preparing all of your meals for the upcoming week. While most meal preppers do their grocery shopping and cooking on Sundays, to keep their meals the freshest, you can choose to cook on a Saturday if that works better with your schedule. Meal prep each week uses one large grocery list of bulk ingredients to get all the supplies you need to make four dinners and four lunches of your choice. This means that you might have to do a bit of mental math quadrupling the serving size, but all you have to do is multiply each ingredient by four. Although you don't have to meal prep more than one meal with four portions each week, if you're already in the kitchen, you most likely have cooking time to work on something else.

Tracking Your Macronutrients

Wouldn't it be nice if you could have a full nutritional label for each of your home-cooked meals, just to make sure that your numbers are adding up in favor of weight loss? Oddly enough, tracking your macronutrients in order to calculate the nutritional value of each of your meals and portions is as easy as stepping on the scale. Not the scale in your bathroom, however. A food scale! If you've never had a good relationship with your weight and numbers, you might suddenly find that they aren't too bad after all. Food scales are used to measure, well, your food, but there's a slick system of online calculators and fitness applications for your smart phone that can take this number and turn it into magic. When you meal prep each week, keep track of your recipes diligently. Remember how you multiplied each of the ingredients on the list by four to create four servings? You're going to want to remember how much of each vegetable, fruit, grain, nut, and fat you cooked with. While you wait for your meal to finish cooking, find a large enough plastic container to fit all of your meals. Make sure it's clean and dry, and use the empty container to zero out your scale.

Counting Calories and Forming a Deficit

When it comes down to the technical science, there is one way and only one way to lose weight: by eating fewer calories in one day than your body requires to survive. Now, this doesn't mean that you can't lose weight for other reasons – be it water weight, as a result of stress, or simply working out harder. Although counting calories might not be the most fun way to lose weight, a calorie deficit is the only sure-fire way of guaranteeing that you reap all the weight loss benefits of the Mediterranean diet for your efforts. Scientifically, you already know that the healthy rate of weight loss for the average adult is between one and two pounds per week. Get ready for a little bit more math, but it's nothing you can't handle in the name of a smaller waistline. One pound of fat equals around thirty-five hundred Calories, which means that your caloric deficit needs to account for that number, each week, without making too much of a dent on your regular nutrition. For most of us, we're used to eating between fifteen hundred and two thousand calories per day, which gives you a blessedly simply five hundred calorie deficit per day in order to reach your healthy weight loss goals. If you cut out exactly five hundred calories each day, you should be able to lose one pound of fat by the end of seven days. Granted, this estimate does take into account thirty minutes of daily exercise, but the results are still about the same when you rely on the scientific facts. If your age, height, weight, and sex predispose you to eat either more or less calories per day, you might want to consult with your doctor about the healthiest way for you to integrate a caloric deficit into your Mediterranean diet.

Goal Setting to Meet Your Achievements

On the subject of control, there are a few steps and activities that you should go through before you begin your Mediterranean diet just to make sure that you have clear and realistic goals in mind. Sitting down to set goals before embarking on a totally new diet routine will help you stay focused and committed during your Mediterranean diet. While a Mediterranean diet lifestyle certainly isn't as demanding as some of the crazy diet fads you see today, it can be a struggle to focus on eating natural fruits and vegetables that are more "salt of the Earth" foods than we're used to. You already know that when it comes to weight loss, you shouldn't expect to lose more than one to two pounds per week healthily while you're dieting. You are still welcome to set a weight loss goal with time in mind, but when it comes to the Mediterranean diet, you should set your goals for one month in the future.

2-WEEKS MEAL PLAN

DAY	BREAKFAST	LUNCH/DINNER	DESSERT
1.	Avocado Egg Scramble	Delicious Pasta Primavera	Mediterranean Baked Apples
2.	Breakfast Tostadas	Beef with Tomatoes	Mediterranean Diet Cookie Recipe
3.	Parmesan Omelet	Italian Beef	Mediterranean Style Fruit Medley
4.	Menemen	Coriander and Coconut Chicken	Mediterranean Watermelon Salad
5.	Watermelon Pizza	Sage Turkey Mix	Melon Cucumber Smoothie
6.	Ham Muffins	Tasty Greek Rice	Peanut Banana Yogurt Bowl
7.	Baked Oatmeal with Cinnamon	Bulgur salad	Pomegranate and Lychee Sorbet
8.	Creamy Oatmeal with Figs	Lemon Artichokes	Pomegranate Granita with Lychee
9.	Cauliflower Fritters	Turkey and Quinoa Stuffed Peppers	Sweet Tropical Medley Smoothie
10.	Egg Casserole with Paprika	Garlicky Clams	Strawberry Banana Greek Yogurt Parfaits
11.	Avocado Milk Shake	Shrimp, Lemon and Basil Pasta	Summertime Fruit Salad
12.	Banana Quinoa	Quick & Easy Shrimp	Strawberry and Avocado Medley
13.	Morning Pizza with Sprouts	Delicious Pepper Zucchini	Smoothie Bowl with Dragon Fruit
14.	Almond Chia Porridge	Salmon and Watermelon Gazpacho	Roasted Berry and Honey Yogurt Pops

SMOOTHIES & BREAKFASTS RECIPES

1. Avocado Egg Scramble

Preparation time: 8 minutes | Cooking time: 15 minutes | Servings: 4

4 eggs, beaten
1 tablespoon avocado oil
½ teaspoon chili flakes
½ teaspoon salt

1 white onion, diced
1 avocado, finely chopped
1 oz Cheddar cheese, shredded
1 tablespoon fresh parsley

1. Pour avocado oil in the skillet and bring it to boil.
2. Then add diced onion and roast it until it is light brown.
3. Meanwhile, mix up together chili flakes, beaten eggs, and salt.
4. Pour the egg mixture over the cooked onion and cook the mixture for 1 minute over the medium heat.
5. After this, scramble the eggs well with the help of the fork or spatula. Cook the eggs until they are solid but soft.
6. After this, add chopped avocado and shredded cheese.
7. Stir the scramble well and transfer in the serving plates.
8. Sprinkle the meal with fresh parsley.

NUTRITION:
Calories 236, Fat 20.1, Fiber 4, Carbs 7.4, Protein 8.6

2. Breakfast Tostadas

Preparation time: 15 minutes | Cooking time: 6 minutes | Servings: 6

½ white onion, diced
1 cucumber, chopped
½ jalapeno pepper, chopped
6 corn tortillas
2 oz Cheddar cheese, shredded
6 eggs
½ teaspoon Sea salt

1 tomato, chopped
1 tablespoon fresh cilantro, hopped
1 tablespoon lime juice
1 tablespoon canola oil
½ cup white beans, canned, drained
½ teaspoon butter

1. Make Pico de Galo: in the salad bowl combine together diced white onion, tomato, cucumber, fresh cilantro, and jalapeno pepper.
2. Then add lime juice and a ½ tablespoon of canola oil. Mix up the mixture well. Pico de Galo is cooked.
3. After this, preheat the oven to 390F.
4. Line the tray with baking paper.
5. Arrange the corn tortillas on the baking paper and brush with remaining canola oil from both sides.
6. Bake the tortillas for 10 minutes or until they start to be crunchy.
7. Chill the cooked crunchy tortillas well.
8. Meanwhile, toss the butter in the skillet.
9. Crack the eggs in the melted butter and sprinkle them with sea salt.
10. Fry the eggs until the egg whites become white (cooked). Approximately for 3-5 minutes over the medium heat.
11. After this, mash the beans until you get puree texture.
12. Spread the bean puree on the corn tortillas.
13. Add fried eggs.
14. Then top the eggs with Pico de Galo and shredded Cheddar cheese.

NUTRITION:
Calories 246, fat 11.1, fiber 4.7, carbs 24.5, protein 13.7

3. Parmesan Omelet

Preparation time: 5 minutes | Cooking time: 10 minutes | Servings: 2

1 tablespoon cream cheese
¼ teaspoon paprika
¼ teaspoon dried dill
1 teaspoon coconut oil

2 eggs, beaten
½ teaspoon dried oregano
1 oz Parmesan, grated

1. Mix up together cream cheese with eggs, dried oregano, and dill.
2. Place coconut oil in the skillet and heat it up until it will coat all the skillet.

3. Then pour the egg mixture in the skillet and flatten it.
4. Add grated Parmesan and close the lid.
5. Cook omelet for 10 minutes over the low heat.
6. Then transfer the cooked omelet in the serving plate and sprinkle with paprika.

NUTRITION:
Calories 148, fat 11.5, fiber 0.3, carbs 1.4, protein 10.6

4. Menemen

Preparation time: 6 minutes | Cooking time: 15 minutes | Servings: 4

2 tomatoes, chopped
1 bell pepper, chopped
¼ cup of water
½ white onion, diced
1/3 teaspoon sea salt

2 eggs, beaten
1 teaspoon tomato paste
1 teaspoon butter
½ teaspoon chili flakes

1. Put butter in the pan and melt it.
2. Add bell pepper and cook it for 3 minutes over the medium heat. Stir it from time to time.
3. After this, add diced onion and cook it for 2 minutes more.
4. Stir the vegetables and add tomatoes.
5. Cook them for 5 minutes over the medium-low heat.
6. Then add water and tomato paste. Stir well.
7. Add beaten eggs, chili flakes, and sea salt.
8. Stir well and cook menemen for 4 minutes over the medium-low heat.
9. The cooked meal should be half runny.

NUTRITION:
Calories 67, fat 3.4, fiber 1.5, carbs 6.4, protein 3.8

5. Watermelon Pizza

Preparation time: 10 minutes | Servings: 2

9 oz watermelon slice
2 oz Feta cheese, crumbled

1 tablespoon Pomegranate sauce
1 tablespoon fresh cilantro, chopped

1. Place the watermelon slice in the plate and sprinkle with crumbled Feta cheese.
2. Add fresh cilantro.
3. After this, sprinkle the pizza with Pomegranate juice generously.
4. Cut the pizza into the servings.

NUTRITION:
Calories 143, fat 6.2, fiber 0.6, carbs 18.4, protein 5.1

6. Ham Muffins

Preparation time: 10 minutes | Cooking time: 15 minutes | Servings: 4

3 oz ham, chopped
2 tablespoons coconut flour
¼ teaspoon dried cilantro

4 eggs, beaten
½ teaspoon dried oregano
Cooking spray

1. Spray the muffin's molds with cooking spray from inside.
2. In the bowl mix up together beaten eggs, coconut flour, dried oregano, cilantro, and ham.
3. When the liquid is homogenous, pour it in the prepared muffin molds.
4. Bake the muffins for 15 minutes at 360F.
5. Chill the cooked meal well and only after this remove from the molds.

NUTRITION:
Calories 128, fat 7.2, fiber 2.9, carbs 5.3, protein 10.1

7. Morning Pizza with Sprouts

Preparation time: 15 minutes | Cooking time: 20 minutes | Servings: 6

½ cup wheat flour, whole grain	2 tablespoons butter, softened
¼ teaspoon baking powder	¾ teaspoon salt
5 oz chicken fillet, boiled	2 oz Cheddar cheese, shredded
1 teaspoon tomato sauce	1 oz bean sprouts

1. Make the pizza crust: mix up together wheat flour, butter, baking powder, and salt. Knead the soft and non-sticky dough. Add more wheat flour if needed.
2. Leave the dough for 10 minutes to chill.
3. Then place the dough on the baking paper. Cover it with the second baking paper sheet.
4. Roll up the dough with the help of the rolling pin to get the round pizza crust.
5. After this, remove the upper baking paper sheet.
6. Transfer the pizza crust in the tray.
7. Spread the crust with tomato sauce.
8. Then shred the chicken fillet and arrange it over the pizza crust.
9. Add shredded Cheddar cheese.
10. Bake pizza for 20 minutes at 355F.
11. Then top the cooked pizza with bean sprouts and slice into the servings.

NUTRITION:
Calories 157, fat 8.8, fiber 0.3, carbs 8.4, protein 10.5

8. Banana Quinoa

Preparation time: 10 minutes | Cooking time: 12 minutes | Servings: 4

1 cup quinoa	2 cup milk
1 teaspoon vanilla extract	1 teaspoon honey
2 bananas, sliced	¼ teaspoon ground cinnamon

1. Pour milk in the saucepan and add quinoa.
2. Close the lid and cook it over the medium heat for 12 minutes or until quinoa will absorb all liquid.
3. Then chill the quinoa for 10-15 minutes and place in the serving mason jars.
4. Add honey, vanilla extract, and ground cinnamon.
5. Stir well.
6. Top quinoa with banana and stir it before serving.

NUTRITION:
Calories 279, fat 5.3, fiber 4.6, carbs 48.4, protein 10.7

9. Avocado Milk Shake

Preparation time: 10 minutes | Servings: 3

1 avocado, peeled, pitted	2 tablespoons of liquid honey
½ teaspoon vanilla extract	½ cup heavy cream
1 cup milk	1/3 cup ice cubes

DIRECTIONS
1. Chop the avocado and put in the food processor.
2. Add liquid honey, vanilla extract, heavy cream, milk, and ice cubes.
3. Blend the mixture until it smooth.
4. Pour the cooked milkshake in the serving glasses.
NUTRITION: Calories 291, fat 22.1, fiber 4.5, carbs 22, protein 4.4

10. Egg Casserole with Paprika

Preparation time: 10 minutes | Cooking time: 28 minutes | Servings: 4

2 eggs, beaten	1 red bell pepper, chopped
1 chili pepper, chopped	½ red onion, diced
1 teaspoon canola oil	½ teaspoon salt
1 teaspoon paprika	1 tablespoon fresh cilantro, chopped
1 garlic clove, diced	1 teaspoon butter, softened
¼ teaspoon chili flakes	

1. Brush the casserole mold with canola oil and pour beaten eggs inside.

2. After this, toss the butter in the skillet and melt it over the medium heat.
3. Add chili pepper and red bell pepper.
4. After this, add red onion and cook the vegetables for 7-8 minutes over the medium heat. Stir them from time to time.
5. Transfer the vegetables in the casserole mold.
6. Add salt, paprika, cilantro, diced garlic, and chili flakes. Stir gently with the help of a spatula to get a homogenous mixture.
7. Bake the casserole for 20 minutes at 355F in the oven.
8. Then chill the meal well and cut into servings. Transfer the casserole in the serving plates with the help of the spatula.

NUTRITION:
Calories 68, fat 4.5, fiber 1, carbs 4.4, protein 3.4

11. Cauliflower Fritters

Preparation time: 10 minutes | Cooking time: 10 minutes | Servings: 2

1 cup cauliflower, shredded	1 egg, beaten
1 tablespoon wheat flour, whole grain	1 oz Parmesan, grated
½ teaspoon ground black pepper	1 tablespoon canola oil

1. In the mixing bowl mix up together shredded cauliflower and egg.
2. Add wheat flour, grated Parmesan, and ground black pepper.
3. Stir the mixture with the help of the fork until it is homogenous and smooth.
4. Pour canola oil in the skillet and bring it to boil.
5. Make the fritters from the cauliflower mixture with the help of the fingertips or use spoon and transfer in the hot oil.
6. Roast the fritters for 4 minutes from each side over the medium-low heat.

NUTRITION:
Calories 167, fat 12.3, fiber 1.5, carbs 6.7, protein 8.8

12. Creamy Oatmeal with Figs

Preparation time: 10 minutes | Cooking time: 20 minutes | Servings: 5

2 cups oatmeal	1 ½ cup milk
1 tablespoon butter	3 figs, chopped
1 tablespoon honey	

1. Pour milk in the saucepan.
2. Add oatmeal and close the lid.
3. Cook the oatmeal for 15 minutes over the medium-low heat.
4. Then add chopped figs and honey.
5. Add butter and mix up the oatmeal well.
6. Cook it for 5 minutes more.
7. Close the lid and let the cooked breakfast rest for 10 minutes before serving.

NUTRITION:
Calories 222, fat 6, fiber 4.4, carbs 36.5, protein 7.1

13. Baked Oatmeal with Cinnamon

Preparation time: 10 minutes | Cooking time: 25 minutes | Servings: 4

1 cup oatmeal	1/3 cup milk
1 pear, chopped	1 teaspoon vanilla extract
1 tablespoon Splenda	1 teaspoon butter
½ teaspoon ground cinnamon	1 egg, beaten

1. In the big bowl mix up together oatmeal, milk, egg, vanilla extract, Splenda, and ground cinnamon.
2. Melt butter and add it in the oatmeal mixture.
3. Then add chopped pear and stir it well.
4. Transfer the oatmeal mixture in the casserole mold and flatten gently. Cover it with the foil and secure edges.
5. Bake the oatmeal for 25 minutes at 350F.

NUTRITION:
Calories 151, fat 3.9, fiber 3.3, carbs 23.6, protein 4.9

14. Almond Chia Porridge

Preparation time: 10 minutes | Cooking time: 30 minutes | Servings: 4

3 cups organic almond milk
1 teaspoon vanilla extract
¼ teaspoon ground cardamom

1/3 cup chia seeds, dried
1 tablespoon honey

1. Pour almond milk in the saucepan and bring it to boil.
2. Then chill the almond milk to the room temperature (or appx. For 10-15 minutes).
3. Add vanilla extract, honey, and ground cardamom. Stir well.
4. After this, add chia seeds and stir again.
5. Close the lid and let chia seeds soak the liquid for 20-25 minutes.
6. Transfer the cooked porridge into the serving ramekins.

NUTRITION:
Calories 150, fat 7.3, fiber 6.1, carbs 18, protein 3.7

15. Cocoa Oatmeal

Preparation time: 10 minutes | Cooking time: 15 minutes | Servings: 2

1 ½ cup oatmeal
½ cup heavy cream
1 teaspoon vanilla extract
2 tablespoons Splenda

1 tablespoon cocoa powder
¼ cup of water
1 tablespoon butter

1. Mix up together oatmeal with cocoa powder and Splenda.
2. Transfer the mixture in the saucepan.
3. Add vanilla extract, water, and heavy cream. Stir it gently with the help of the spatula.
4. Close the lid and cook it for 10-15 minutes over the medium-low heat.
5. Remove the cooked cocoa oatmeal from the heat and add butter. Stir it well.

NUTRITION:
Calories 230, fat 10.6, fiber 3.5, carbs 28.1, protein 4.6

16. Cinnamon Roll Oats

Preparation time: 7 minutes | Cooking time: 10 minutes | Servings: 4

½ cup rolled oats
1 teaspoon vanilla extract
2 teaspoon honey
1 teaspoon butter

1 cup milk
1 teaspoon ground cinnamon
2 tablespoons Plain yogurt

1. Pour milk in the saucepan and bring it to boil.
2. Add rolled oats and stir well.
3. Close the lid and simmer the oats for 5 minutes over the medium heat. The cooked oats will absorb all milk.
4. Then add butter and stir the oats well.
5. In the separated bowl, whisk together Plain yogurt with honey, cinnamon, and vanilla extract.
6. Transfer the cooked oats in the serving bowls.
7. Top the oats with the yogurt mixture in the shape of the wheel.

NUTRITION:
Calories 243, fat 20.2, fiber 1, carbs 2.8, protein 13.3

17. Pumpkin Oatmeal with Spices

Preparation time: 10 minutes | Cooking time: 13 minutes | Servings: 6

2 cups oatmeal
1 cup milk
2 tablespoons pumpkin puree
½ teaspoon butter

1 cup of coconut milk
1 teaspoon Pumpkin pie spices
1 tablespoon Honey

1. Pour coconut milk and milk in the saucepan. Add butter and bring the liquid to boil.
2. Add oatmeal, stir well with the help of a spoon and close the lid.
3. Simmer the oatmeal for 7 minutes over the medium heat.
4. Meanwhile, mix up together honey, pumpkin pie spices, and pumpkin puree.

5. When the oatmeal is cooked, add pumpkin puree mixture and stir well.
6. Transfer the cooked breakfast in the serving plates.

NUTRITION:
Calories 232, fat 12.5, fiber 3.8, carbs 26.2, protein 5.9

18. Zucchini Oats

Preparation time: 10 minutes | Cooking time: 10 minutes | Servings: 4

2 cups rolled oats
½ teaspoon salt
1 zucchini, grated

2 cups of water
1 tablespoon butter
¼ teaspoon ground ginger

1. Pour water in the saucepan.
2. Add rolled oats, butter, and salt.
3. Stir gently and start to cook the oats for 4 minutes over the high heat.
4. When the mixture starts to boil, add ground ginger and grated zucchini. Stir well.
5. Cook the oats for 5 minutes more over the medium-low heat.

NUTRITION:
Calories 189, fat 5.7, fiber 4.7, carbs 29.4, protein 6

19. Breakfast Spanakopita

Preparation time: 15 minutes | Cooking time: 1 hour | Servings: 6

2 cups spinach
½ cup fresh parsley
3 oz Feta cheese, crumbled
2 eggs, beaten
2 oz Phyllo dough

1 white onion, diced
1 teaspoon minced garlic
1 teaspoon ground paprika
1/3 cup butter, melted

1. Separate Phyllo dough into 2 parts.
2. Brush the casserole mold with butter well and place 1 part of Phyllo dough inside.
3. Brush its surface with butter too.
4. Put the spinach and fresh parsley in the blender. Blend it until smooth and transfer in the mixing bowl.
5. Add minced garlic, Feta cheese, ground paprika, eggs, and diced onion. Mix up well.
6. Place the spinach mixture in the casserole mold and flatten it well.
7. Cover the spinach mixture with remaining Phyllo dough and pour remaining butter over it.
8. Bake spanakopita for 1 hour at 350F.
9. Cut it into the servings.

NUTRITION:
Calories 190, fat 15.4, fiber 1.1, carbs 8.4, protein 5.4

20. Quinoa Bowl

Preparation time: 10 minutes | Cooking time: 20 minutes | Servings: 4

1 sweet potato, peeled, chopped
½ teaspoon chili flakes
1 cup quinoa
1 teaspoon butter

1 tablespoon olive oil
½ teaspoon salt
2 cups of water
1 tablespoon fresh cilantro, chopped

1. Line the baking tray with parchment.
2. Arrange the chopped sweet potato in the tray and sprinkle it with chili flakes, salt, and olive oil.
3. Bake the sweet potato for 20 minutes at 355F.
4. Meanwhile, pour water in the saucepan.
5. Add quinoa and cook it over the medium heat for 7 minutes or until quinoa will absorb all liquid.
6. Add butter in the cooked quinoa and stir well.
7. Transfer it in the bowls, add baked sweet potato and chopped cilantro.

NUTRITION:
Calories 221, fat 7.1, fiber 3.9, carbs 33.2, protein 6.6

21. Overnight Oats with Nuts

Preparation time: 10 minutes | Cooking time: 8 hours | Servings: 2

½ cup oats
1 tablespoon almond, chopped
1 cup skim milk
½ teaspoon vanilla extract

2 teaspoons chia seeds, dried
½ teaspoon walnuts, chopped
2 teaspoons honey

1. In the big bowl mix up together chia seeds, oats, honey, and vanilla extract.
2. Then add skim milk, walnuts, and almonds. Stir well.
3. Transfer the prepared mixture into the mason jars and close with lids.
4. Put the mason jars in the fridge and leave overnight.
5. Store the meal in the fridge up to 2 days.

NUTRITION:
Calories 202, fat 5.4, fiber 4.9, carbs 29.4, protein 8.7

22. Stuffed Figs

Preparation time: 10 minutes | Cooking time: 15 minutes | Servings: 2

7 oz fresh figs
½ teaspoon walnuts, chopped
¼ teaspoon paprika
½ teaspoon canola oil

1 tablespoon cream cheese
4 bacon slices
¼ teaspoon salt
½ teaspoon honey

1. Make the crosswise cuts in every fig.
2. In the shallow bowl mix up together cream cheese, walnuts, paprika, and salt.
3. Fill the figs with cream cheese mixture and wrap in the bacon.
4. Secure the fruits with toothpicks and sprinkle with honey.
5. Line the baking tray with baking paper.
6. Place the prepared figs in the tray and sprinkle them with olive oil gently.
7. Bake the figs for 15 minutes at 350F.

NUTRITION:
Calories 299, fat 19.4, fiber 2.3, carbs 16.7, protein 15.2

23. Poblano Fritatta

Preparation time: 10 minutes | Cooking time: 15 minutes | Servings: 4

5 eggs, beaten
1 oz scallions, chopped
½ teaspoon butter
½ teaspoon chili flakes

1 poblano chile, chopped, raw
1/3 cup heavy cream
½ teaspoon salt
1 tablespoon fresh cilantro, chopped

1. Mix up together eggs with heavy cream and whisk until homogenous.
2. Add chopped poblano chile, scallions, salt, chili flakes, and fresh cilantro.
3. Toss butter in the skillet and melt it.
4. Add egg mixture and flatten it in the skillet if needed.
5. Close the lid and cook the frittata for 15 minutes over the medium-low heat.
6. When the frittata is cooked, it will be solid.

NUTRITION:
Calories 131, fat 10.4, fiber 0.2, carbs 1.3, protein 8.2

24. Mushroom-Egg Casserole

Preparation time: 7 minutes | Cooking time: 25 minutes | Servings: 3

½ cup mushrooms, chopped
4 eggs, beaten
½ teaspoon chili pepper
1 teaspoon canola oil

½ yellow onion, diced
1 tablespoon coconut flakes
1 oz Cheddar cheese, shredded

1. Pour canola oil in the skillet and preheat well.
2. Add mushrooms and onion and roast for 5-8 minutes or until the vegetables are light brown.
3. Transfer the cooked vegetables in the casserole mold.
4. Add coconut flakes, chili pepper, and Cheddar cheese.

5. Then add eggs and stir well.
6. Bake the casserole for 15 minutes at 360F.

NUTRITION:
Calories 152, fat 11.1, fiber 0.7, carbs 3, protein 10.4

25. Vegetable Breakfast Bowl

Preparation time: 10 minutes | Cooking time: 35 minutes | Servings: 4

1 cup sweet potatoes, peeled, chopped
1 red onion, sliced
½ teaspoon garlic powder
1 tablespoon olive oil
1 tablespoon coconut milk

1 russet potato, chopped
2 bell pepper, trimmed
¾ teaspoon onion powder
1 tablespoon Sriracha sauce

1. Line the baking tray with baking paper.
2. Place the chopped russet potato and sweet potato in the tray.
3. Add onion, bell peppers, and sprinkle the vegetables with olive oil, onion powder, and garlic powder.
4. Mix up the vegetables well with the help of the fingertips and transfer in the preheated to the 360F oven.
5. Bake the vegetables for 45 minutes.
6. Meanwhile, make the sauce: mix up together Sriracha sauce and coconut milk.
7. Transfer the cooked vegetables in the serving plates and sprinkle with Sriracha sauce.

NUTRITION:
Calories 213, fat 7.2, fiber 4.8, carbs 34.6, protein 3.6

26. Breakfast Green Smoothie

Preparation time: 7 minutes | Servings: 2

2 cups spinach
1 cup bok choy
1 tablespoon almonds, chopped

2 cups kale
1 ½ cup organic almond milk
½ cup of water

1. Place all ingredients in the blender and blend until you get a smooth mixture.
2. Pour the smoothie in the serving glasses.
3. Add ice cubes if desired.

NUTRITION:
Calories 107, fat 3.6, fiber 2.4, carbs 15.5, protein 4.8

27. Simple and Quick Steak

Preparation time: 15 minutes | Cooking time: 10 minutes | Servings: 2

½ lb steak, quality - cut

Salt and freshly cracked black pepper

1. Switch on the air fryer, set frying basket in it, then set its temperature to 385°F and let preheat.
2. Meanwhile, prepare the steaks, and for this, season steaks with salt and freshly cracked black pepper on both sides.
3. When air fryer has preheated, add prepared steaks in the fryer basket, shut it with lid and cook for 15 minutes.
4. When done, transfer steaks to a dish and then serve immediately.
5. For meal prepping, evenly divide the steaks between two heatproof containers, close them with lid and refrigerate for up to 3 days until ready to serve.
6. When ready to eat, reheat steaks into the microwave until hot and then serve.

NUTRITION:
Calories 301, Total Fat 25.1, Protein 19.1g, Sodium 65mg

28. Almonds Crusted Rack of Lamb with Rosemary

Preparation time: 10 minutes | Cooking time: 35 minutes | Servings: 2

1 garlic clove, minced	½ tbsp olive oil
Salt and freshly cracked black pepper	¾ lb rack of lamb
1 small organic egg	1 tbsp breadcrumbs
2 oz almonds, finely chopped	½ tbsp fresh rosemary, chopped

1. Switch on the oven and set its temperature to 350°F, and let it preheat.
2. Meanwhile, take a baking tray, grease it with oil, and set aside until required.
3. Mix garlic, oil, salt, and freshly cracked black pepper in a bowl and coat the rack of lamb with this garlic, rub on all sides.
4. Crack the egg in a bowl, whisk until blended, and set aside until required.
5. Place breadcrumbs in another dish, add almonds and rosemary and stir until mixed.
6. Dip the seasoned rack of lamb with egg, dredge with the almond mixture until evenly coated on all sides and then place it onto the prepared baking tray.
7. When the oven has preheated, place the rack of lamb in it, and cook for 35 minutes until thoroughly cooked.
8. When done, take out the baking tray, transfer rack of lamb onto a dish, and serve straight away.
9. For meal prep, cut rack of lamb into pieces, evenly divide the lamb between two heatproof containers, close them with lid and refrigerate for up to 3 days until ready to serve.
10. When ready to eat, reheat rack of lamb in the microwave until hot and then serve.

NUTRITION:
Calories 471, Total Fat 31.6g, Total Carbs 8.5g, Protein 39g, Sugar 1.5g, Sodium 145mg

29. Cheesy Eggs in Avocado

Preparation time: 20 minutes | Cooking time: 15 minutes | Servings: 2

1 medium avocado	2 organic eggs
¼ cup shredded cheddar cheese	Salt and freshly cracked black pepper
1 tbsp olive oil	

1. Switch on the oven, then set its temperature to 425°F, and let preheat.
2. Meanwhile, prepare the avocados and for this, cut the avocado in half and remove its pit.
3. Take two muffin tins, grease them with oil, and then add an avocado half into each tin.
4. Crack an egg into each avocado half, season well with salt and freshly cracked black pepper, and then sprinkle cheese on top.
5. When the oven has preheated, place the muffin tins in the oven and bake for 15 minutes until cooked.
6. When done, take out the muffin tins, transfer the avocados baked organic eggs to a dish, and then serve them.

NUTRITION:
Calories 210, Total Fat 16.6g, Total Carbs 6.4g, Protein 10.7g, Sugar 2.2g, Sodium 151mg

30. Bacon, Vegetable and Parmesan Combo

Preparation time: 10 minutes | Cooking time: 25 minutes | Servings: 2

- 2 slices of bacon, thick-cut
- ½ tbsp mayonnaise
- ½ of medium green bell pepper, deseeded, chopped
- 1 scallion, chopped
- ¼ cup grated Parmesan cheese
- 1 tbsp olive oil

1. Switch on the oven, then set its temperature to 375°F and let it preheat.

2. Meanwhile, take a baking dish, grease it with oil, and add slices of bacon in it.
3. Spread mayonnaise on top of the bacon, then top with bell peppers and scallions, sprinkle with Parmesan cheese and bake for about 25 minutes until cooked thoroughly.
4. When done, take out the baking dish and serve immediately.
5. For meal prepping, wrap bacon in a plastic sheet and refrigerate for up to 2 days.
6. When ready to eat, reheat bacon in the microwave and then serve.

NUTRITION:
Calories 197, Total Fat 13.8g, Total Carbs 4.7g, Protein 14.3g, Sugar 1.9g, Sodium 662mg

31. Four-Cheese Zucchini Noodles with Basil Pesto

Preparation time: 10 minutes | Cooking time: 15 minutes | Servings: 2

4 cups zucchini noodles	4 oz Mascarpone cheese
1/8 cup Romano cheese	2 tbsp grated parmesan cheese
¼ tsp salt	½ tsp cracked black pepper
2 1/8 tsp ground nutmeg	1/8 cup basil pesto
½ cup shredded mozzarella cheese	1 tbsp olive oil

1. Switch on the oven, then set its temperature to 400°F and let it preheat.
2. Meanwhile, place zucchini noodles in a heatproof bowl and microwave at high heat setting for 3 minutes, set aside until required.
3. Take another heatproof bowl, add all cheeses in it, except for mozzarella, season with salt, black pepper and nutmeg, and microwave at high heat setting for 1 minute until cheese has melted.
4. Whisk the cheese mixture, add cooked zucchini noodles in it along with basil pesto and mozzarella cheese and fold until well mixed.
5. Take a casserole dish, grease it with oil, add zucchini noodles mixture in it, and then bake for 10 minutes until done.
6. Serve straight away.

NUTRITION:
Calories 139, Total Fat 9.7g, Total Carbs 3.3, Protein 10.2g, Sodium 419mg, Sugar 0.2g

32. Baked Eggs with Cheddar and Beef

Preparation time: 10 minutes | Cooking time: 20 minutes | Servings: 2

3 oz ground beef, cooked	2 organic eggs
2oz shredded cheddar cheese	1 tbsp olive oil

1. Switch on the oven, then set its temperature to 390°F and let it preheat.
2. Meanwhile, take a baking dish, grease it with oil, add spread cooked beef in the bottom, then make two holes in it and crack an organic egg into each hole.
3. Sprinkle cheese on top of beef and eggs and bake for 20 minutes until beef has cooked and eggs have set.
4. When done, let baked eggs cool for 5 minutes and then serve straight away.
5. For meal prepping, wrap baked eggs in foil and refrigerate for up to two days.
6. When ready to eat, reheat baked eggs in the microwave and then serve.

NUTRITION:
Calories 512, Total Fat 32.8g, Total Carbs 1.4g, Protein 51g, Sugar 1g, Sodium 531mg

33. Heavenly Egg Bake with Blackberry

Preparation time: 10 minutes | Cooking time: 15 minutes | Servings: 4

Chopped rosemary	1 tsp lime zest
½ tsp salt	¼ tsp vanilla extract, unsweetened
1 tsp grated ginger	3 tbsp coconut flour
1 tbsp unsalted butter	5 organic eggs
1 tbsp olive oil	½ cup fresh blackberries
Black pepper to taste	

1. Switch on the oven, then set its temperature to 350°F and let it preheat.
2. Meanwhile, place all the ingredients in a blender, reserving the berries and pulse for 2 to 3 minutes until well blended and smooth.
3. Take four silicon muffin cups, grease them with oil, evenly distribute the blended batter in the cups, top with black pepper and bake for 15 minutes until cooked through and the top has golden brown.
4. When done, let blueberry egg bake cool in the muffin cups for 5 minutes, then take them out, cool them on a wire rack and then serve.
5. For meal prepping, wrap each egg bake with aluminum foil and freeze for up to 3 days.
6. When ready to eat, reheat blueberry egg bake in the microwave and then serve.

NUTRITION:
Calories 144, Total Fat 10g, Total Carbs 2g, Protein 8.5g

34. Protein-Packed Blender Pancakes

Preparation time: 5 minutes | Cooking time: 10 minutes | Servings: 1

2 organic eggs	1 scoop protein powder
Salt to taste	¼ tsp cinnamon
2oz cream cheese, soften	1 tsp unsalted butter

1. Crack the eggs in a blender, add remaining ingredients except for butter and pulse for 2 minutes until well combined and blended.
2. Take a skillet pan, place it over medium heat, add butter and when it melts, pour in prepared batter, spread it evenly, and cook for 4 to 5 minutes per side until cooked through and golden brown.
3. Serve straight away.

NUTRITION:
Calories 450, Total Fat 29g, Total Carbs 4g, Protein 41g

35. Blueberry and Vanilla Scones

Preparation time: 10 minutes | Cooking time: 10 minutes | Servings: 12

1½ cup almond flour	3 organic eggs, beaten
2 tsp baking powder	½ cup stevia
2 tsp vanilla extract, unsweetened	¾ cup fresh raspberries
1 tbsp olive oil	

1. Switch on the oven, then set its temperature to 375 °F and let it preheat.
2. Take a large bowl, add flour and eggs in it, stir in baking powder, stevia, and vanilla until combined and then fold in berries until mixed.
3. Take a baking dish, grease it with oil, scoop the prepared batter on it with an ice cream scoop and bake for 10 minutes until done.
4. When done, transfer scones on a wire rack, cool them completely, and then serve.

NUTRITION:
Calories 133, Total Fat 8g, Total Carbs 4g, Protein 2g

36. Healthy Blueberry and Coconut Smoothie

Preparation time: 5 minutes | Servings: 2

1 cup fresh blueberries	1 tsp vanilla extract, unsweetened
28 oz coconut milk, unsweetened	2 tbsp lemon juice

1. Add berries in a blender or food processor, then add remaining ingredients and pulse for 2 minutes until smooth and creamy.

2. Divide the smoothie between two glasses and serve.

NUTRITION:
Calories 152, Total Fat 13.1g, Total Carbs 6.9g, Protein 1.5g, Sugar 4.5g, Sodium 1mg

37. Avocado and Eggs Breakfast Tacos

Preparation time: 10 minutes | Cooking time: 13 minutes | Servings: 2

4 organic eggs	1 tbsp unsalted butter
2 low-carb tortillas	2 tbsp mayonnaise
4 sprigs of cilantro	½ of an avocado, sliced
Salt and freshly cracked black pepper, to taste	1 tbsp Tabasco sauce

1. Take a bowl, crack eggs in it and whisk well until smooth.
2. Take a skillet pan, place it over medium heat, add butter and when it melts, pour in eggs, spread them evenly in the pan and cook for 4 to 5 minutes until done.
3. When done, transfer eggs to a plate and set aside until required.
4. Add tortillas into the pan, cook for 2 to 3 minutes per side until warm through, and then transfer them onto a plate.
5. Assemble tacos and for this, spread mayonnaise on the side of each tortilla, then distribute cooked eggs, and top with cilantro and sliced avocado.
6. Season with salt and black pepper, drizzle with tabasco sauce, and roll up the tortillas.
7. Serve straight away or store in the refrigerator for up to 2 days until ready to eat.

NUTRITION:
Calories 289, Total Fat 27g, Total Carbs 6g, Protein 7g

38. Delicious Frittata with Brie and Bacon

Preparation time: 10 minutes | Cooking time: 20 minutes | Servings: 2

4 slices of bacon	4 organic eggs, beaten
½ cup heavy cream	Salt and freshly cracked black pepper, to taste
4 oz brie, diced	1 ½ cup of water
1 tbsp olive oil	

1. Switch on the instant pot, insert its inner pot, press the 'sauté' button, and when hot, add bacon slices and cook for 5 to 7 minutes until crispy.
2. Then transfer bacon to a plate lined with paper towels to drain grease and set aside until required.
3. Crack eggs in a bowl, add cream, season with salt and black pepper and whisk until combined.
4. Chop the cooked bacon, add to the eggs along with brie and stir until mixed.
5. Take a baking dish, grease it with oil, pour in the egg mixture, and spread evenly.
6. Carefully pour water into the instant pot, insert a trivet stand, place baking dish on it, shut with lid, then press the 'manual' button and cook the frittata for 20 minutes at high-pressure setting.
7. When the timer beeps, press the 'cancel' button, allow pressure to release naturally until pressure valve drops, then open the lid and take out the baking dish.
8. Wipe clean moisture on top of the frittata with a paper towel and let it cool completely.
9. For meal prep, cut frittata into six slices, then place each slice in a plastic bag or airtight container and store in the refrigerator for up to three days or store in the freezer until ready to eat.

NUTRITION:
Calories 210, Total Fat 19g, Saturated Fat 8g, Total Carbs 3g, Protein 13g, Fiber 0g

39. Awesome Coffee with Butter

Preparation time: 5 minutes | Cooking time: 5 minutes | Servings: 1

1 cup of water

1 tbsp unsalted butter

1 tbsp coconut oil

2 tbsp coffee

1. Take a small pan, place it over medium heat, pour in water, and bring to boil.
2. Then add remaining ingredients, stir well, and cook until butter and oil have melted.
3. Remove pan from heat, pass the coffee through a strainer, and serve immediately.

NUTRITION:

Calories 230, Total Fat 25g, Total Carbs 0g, Protein 0g

40. Buttered Thyme Scallops

Preparation time: 10 minutes | Cooking time: 5 minutes | Servings: 2

¾ lb sea scallops

Salt and freshly cracked black pepper, to taste

1 tbsp olive oil

½ tbsp fresh minced thyme

1 tbsp unsalted butter, melted

1. Switch on the oven, then set its temperature to 390°F and let it preheat.
2. Take a large bowl, add all the ingredients in it and toss until well coated.
3. Take a baking dish, grease it with oil, add prepared scallop mixture in it and bake for 5 minutes until thoroughly cooked.
4. When done, take out the baking dish, then scallops cool for 5 minutes and then serve.
5. For meal prepping, transfer scallops into an airtight container and store in the refrigerator for up to two days.
6. When ready to eat, reheat scallops in the microwave until hot and then serve.

NUTRITION:

Calories 202, Total Fat 7.1g, Total Carbs 4.4g, Protein 28.7g, Sugar 0g, Sodium 315mg

41. Cheesy Caprese Style Portobellos Mushrooms

Preparation time: 5 minutes | Cooking time: 15 minutes | Servings: 2

2 large caps of Portobello mushroom, gills removed

Salt and freshly cracked black pepper, to taste

4 tbsp olive oil

4 tomatoes, halved

¼ cup fresh basil

¼ cup shredded Mozzarella cheese

1. Switch on the oven, then set its temperature to 400°F and let it preheat.
2. Meanwhile, prepare mushrooms, and for this, brush them with olive oil and set aside until required.
3. Place tomatoes in a bowl, season with salt and black pepper, add basil, drizzle with oil and toss until mixed.
4. Distribute cheese evenly in the bottom of each mushroom cap and then top with prepared tomato mixture.
5. Take a baking sheet, line it with aluminum foil, place prepared mushrooms on it and bake for 15 minutes until thoroughly cooked.

NUTRITION:

Calories 315, Total Fat 29.2g, Total Carbs 14.2g, Protein 4.7g, Sugar 10.4g, Sodium 55mg

42. Persimmon Toast with Cream Cheese

Preparation time: 5 minutes | Cooking time: 3 minutes | Servings: 2

2 slices whole-grain bread

2 teaspoons cream cheese

1 persimmon

1 teaspoon honey

1. Toast the bread with the help of the toaster. You should get light brown bread slices.
2. After this, slice persimmon.
3. Spread the cream cheese on the toasted bread and top it with sliced persimmon.
4. Then sprinkle very toast with honey.

NUTRITION:

Calories 107, fat 2.2, fiber 1.9, carbs 18.7, protein 4

43. Scrambled Eggs

Servings: 2 | Preparation time: 25 mins

1 tablespoon butter

Salt and black pepper, to taste

4 eggs

1. Combine together eggs, salt and black pepper in a bowl and keep aside.
2. Heat butter in a pan over medium-low heat and slowly add the whisked eggs.
3. Stir the eggs continuously in the pan with the help of a fork for about 4 minutes.
4. Dish out in a plate and serve immediately.
5. You can refrigerate this scramble for about 2 days for meal prepping and reuse by heating it in microwave oven.

NUTRITION:

Calories: 151 , Fat: 11.6g Carbohydrates: 0.7g Protein: 11.1g Sodium: 144mg Sugar: 0.7g

44. Bacon Veggies Combo

Servings: 2 | Preparation time: 35 mins

½ green bell pepper, seeded and chopped

¼ cup Parmesan Cheese

1 scallion, chopped

2 bacon slices

½ tablespoon mayonnaise

1. Preheat the oven to 375 degrees F and grease a baking dish.
2. Place bacon slices on the baking dish and top with mayonnaise, bell peppers, scallions and Parmesan Cheese.
3. Transfer in the oven and bake for about 25 minutes.
4. Dish out to serve immediately or refrigerate for about 2 days wrapped in a plastic sheet for meal prepping.

NUTRITION:

Calories: 197 Fat: 13.8g Carbohydrates: 4.7g Protein: 14.3g Sugar: 1.9g Sodium: 662mg

45. Tofu with Mushrooms

Servings: 2 | Preparation time: 25 mins

1 cup fresh mushrooms, chopped finely

4 tablespoons butter

4 tablespoons Parmesan cheese, shredded

1 block tofu, pressed and cubed into 1-inch pieces

Salt and black pepper, to taste

1. Season the tofu with salt and black pepper.
2. Put butter and seasoned tofu in a pan and cook for about 5 minutes.
3. Add mushrooms and Parmesan cheese and cook for another 5 minutes, stirring occasionally.
4. Dish out and serve immediately or refrigerate for about 3 days wrapped in a foil for meal prepping and microwave it to serve again.

NUTRITION:

Calories: 423 Fat: 37g Carbohydrates: 4g Protein: 23.1g Sugar: 0.9g Sodium: 691mg

46. Ham Spinach Ballet

Servings: 2 | Preparation time: 40 mins

4 teaspoons cream

7-ounce ham, sliced

1 tablespoon unsalted butter, melted

¾ pound fresh baby spinach

Salt and black pepper, to taste

1. Preheat the oven to 360 degrees F. and grease 2 ramekins with butter.
2. Put butter and spinach in a skillet and cook for about 3 minutes.
3. Add cooked spinach in the ramekins and top with ham slices, cream, salt and black pepper.
4. Bake for about 25 minutes and dish out to serve hot.

5. For meal prepping, you can refrigerate this ham spinach ballet for about 3 days wrapped in a foil.

NUTRITION:
Calories: 188 Fat: 12.5g Carbohydrates: 4.9g Protein: 14.6g Sugar: 0.3g Sodium: 1098mg

47. Creamy Parsley Soufflé

Servings: 2 | Preparation time: 25 mins

2 fresh red chili peppers, chopped	Salt, to taste
4 eggs	4 tablespoons light cream
2 tablespoons fresh parsley, chopped	

1. Preheat the oven to 375 degrees F and grease 2 soufflé dishes.
2. Combine all the ingredients in a bowl and mix well.
3. Put the mixture into prepared soufflé dishes and transfer in the oven.
4. Cook for about 6 minutes and dish out to serve immediately.
5. For meal prepping, you can refrigerate this creamy parsley soufflé in the ramekins covered in a foil for about 2-3 days.

NUTRITION:
Calories: 108 Fat: 9g Carbohydrates: 1.1g Protein: 6g Sugar: 0.5g Sodium: 146mg

48. Vegetarian Three Cheese Quiche Stuffed Peppers

Servings: 2 | Preparation time: 50 mins

2 large eggs	¼ cup mozzarella, shredded
1 medium bell peppers, sliced in half and seeds removed	¼ cup ricotta cheese
¼ cup grated Parmesan cheese	½ teaspoon garlic powder
1/8 cup baby spinach leaves	¼ teaspoon dried parsley
1 tablespoon Parmesan cheese, to garnish	

1. Preheat oven to 375 degrees F.
2. Blend all the cheeses, eggs, garlic powder and parsley in a food processor and process until smooth.
3. Pour the cheese mixture into each sliced bell pepper and top with spinach leaves.
4. Stir with a fork, pushing them under the cheese mixture and cover with foil.
5. Bake for about 40 minutes and sprinkle with Parmesan cheese.
6. Broil for about 5 minutes and dish out to serve.

NUTRITION:
Calories: 157 Carbs: 7.3g Fats: 9g Proteins: 12.7g Sodium: 166mg Sugar: 3.7g

49. Spinach Artichoke Egg Casserole

Servings: 2 | Preparation time: 45 mins

1/8 cup milk	2.5-ounce frozen chopped spinach, thawed and drained well
1/8 cup parmesan cheese	1/8 cup onions, shaved
¼ teaspoon salt	¼ teaspoon crushed red pepper
4 large eggs	3.5-ounce artichoke hearts, drained
¼ cup white cheddar, shredded	1/8 cup ricotta cheese
½ garlic clove, minced	¼ teaspoon dried thyme

1. Preheat the oven to 350 degrees F and grease a baking dish with non-stick cooking spray.
2. Whisk eggs and milk together and add artichoke hearts and spinach.
3. Mix well and stir in rest of the ingredients, withholding the ricotta cheese.
4. Pour the mixture into the baking dish and top evenly with ricotta cheese.
5. Transfer in the oven and bake for about 30 minutes.
6. Dish out and serve warm.

NUTRITION:
Calories: 228 Carbs: 10.1g Fats: 13.3g Proteins: 19.1g Sodium: 571mg Sugar: 2.5g

50. Avocado Baked Eggs

Servings: 2 | Preparation time: 25 mins

2 eggs	1 medium sized avocado, halved and pit removed
¼ cup cheddar cheese, shredded	Kosher salt and black pepper, to taste

1. Preheat oven to 425 degrees and grease a muffin pan.
2. Crack open an egg into each half of the avocado and season with salt and black pepper.
3. Top with cheddar cheese and transfer the muffin pan in the oven.
4. Bake for about 15 minutes and dish out to serve.

NUTRITION:
Calories: 210 Carbs: 6.4g Fats: 16.6g Proteins: 10.7g Sodium: 151mg Sugar: 2.2g

51. Cinnamon Faux-St Crunch Cereal

Servings: 2 | Preparation time: 35 mins

¼ cup hulled hemp seeds	½ tablespoon coconut oil
¼ cup milled flax seed	1 tablespoon ground cinnamon
¼ cup apple juice	

1. Preheat the oven to 300 degrees F and line a cookie sheet with parchment paper.
2. Put hemp seeds, flax seed and ground cinnamon in a food processor.
3. Add coconut oil and apple juice and blend until smooth.
4. Pour the mixture on the cookie sheet and transfer in the oven.
5. Bake for about 15 minutes and lower the temperature of the oven to 250 degrees F.
6. Bake for another 10 minutes and dish out from the oven, turning it off.
7. Cut into small squares and place in the turned off oven.
8. Place the cereal in the oven for 1 hour until it is crisp.
9. Dish out and serve with unsweetened almond milk.

NUTRITION:
Calories: 225 Carbs: 9.2g Fats: 18.5g Proteins: 9.8g Sodium: 1mg Sugar: 1.6g

52. Quick Keto McMuffins

Servings: 2 | Preparation time: 15 mins

Muffins	¼ cup flaxmeal
¼ cup almond flour	¼ teaspoon baking soda
1 large egg, free-range or organic	2 tablespoons water
1 pinch salt	2 tablespoons heavy whipping cream
¼ cup cheddar cheese, grated	**Filling:**
1 tablespoon ghee	2 slices cheddar cheese
Salt and black pepper, to taste	2 large eggs
1 tablespoon butter	1 teaspoon Dijon mustard

For Muffins:
1. Mix together all the dry ingredients for muffins in a small bowl and add egg, cream, cheese and water.
2. Combine well and pour in 2 single-serving ramekins.
3. Microwave on high for about 90 seconds.

For Filling:
4. Fry the eggs on ghee and season with salt and black pepper.
5. Cut the muffins in half and spread butter on the inside of each half.
6. Top each buttered half with cheese slices, eggs and Dijon mustard.
7. Serve immediately.

NUTRITION:
Calories: 299 Carbs: 8.8g Fats: 24.3g Proteins: 13g Sodium: 376mg Sugar: 0.4g

53. Keto Egg Fast Snickerdoodle Crepes

Servings: 2 | Preparation time: 15 mins

For the crepes:
6 eggs
Butter, for frying
For the filling:
8 tablespoons butter, softened

5 oz cream cheese, softened
1 teaspoon cinnamon
1 tablespoon Swerve
2 tablespoons granulated Swerve
1 tablespoon cinnamon

1. For the crepes: Put all the ingredients together in a blender except the butter and process until smooth.
2. Heat butter on medium heat in a non-stick pan and pour some batter in the pan.
3. Cook for about 2 minutes, then flip and cook for 2 more minutes.
4. Repeat with the remaining mixture.
5. Mix Swerve, butter and cinnamon in a small bowl until combined.
6. Spread this mixture onto the centre of the crepe and serve rolled up.

NUTRITION:
Calories: 543 Carbs: 8g Fats: 51.6g Proteins: 15.7g Sodium: 455mg Sugar: 0.9g

54. Cauliflower Hash Brown Breakfast Bowl

Servings: 2 - Preparation time: 30 mins

1 tablespoon lemon juice
1 avocado
2 tablespoons extra virgin olive oil
½ green onion, chopped
¾ cup cauliflower rice
Salt and black pepper, to taste

1 egg
1 teaspoon garlic powder
2 oz mushrooms, sliced
¼ cup salsa
½ small handful baby spinach

1. Mash together avocado, lemon juice, garlic powder, salt and black pepper in a small bowl.
2. Whisk eggs, salt and black pepper in a bowl and keep aside.
3. Heat half of olive oil over medium heat in a skillet and add mushrooms.
4. Sauté for about 3 minutes and season with garlic powder, salt, and pepper.
5. Sauté for about 2 minutes and dish out in a bowl.
6. Add rest of the olive oil and add cauliflower, garlic powder, salt and pepper.
7. Sauté for about 5 minutes and dish out.
8. Return the mushrooms to the skillet and add green onions and baby spinach.
9. Sauté for about 30 seconds and add whisked eggs.
10. Sauté for about 1 minute and scoop on the sautéed cauliflower hash browns.
11. Top with salsa and mashed avocado and serve.

NUTRITION:
Calories: 400 Carbs: 15.8g Fats: 36.7g Proteins: 8g Sodium: 288mg Sugar: 4.2g

55. Cheesy Thyme Waffles

Servings: 2 | Preparation time: 15 mins

½ cup mozzarella cheese, finely shredded
¼ large head cauliflower
1 large egg
½ tablespoon olive oil
¼ teaspoon salt
1 teaspoon fresh thyme, chopped

¼ cup Parmesan cheese
½ cup collard greens
1 stalk green onion
½ teaspoon garlic powder
½ tablespoon sesame seed
¼ teaspoon ground black pepper

1. Put cauliflower, collard greens, spring onion and thyme in a food processor and pulse until smooth.
2. Dish out the mixture in a bowl and stir in rest of the ingredients.
3. Heat a waffle iron and transfer the mixture evenly over the griddle.
4. Cook until a waffle is formed and dish out in a serving platter.

NUTRITION:
Calories: 144 Carbs: 8.5g Fats: 9.4g Proteins: 9.3g Sodium: 435mg Sugar: 3g

56. Baked Eggs and Asparagus with Parmesan

Servings: 2 Preparation time: 30 mins

4 eggs

2 teaspoons olive oil
Salt and black pepper, to taste

8 thick asparagus spears, cut into bite-sized pieces
2 tablespoons Parmesan cheese

1. Preheat the oven to 400 degrees F and grease two gratin dishes with olive oil.
2. Put half the asparagus into each gratin dish and place in the oven.
3. Roast for about 10 minutes and dish out the gratin dishes.
4. Crack eggs over the asparagus and transfer into the oven.
5. Bake for about 5 minutes and dish out the gratin dishes.
6. Sprinkle with Parmesan cheese and put the dishes back in the oven.
7. Bake for another 3 minutes and dish out to serve hot.

NUTRITION:
Calories: 336 Carbs: 13.7g Fats: 19.4g Proteins: 28.1g Sodium: 2103mg Sugar: 4.7g

57. Low Carb Green Smoothie

Servings: 2 Preparation time: 15 mins

1/3 cup romaine lettuce

1½ cups filtered water
¾ tablespoon fresh parsley

¼ Hass avocado

1/3 tablespoon Swerve

1/3 tablespoon fresh ginger, peeled and chopped
1/8 cup fresh pineapple, chopped
1/3 cup raw cucumber, peeled and sliced
¼ cup kiwi fruit, peeled and chopped

1. Put all the ingredients in a blender and blend until smooth.
2. Pour into 2 serving glasses and serve chilled.

NUTRITION:
Calories: 108 Carbs: 7.8g Fats: 8.9g Proteins: 1.6g Sodium: 4mg Sugar: 2.2

58. Lentil Salmon Salad
Servings 4 | Preparation and Cooking Time 25 minutes

Vegetable stock	2 cups
Green lentils	1, rinsed
Red onion	1, chopped
Parsley	1 2 cup, chopped
Smoked salmon	4 oz., shredded
Cilantro	2 tbsp., chopped
Red pepper	1, chopped
Lemon	1, juiced
Salt and pepper	to taste

1. Cook vegetable stock and lentils in a sauce pan for 15 to 20 minutes, on low heat. Ensure all liquid has been absorbed and then remove from heat.
2. Pour into a salad bowl and top with red pepper, parsley, cilantro and salt and pepper (to suit your taste) and mix.
3. Mix in lemon juice and shredded salmon.
4. This salad should be served fresh.

59. Peppy Pepper Tomato Salad
Servings 4 | Preparation Time 20 minutes

Yellow bell pepper - 1, cored and diced	Cucumbers - 4, diced
Red onion - 1, chopped	Balsamic vinegar – 1 tbsp.
Extra virgin olive oil – 2 tbsp.	Tomatoes - 4, diced
Red bell peppers - 2, cored and diced	Chili flakes - 1 pinch
Salt and pepper - to taste	

1. Mix all above Ingredients in a salad bowl, except salt and pepper.
2. Season with salt and pepper to suit your taste and mix well.
3. Eat while fresh.

60. Bulgur Salad
Servings 4 | Preparation and Cooking Time 30 minutes

Vegetable stock	2 cups
Bulgur	2 3 cup
Garlic clove	1, minced
Cherry tomatoes	1 cup, halved
Almonds	2 tbsp., sliced
Dates	1 4 cup, pitted and chopped
Lemon juice	1 tbsp.
Baby spinach	8 oz.
Cucumber	1, diced
Balsamic vinegar	1 tbsp.
Salt and pepper	to taste
Mixed seeds	2 tbsp.

1. Pour stock into sauce pan and heat until hot, then stir in bulgur and cook until bulgur has absorbed all stock.
2. Put in salad bowl and add remaining Ingredients:, stir well.
3. Add salt and pepper to suit your taste.
4. Serve and eat immediately.

61. Tasty Tuna Salad
Servings 4 | Preparation Time 15 minutes

Green olives - 1 4 cup, sliced	Tuna in water - 1 can, drained
Pine nuts - 2 tbsp.	Artichoke hearts – 1 jar, drained and chopped
Extra virgin olive oil - 2 tbsp.	Lemon – 1, juiced
Arugula - 2 leaves	Dijon mustard - 1 tbsp.
Salt and pepper - to taste	

1. Mix mustard, oil and lemon juice in a bowl to make a dressing. Combine the artichoke hearts, tuna, green olives, arugula and pine nuts in a salad bowl.
2. In a separate salad bowl, mix tuna, arugula, pine nuts, artichoke hearts and tuna.
3. Pour dressing mix onto salad and serve fresh.

62. Sweet and Sour Spinach Salad
Servings 4 | Preparation Time 15 minutes

Red onions	2, sliced
Baby spinach leaves	4
Sesame oil	1 2 tsp.
Apple cider vinegar	2 tbsp.
Honey	1 tsp.
Sesame seeds	2 tbsp.
Salt and pepper	to taste

1. Mix together honey, sesame oil, vinegar and sesame seeds in a small bowl to make a dressing. Add in salt and pepper to suit your taste.
2. Add red onions and spinach together in a salad bowl.
3. Pour dressing over the salad and serve while cool and fresh.

63. Easy Eggplant Salad
Servings 4 | Preparation Time 30 minutes

Salt and pepper	to taste
Eggplant	2, sliced
Smoked paprika	1 tsp.
Extra virgin olive oil	2 tbsp.
Garlic cloves	2, minced
Mixed greens	2 cups
Sherry vinegar	2 tbsp.

1. Mix together garlic, paprika and oil in a small bowl.
2. Place eggplant on a plate and sprinkle with salt and pepper to suit your taste. Next, brush oil mixture onto the eggplant.
3. Cook eggplant on a medium heated grill pan until brown on both sides. Once cooked, put eggplant into a salad bowl.
4. Top with greens and vinegar, serve and eat.

64. Sweetest Sweet Potato Salad
Servings 4 | Preparation and Cooking Time 30 minutes

Honey - 2 tbsp.	Sumac spice - 1 tsp.
Sweet potato - 2, finely sliced	Extra virgin olive oil - 3 tbsp.
Dried mint - 1 tsp.	Balsamic vinegar – 1 tbsp.
Salt and pepper - to taste	Pomegranate - 1, seeded
Mixed greens - 3 cups	

1. Place sweet potato slices on a plate and add sumac, mint, salt and pepper on both sides. Next, drizzle oil and honey over both sides.
2. Add oil to a grill pan and heat. Grill sweet potatoes on medium heat until brown on both sides.
3. Put sweet potatoes in a salad bowl and top with pomegranate and mixed greens.
4. Stir and eat right away.

65. Delicious Chickpea Salad

Servings 4 | Preparation Time 15 minutes

Chickpeas	1 can, drained
Cherry tomatoes	1 cup, quartered
Parsley	1 2 cup, chopped
Red seedless grapes	1 2 cup, halved
Feta cheese	4 oz., cubed
Salt and pepper	to taste
Lemon juice	1 tbsp.
Greek yogurt	1 4 cup
Extra virgin olive oil	2 tbsp.

1. In a salad bowl, mix together parsley, chickpeas, grapes, feta cheese and tomatoes.
2. Add in remaining ingredients, seasoning with salt and pepper to suit your taste.
3. This fresh salad is best when served right away.

66. Couscous Arugula Salad

Servings 4 | Preparation and Cooking Time 20 minutes

Couscous	1 2 cup
Vegetable stock	1 cup
Asparagus	1 bunch, peeled
Lemon	1, juiced
Dried tarragon	1 tsp.
Arugula	2 cups
Salt and pepper	to taste

1. Heat vegetable stock in a pot until hot. Remove from heat and add in couscous. Cover until couscous has absorbed all the stock.
2. Pour in a bowl and fluff with a fork and then set aside to cool.
3. Peel asparagus with a vegetable peeler, making them into ribbons and put into a bowl with couscous.
4. Add remaining Ingredients and add salt and pepper to suit your taste.
5. Serve the salad immediately.

67. Spinach and Grilled Feta Salad

Servings 6 | Preparation and Cooking Time 20 minutes

Feta cheese	8 oz., sliced
Black olives	1 4 cup, sliced
Green olives	1 4 cup, sliced
Baby spinach	4 cups
Garlic cloves	2, minced
Capers	1 tsp., chopped
Extra virgin olive oil	2 tbsp.
Red wine vinegar	1 tbsp.

1. Grill feta cheese slices over medium to high flame until brown on both sides.
2. In a salad bowl, mix green olives, black olives and spinach.
3. In a separate bowl, mix vinegar, capers and oil together to make a dressing.
4. Top salad with the dressing and cheese and it's is ready to serve.

68. Creamy Cool Salad

Servings 4 | Preparation Time 15 minutes

Greek yogurt	1 2 cup
Dill	2 tbsp., chopped
Lemon juice	1 tsp.
Cucumbers	4, diced
Garlic cloves	2, minced
Salt and pepper	to taste

1. Mix all Ingredients in a salad bowl.
2. Add salt and pepper to suit your taste and eat.

69. Grilled Salmon Summer Salad

Servings 4 | Preparation and Cooking Time 30 minutes

Salmon fillets	2
Salt and pepper	to taste
Vegetable stock	2 cups
Bulgur	1 2 cup
Cherry tomatoes	1 cup, halved
Sweet corn	1 2 cup
Lemon	1, juiced
Green olives	1 2 cup, sliced
Cucumber	1, cubed
Green onion	1, chopped
Red pepper	1, chopped
Red bell pepper	1, cored and diced

1. Heat a grill pan on medium and then place salmon on, seasoning with salt and pepper. Grill both sides of salmon until brown and set aside.
2. Heat stock in sauce pan until hot and then add in bulgur and cook until liquid is completely soaked into bulgur.
3. Mix salmon, bulgur and all other Ingredients in a salad bowl and again add salt and pepper, if desired, to suit your taste.
4. Serve salad as soon as completed.

70. Broccoli Salad with Caramelized Onions

Servings 4 | Preparation and Cooking Time 25 minutes

Extra virgin olive oil	3 tbsp.
Red onions	2, sliced
Dried thyme	1 tsp.
Balsamic vinegar	2 tbsp. vinegar
Broccoli	1 lb., cut into florets
Salt and pepper	to taste

1. Heat extra virgin olive oil in a pan over high heat and add in sliced onions. Cook for approximately 10 minutes or until the onions are caramelized. Stir in vinegar and thyme and then remove from stove.
2. Mix together the broccoli and onion mixture in a bowl, adding salt and pepper if desired. Serve and eat salad as soon as possible.

71. Baked Cauliflower Mixed Salad

Servings 4 | Preparation and Cooking Time 30 minutes

Cauliflower - 1 lb., cut into florets	Extra virgin olive oil - 2 tbsp.
Dried mint - 1 tsp.	Dried oregano - 1 tsp.
Parsley - 2 tbsp., chopped	Red pepper - 1, chopped
Lemon - 1, juiced	Green onion - 1, chopped
Cilantro - 2 tbsp., chopped	Salt and pepper to taste

1. Heat oven to 350 degrees.
2. In a deep baking pan, combine olive oil, mint, cauliflower and oregano and bake for 15 minutes.
3. Once cooked, pour into a salad bowl and add remaining Ingredients:, stirring together.
4. Plate the salad and eat fresh and warm.

72. Quick Arugula Salad

Servings 4 | Preparation Time 15 minutes

Roasted red bell peppers - 6, sliced	Pine nuts - 2 tbsp.
Dried raisins - 2 tbsp.	Red onion - 1, sliced
Arugula - 3 cups	Balsamic vinegar - 2 tbsp.
Feta cheese - 4 oz., crumbled	Extra virgin olive oil – 2 tbsp.
Feta cheese - 4 oz., crumbled	Salt and pepper - to taste

1. Using a salad bowl, combine vinegar, olive oil, pine nuts, raisins, peppers and onions.
2. Add arugula and feta cheese to the mix and serve.

73. Bell Pepper and Tomato Salad
Servings 4 | Preparation Time 15 minutes

Roasted red bell pepper	8, sliced
Extra virgin olive oil	2 tbsp.
Chili flakes	1 pinch
Garlic cloves	4, minced
Pine nuts	2 tbsp.
Shallot	1, sliced
Cherry tomatoes	1 cup, halved
Parsley	2 tbsp., chopped
Balsamic vinegar	1 tbsp.
Salt and pepper	to taste

1. Mix all Ingredients except salt and pepper in a salad bowl.
2. Season with salt and pepper if you want, to suit your taste.
3. Eat once freshly made.

74. One Bowl Spinach Salad
Servings 4 | Preparation Time 20 minutes

Red beets	2, cooked and diced
Apple cider vinegar	1 tbsp.
Baby spinach	3 cups
Greek yogurt	1 4 cup
Horseradish	1 tbsp.
Salt and pepper	to taste

1. Mix beets and spinach in a salad bowl.
2. Add in yogurt, horseradish, and vinegar. You can also add salt and pepper if you wish.
3. Serve salad as soon as mixed.

75. Olive and Red Bean Salad
Servings 4 | Preparation Time 20 minutes

Red onions	2, sliced
Garlic cloves	2, minced
Balsamic vinegar	2 tbsp.
Green olives	1 4 cup, sliced
Salt and pepper	to taste
Mixed greens	2 cups
Red beans	1 can, drained
Chili flakes	1 pinch
Extra virgin olive oil	2 tbsp.
Parsley	2 tbsp., chopped

1. In a salad bowl, mix all Ingredients
2. Add salt and pepper, if desired, and serve right away.

76. Fresh and Light Cabbage Salad
Servings 4 | Preparation Time 25 minutes

Mint - 1 tbsp., chopped	Ground coriander - 1 2 tsp.
Savoy cabbage - 1, shredded	Greek yogurt - 1 2 cup
Cumin seeds - 1 4 tsp.	Extra virgin olive oil - 2 tbsp.
Carrot - 1, grated	Red onion – 1, sliced
Honey - 1 tsp.	Lemon zest - 1 tsp.
Lemon juice - 2 tbsp.	Salt and pepper - to taste

1. In a salad bowl, mix all Ingredients
2. You can add salt and pepper to suit your taste and then mix again.
3. This salad is best when cool and freshly made.

77. Vegetable Patch Salad
Servings 6 | Preparation and Cooking Time 30 minutes

Cauliflower - 1 bunch, cut into florets	Zucchini - 1, sliced
Sweet potato - 1, peeled and cubed	Baby carrots - 1 2 lb.
Salt and pepper - to taste	Dried basil - 1 tsp.
Red onions - 2, sliced	Eggplant - 2, cubed

Endive - 1, sliced	Extra virgin olive oil - 3 tbsp.
Lemon – 1, juiced	Balsamic vinegar - 1 tbsp.

1. Preheat oven to 350 degrees. Mix together all vegetables, basil, salt, pepper and oil in a baking dish and cook for 25 – 30 minutes.
2. After cooked, pour into salad bowl and stir in vinegar and lemon juice.
3. Dish up and serve.

78. Cucumber Greek yoghurt Salad
Serves:6 | Preparation time: 5 minutes | Cooking Time: 0 minutes

4tbsp Greek yoghurt	4 large cucumbers peeled seeded and sliced
1 tbsp dried dill	1 tbsp apple cider vinegar
1/4 tsp garlic powder	1/4 tsp ground black pepper
1/2 tsp sugar	1/2 tsp salt

1. Place all the Ingredients leaving out the cucumber into a bowl and whisk this until all is incorporated. Add your cucumber slices and toss until all is well mixed.
2. Let the salad chill 10 minutes in the refrigerator and then serve.

79. Chickpea Salad Recipe
Servings: 4 Duration: 15 minutes

Drained chickpeas: 1 can	Halved cherry tomatoes: 1 cup
Sun-dried chopped tomatoes: 1 2 cups	Arugula: 2 cups
Cubed pita bread: 1	Pitted black olives: 1 2 cups
1 sliced shallot	Cumin seeds: 1 2 teaspoon
Coriander seeds: 1 2 teaspoon	Chili powder: 1 4 teaspoon
Chopped mint: 1 teaspoon	Pepper and salt to taste
Crumbled goat cheese: 4 oz.	

1. In a salad bowl, mix the tomatoes, chickpeas, pita bread, arugula, olives, shallot, spices and mint.
2. Stir in pepper and salt as desired to the cheese and stir.
3. You can now serve the fresh Salad.

80. Orange salad
Servings: 4 | Cooking Time: 15 minutes

4 sliced endives	1 sliced red onion
2 oranges already cut into segments	Extra virgin olive oil: 2 tablespoon
Pepper and salt to taste	

1. Mix all the Ingredients in a salad bowl
2. Sprinkle pepper and salt to taste.
3. You can now serve the salad fresh.

81. Yogurt lettuce salad recipe
Servings: 4 | Cooking Time: 20 minutes

Shredded Romaine lettuce: 1 head	Sliced cucumbers: 2
2 minced garlic cloves	Greek yogurt: 1 2 cup
Dijon mustard: 1 teaspoon	Chili powder: 1 pinch
Extra virgin olive oil: 2 tablespoon	Lemon juice: 1 tablespoon
Chopped dill: 2 tablespoon	4 chopped mint leaves
Pepper and salt to taste	

1. In a salad bowl, combine the lettuce with the cucumbers.
2. Add the yogurt, chili, mustard, lemon juice, dill, mint, garlic and oil in a mortar with pepper and salt as desired. Then, mix well into paste, this is the dressing for the salad .
3. Top the Salad with the dressing then serve fresh.

82. Fruit de salad recipe
Servings: 4 | Cooking Time: 20 minutes

Cubed seedless watermelon: 8 oz.	Halved red grapes: 4 oz.
2 Sliced cucumbers	Halved strawberries: 1 cup
Cubed feta cheese: 6 oz.	Balsamic vinegar: 2 tablespoon
Arugula: 2 cups	

1. In a salad bowl, mix the strawberries, grapes, arugula, cucumbers, feta cheese and watermelon together.
2. Top the salad with vinegar and serve fresh.

83. Chickpea with mint salad recipe
Servings: 6 Duration: 20 minutes

1 diced cucumber	Sliced black olives:1 4 cup
Chopped mint: 2 tablespoon	Cooked and drained short pasta: 4 oz.
Arugula: 2 cups	Drained chickpeas: 1 can
1 sliced shallot	Chopped Parsley: 1 2 cup
Halved cherry tomatoes: 1 2 pound	Sliced green olives: 1 4 cup
1 juiced lemon	Extra virgin olive oil: 2 tablespoon
Chopped walnut: 1 2 cup	Pepper and salt to taste

1. Mix the chickpeas with the other Ingredients in a salad bowl
2. Top with oil and lemon juice, sprinkle pepper and salt then mix well.
3. Refrigerate the Salad (can last in a sealed container for about 2 days) or serve fresh.

84. Grapy Fennel salad
Servings: 2 Time to prepare : 15 minutes

Grape seed oil: 1 tablespoon	Chopped dill: 1 tablespoon
1 finely sliced fennel bulb	Toasted almond slices: 2 tablespoon
Chopped mint: 1 teaspoon	1 grapefruit already cut into segments
1 orange already cut into segments	Pepper and salt as desired

1. Using a platter, mix the grapefruit and orange segments with the fennel bulb
2. Add the mint, almond slices and dill, top with the oil and add pepper and salt as desired.
3. You can now serve the Salad fresh.

85. Greenie salad recipe
Servings: 4   Cooking time: 15 minutes

Extra virgin olive oil: 2 tablespoon	Mixed greens: 12 oz.
Pitted black olives: 1 2 cup	Pitted green olives: 1 4 cup
Sherry vinegar: 2 tablespoon	Pitted Kalamata olives: 1 2 cup
Almond slices: 2 tablespoon	Parmesan shavings: 2 oz.
Sliced Parma ham: 2 oz.	Pepper and salt as desired

1. Stir the almonds, olives and mixed greens together in a salad bowl
2. Drizzle the oil and vinegar then sprinkle pepper and salt as you want.
3. Top with the Parma ham and Parmesan shavings before serving.
4. You can now serve fresh.

86. A Refreshing Detox Salad
Servings: 4 | Cooking Time: 0 minutes

1 large apple, diced	1 large beet, coarsely grated
1 large carrot, coarsely grated	1 tbsp chia seeds
2 tbsp almonds, chopped	2 tbsp lemon juice
2 tbsp pumpkin seed oil	4 cups mixed greens

1. In a medium salad bowl, except for mixed greens, combine all ingredients thoroughly.
2. Into 4 salad plates, divide the mixed greens.
3. Evenly top mixed greens with the salad bowl mixture.
4. Serve and enjoy.

NUTRITION:
Calories: 136.4; Protein: 1.93g; Carbs: 14.4g; Fat: 7.9g

87. Amazingly Fresh Carrot Salad
Servings: 4 | Cooking Time: 0 minutes

¼ tsp chipotle powder	1 bunch scallions, sliced
1 cup cherry tomatoes, halved	1 large avocado, diced
1 tbsp chili powder	1 tbsp lemon juice
2 tbsp olive oil	3 tbsp lime juice
4 cups carrots, spiralized	salt to taste

1. In a salad bowl, mix and arrange avocado, cherry tomatoes, scallions and spiralized carrots. Set aside.
2. In a small bowl, whisk salt, chipotle powder, chili powder, olive oil, lemon juice and lime juice thoroughly.
3. Pour dressing over noodle salad. Toss to coat well.
4. Serve and enjoy at room temperature.

NUTRITION:
Calories: 243.6; Fat: 14.8g; Protein: 3g; Carbs: 24.6g

88. Anchovy and Orange Salad
Servings: 4 | Cooking Time: 0 minutes

1 small red onion, sliced into thin rounds	1 tbsp fresh lemon juice
1/8 tsp pepper or more to taste	16 oil cure Kalamata olives
2 tsp finely minced fennel fronds for garnish	3 tbsp extra virgin olive oil
4 small oranges, preferably blood oranges	6 anchovy fillets

1. With a paring knife, peel oranges including the membrane that surrounds it.
2. In a plate, slice oranges into thin circles and allow plate to catch the orange juices.
3. On serving plate, arrange orange slices on a layer.
4. Sprinkle oranges with onion, followed by olives and then anchovy fillets.
5. Drizzle with oil, lemon juice and orange juice.
6. Sprinkle with pepper.
7. Allow salad to stand for 30 minutes at room temperature to allow the flavors to develop.
8. To serve, garnish with fennel fronds and enjoy.

NUTRITION:
Calories: 133.9; Protein: 3.2 g; Carbs: 14.3g; Fat: 7.1g

89. Arugula with Blueberries 'n Almonds
Servings: 2 | Cooking Time: 0 minutes

½ cup slivered almonds	½ cup blueberries, fresh
1 ripe red pear, sliced	1 shallot, minced
1 tsp minced garlic	1 tsp whole grain mustard
2 tbsp fresh lemon juice	3 tbsp extra virgin olive oil
6 cups arugula	

1. In a big mixing bowl, mix garlic, olive oil, lemon juice and mustard.
2. Once thoroughly mixed, add remaining ingredients.
3. Toss to coat.
4. Equally divide into two bowls, serve and enjoy.

NUTRITION:
Calories: 530.4; Protein: 6.1g; Carbs: 39.2g; Fat: 38.8g

90. Asian Peanut Sauce Over Noodle Salad

Servings: 4 | Cooking Time: 0 minutes

1 cup shredded green cabbage	1 cup shredded red cabbage
1/4 cup chopped cilantro	1/4 cup chopped peanuts
1/4 cup chopped scallions	4 cups shiritake noodles (drained and rinsed)
Asian Peanut Sauce Ingredients	1/4 cup sugar free peanut butter
¼ teaspoon cayenne pepper	½ cup filtered water
½ teaspoon kosher salt	1 tablespoon fish sauce (or coconut aminos for vegan)
1 tablespoon granulated erythritol sweetener	1 tablespoon lime juice
1 tablespoon toasted sesame oil	1 tablespoon wheat-free soy sauce
1 teaspoon minced garlic	2 tablespoons minced ginger

1. In a large salad bowl, combine all noodle salad ingredients and toss well to mix.
2. In a blender, mix all sauce ingredients and pulse until smooth and creamy.
3. Pour sauce over the salad and toss well to coat.
4. Evenly divide into four equal servings and enjoy.

NUTRITION:
Calories: 104; Protein: 7.0g; Carbs: 12.0g; Fat: 16.0g

91. Asian Salad with pistachios

Servings: 6 | Cooking Time: 0

¼ cup chopped pistachios	¼ cup green onions, sliced
1 bunch watercress, trimmed	1 cup red bell pepper, diced
2 cups medium sized fennel bulb, thinly sliced	2 tbsp vegetable oil
3 cups Asian pears, cut into matchstick size	3 tbsp fresh lime juice

1. In a large salad bowl, mix pistachios, green onions, bell pepper, fennel, watercress and pears.
2. In a small bowl, mix vegetable oil and lime juice. Season with pepper and salt to taste.
3. Pour dressing to salad and gently mix before serving.

NUTRITION:
Calories: 160; Protein: 3g; Fat: 1g; Carbs: 16g

92. Balela Salad from the Middle East

Servings: 6 | Cooking Time: 0 minutes

1 jalapeno, finely chopped (optional)	1/2 green bell pepper, cored and chopped
2 1/2 cups grape tomatoes, slice in halves	1/2 cup sun-dried tomatoes
1/2 cup freshly chopped parsley leaves	1/2 cup freshly chopped mint or basil leaves
1/3 cup pitted Kalamata olives	1/4 cup pitted green olives
3 1/2 cups cooked chickpeas, drained and rinsed	3–5 green onions, both white and green parts, chopped
Dressing Ingredients	1 garlic clove, minced
1 tsp ground sumac	1/2 tsp Aleppo pepper
1/4 cup Early Harvest Greek extra virgin olive oil	1/4 to 1/2 tsp crushed red pepper (optional)
2 tbsp lemon juice	2 tbsp white wine vinegar
Salt and black pepper, a generous pinch to your taste	

1. mix together the salad ingredients in a large salad bowl.
2. In a separate smaller bowl or jar, mix together the dressing ingredients.
3. Drizzle the dressing over the salad and gently toss to coat.
4. Set aside for 30 minutes to allow the flavors to mix.
5. Serve and enjoy.

NUTRITION:
Calories: 257; Carbs: 30.5g; Protein: 8.4g; Fats: 12.6g

93. Blue Cheese and Portobello Salad

Servings: 2 | Cooking Time: 15 minutes

½ cup croutons	1 tbsp merlot wine
1 tbsp water	1 tsp minced garlic
1 tsp olive oil	2 large Portobello mushrooms, stemmed, wiped clean and cut into bite sized pieces
2 pieces roasted red peppers (canned), sliced	2 tbsp balsamic vinegar
2 tbsp crumbled blue cheese	4 slices red onion
6 asparagus stalks cut into 1-inch sections	6 cups Bibb lettuce, chopped
Ground pepper to taste	

1. On medium fire, place a small pan and heat oil. Once hot, add onions and mushrooms. For 4 to 6 minutes, sauté until tender.
2. Add garlic and for a minute continue sautéing.
3. Pour in wine and cook for a minute.
4. Bring an inch of water to a boil in a pot with steamer basket. Once boiling, add asparagus, steam for two to three minutes or until crisp and tender, while covered. Once cooked, remove basket from pot and set aside.
5. In a small bowl whisk thoroughly black pepper, water, balsamic vinegar, and blue cheese.
6. To serve, place 3 cups of lettuce on each plate. Add 1 roasted pepper, ½ of asparagus, ½ of mushroom mixture, whisk blue cheese dressing before drizzling equally on to plates. Garnish with croutons, serve and enjoy.

NUTRITION:
Calories: 660.8; Protein: 38.5g; Carbs: 30.4g; Fat: 42.8g

94. Blue Cheese and Arugula Salad

Servings: 4 | Cooking Time: 0 minutes

¼ cup crumbled blue cheese	1 tsp Dijon mustard
1-pint fresh figs, quartered	2 bags arugula
3 tbsp Balsamic Vinegar	3 tbsp olive oil
Pepper and salt to taste	

1. Whisk thoroughly together pepper, salt, olive oil, Dijon mustard, and balsamic vinegar to make the dressing. Set aside in the ref for at least 30 minutes to marinate and allow the spices to combine.
2. On four serving plates, evenly arrange arugula and top with blue cheese and figs.
3. Drizzle each plate of salad with 1 ½ tbsp of prepared dressing.
4. Serve and enjoy.

NUTRITION:
Calories: 202; Protein: 2.5g; Carbs: 25.5g; Fat: 10g

95. Broccoli Salad Moroccan Style

Servings: 4 | Cooking Time: 0 minutes

¼ tsp sea salt	¼ tsp ground cinnamon
½ tsp ground turmeric	¾ tsp ground ginger
½ tbsp extra virgin olive oil	½ tbsp apple cider vinegar
2 tbsp chopped green onion	1/3 cup coconut cream
½ cup carrots, shredded	1 small head of broccoli, chopped

1. In a large salad bowl, mix well salt, cinnamon, turmeric, ginger, olive oil, and vinegar.
2. Add remaining ingredients, tossing well to coat.
3. Pop in the ref for at least 30 to 60 minutes before serving.

NUTRITION:
Calories: 90.5; Protein: 1.3g; Carbs: 4g; Fat: 7.7g

96. Charred Tomato and Broccoli Salad

Servings: 6 | Cooking Time: minutes

¼ cup lemon juice
1 ½ lbs. boneless chicken breast
1 tsp freshly ground pepper
4 cups broccoli florets

½ tsp chili powder
1 ½ lbs. medium tomato
1 tsp salt
5 tbsp extra virgin olive oil, divided to 2 and 3 tablespoons

1. Place the chicken in a skillet and add just enough water to cover the chicken. Bring to a simmer over high heat. Reduce the heat once the liquid boils and cook the chicken thoroughly for 12 minutes. Once cooked, shred the chicken into bite-sized pieces.
2. On a large pot, bring water to a boil and add the broccoli. Cook for 5 minutes until slightly tender. Drain and rinse the broccoli with cold water. Set aside.
3. Core the tomatoes and cut them crosswise. Discard the seeds and set the tomatoes cut side down on paper towels. Pat them dry.
4. In a heavy skillet, heat the pan over high heat until very hot. Brush the cut sides of the tomatoes with olive oil and place them on the pan. Cook the tomatoes until the sides are charred. Set aside.
5. In the same pan, heat the remaining 3 tablespoon olive oil over medium heat. Stir the salt, chili powder and pepper and stir for 45 seconds. Pour over the lemon juice and remove the pan from the heat.
6. Plate the broccoli, shredded chicken and chili powder mixture dressing.

NUTRITION:
Calories: 210.8; Protein: 27.5g; Carbs: 6.3g; Fat: 8.4g

97. Chopped Chicken on Greek Salad

Servings: 4 | Cooking Time: 0 minutes

¼ tsp pepper
½ cup crumbled feta cheese
½ cup sliced ripe black olives

1 tbsp chopped fresh dill
1/3 cup red wine vinegar
2 medium tomatoes, chopped
6 cups chopped romaine lettuce

¼ tsp salt
½ cup finely chopped red onion
1 medium cucumber, peeled, seeded and chopped
1 tsp garlic powder
2 ½ cups chopped cooked chicken
2 tbsp extra virgin olive oil

1. In a large bowl, whisk well pepper, salt, garlic powder, dill, oil and vinegar.
2. Add feta, olives, onion, cucumber, tomatoes, chicken, and lettuce.
3. Toss well to combine.
4. Serve and enjoy.

NUTRITION:
Calories: 461.9; Protein: 19.4g; Carbs: 10.8g; Fat: 37.9g

98. Classic Greek Salad

Servings: 4 | Cooking Time: 0 minutes

¼ cup extra virgin olive oil, plus more for drizzling
1 4-oz block Greek feta cheese packed in brine
1 lemon, juiced and zested

1 tsp dried oregano
14 small vine-ripened tomatoes, quartered
Fresh oregano leaves for topping, optional
Salt to taste

¼ cup red wine vinegar

1 cup Kalamata olives, halved and pitted
1 small red onion, halved and thinly sliced
1 tsp honey
5 Persian cucumbers

Pepper to taste

1. In a bowl of ice water, soak red onions with 2 tbsp salt.
2. In a large bowl, whisk well ¼ tsp pepper, ½ tsp salt, dried oregano, honey, lemon zest, lemon juice, and vinegar. Slowly pour olive oil in a steady stream as you briskly whisk mixture. Continue whisking until emulsified.
3. Add olives and tomatoes, toss to coat with dressing.

4. Alternatingly peel cucumber leaving strips of skin on. Trim ends slice lengthwise and chop in ½-inch thick cubes. Add into bowl of tomatoes.
5. Drain onions and add into bowl of tomatoes. Toss well to coat and mix.
6. Drain feta and slice into four equal rectangles.
7. Divide Greek salad into serving plates, top each with oregano and feta.
8. To serve, season with pepper and drizzle with oil and enjoy.

NUTRITION:
Calories: 365.5; Protein: 9.6g; Carbs: 26.2g; Fat: 24.7g

99. Cold Zucchini Noodle Bowl

Servings: 4 | Cooking Time: 20 minutes

¼ cup basil leaves, roughly chopped
¼ tsp sea salt
1 lb. peeled and uncooked shrimp
1 tsp lime zest
2 tbsp lemon juice
3 clementine, peeled and separated
pinch of black pepper

¼ cup olive oil
½ tsp salt 1 tsp garlic powder
1 tsp lemon zest
2 tbsp butter
2 tbsp lime juice
4 cups zucchini, spirals or noodles

1. Make zucchini noodles and set aside.
2. On medium fire, place a large nonstick saucepan and heat butter.
3. Meanwhile, pat dry shrimps and season with salt and garlic. Add into hot saucepan and sauté for 6 minutes or until opaque and cooked.
4. Remove from pan, transfer to a bowl and put aside.
5. Right away, add zucchini noodles to still hot pan and stir fry for a minute. Leave noodles on pan as you prepare the dressing.
6. Blend well salt, olive oil, juice and zest in a small bowl.
7. Then place noodles into salad bowl, top with shrimp, pour oil mixture, basil and clementine. Toss to mix well.
8. Refrigerate for an hour before serving.

NUTRITION:
Calories: 353.4; Carbs: 14.8g; Protein: 24.5g; Fat: 21.8g

100. Coleslaw Asian Style

Servings: 10 | Cooking Time: 0 minutes

½ cup chopped fresh cilantro
2 carrots, julienned
2 cups thinly sliced red cabbage
2 tbsp minced fresh ginger root
3 tbsp soy sauce
5 tbsp creamy peanut butter
6 tbsp rice wine vinegar

1 ½ tbsp minced garlic
2 cups shredded napa cabbage
2 red bell peppers, thinly sliced
3 tbsp brown sugar
5 cups thinly sliced green cabbage
6 green onions, chopped
6 tbsp vegetable oil

1. Mix thoroughly the following in a medium bowl: garlic, ginger, brown sugar, soy sauce, peanut butter, oil and rice vinegar.
2. In a separate bowl, blend well cilantro, green onions, carrots, bell pepper, Napa cabbage, red cabbage and green cabbage. Pour in the peanut sauce above and toss to mix well.
3. Serve and enjoy.

NUTRITION:
Calories: 193.8; Protein: 4g; Fat: 12.6g; Carbs: 16.1g

101. Cucumber and Tomato Salad

Servings: 4 | Cooking Time: 0 minutes

Ground pepper to taste
1 tbsp fresh lemon juice
1 cucumber, peeled and diced
4 cups spinach

Salt to taste
1 onion, chopped
2 tomatoes, chopped

1. In a salad bowl, mix onions, cucumbers and tomatoes.
2. Season with pepper and salt to taste.
3. Add lemon juice and mix well.
4. Add spinach, toss to coat, serve and enjoy.

NUTRITION:
Calories: 70.3; Fat: 0.3g; Protein: 1.3g; Carbohydrates: 7.1g

102. Cucumber Salad Japanese Style

Servings: 5 servings | Cooking Time: 0 minutes

1 ½ tsp minced fresh ginger root
1 tsp salt
1/3 cup rice vinegar
2 large cucumbers, ribbon cut
4 tsp white sugar

1. Mix well ginger, salt, sugar and vinegar in a small bowl.
2. Add ribbon cut cucumbers and mix well.
3. Let stand for at least one hour in the ref before serving.

NUTRITION:
Calories: 29; Fat: .2g; Protein: .7g; Carbs: 6.1g

103. Easy Garden Salad with Arugula

Servings: 2 | Cooking Time: 0

¼ cup grated parmesan cheese	¼ cup pine nuts
1 cup cherry tomatoes, halved	1 large avocado, sliced into ½ inch cubes
1 tbsp rice vinegar	2 tbsp olive oil or grapeseed oil
4 cups young arugula leaves, rinsed and dried	Black pepper, freshly ground
Salt to taste	

1. Get a bowl with cover, big enough to hold the salad and mix together the parmesan cheese, vinegar, oil, pine nuts, cherry tomatoes and arugula.
2. Season with pepper and salt according to how you like it. Place the lid and jiggle the covered bowl to combine the salad.
3. Serve the salad topped with sliced avocadoes.

NUTRITION:
Calories: 490.8; Fat: 43.6g; Protein: 9.1g; Carbs: 15.5g

104. Easy Quinoa & Pear Salad

Servings: 6 | Cooking Time: 0 minutes

¼ cup chopped parsley	¼ cup chopped scallions
¼ cup lime juice	¼ cup red onion, diced
½ cup diced carrots	½ cup diced celery
½ cup diced cucumber	½ cup diced red pepper
½ cup dried wild blueberries	½ cup olive oil
½ cup spicy pecans, chopped	1 tbsp chopped parsley
1 tsp honey	1 tsp sea salt
2 fresh pears, cut into chunks	3 cups cooked quinoa

1. In a small bowl mix well olive oil, salt, lime juice, honey, and parsley. Set aside.
2. In large salad bowl, add remaining ingredients and toss to mix well.
3. Pour dressing and toss well to coat.
4. Serve and enjoy.

NUTRITION:
Calories: 382; Protein: 5.6g; Carbs: 31.4g; Fat: 26g

105. Easy-Peasy Club Salad

Servings: 3 | Cooking Time: 0 minutes

½ cup cherry tomatoes, halved	½ teaspoon garlic powder
½ teaspoon onion powder	1 cup diced cucumber
1 tablespoon Dijon mustard	1 tablespoon milk
1 teaspoon dried parsley	2 tablespoons mayonnaise
2 tablespoons sour cream	3 cups romaine lettuce, torn into pieces
3 large hard-boiled eggs, sliced	4 ounces cheddar cheese, cubed

1. Make the dressing by mixing garlic powder, onion powder, dried parsley, mayonnaise, and sour cream in a small bowl. Add a tablespoon

of milk and mix well. If you want the dressing thinner, you can add more milk.
2. In a salad platter, layer salad ingredients with Dijon mustard in the middle.
3. Evenly drizzle with dressing and toss well to coat.
4. Serve and enjoy.

NUTRITION:
Calories: 335.5; Protein: 16.8g; Carbs: 7.9g; Fat: 26.3g

106. Fennel and Seared Scallops Salad

Servings: 4 | Cooking Time: 10 minutes

¼ tsp salt	½ large fennel bulb, halved, cored and very thinly sliced
½ tsp whole fennel seeds, freshly ground	1 large pink grapefruit
1 lb. fresh sea scallops, muscle removed, room temperature	1 tbsp olive oil, divided
1 tsp raw honey	12 whole almonds chopped coarsely and lightly toasted
4 cups red leaf lettuce, cored and torn into bite sized pieces	A pinch of ground pepper

1. To catch the juices, work over a bowl. Peel and segment grapefruit. Strain the juice in a cup.
2. For the dressing, whisk together in a small bowl black pepper, 1/8 tsp salt, 1/8 tsp ground fennel, honey, 2 tsp water, 2 tsp oil and 3 tbsp of pomegranate juice. Set aside 1 tbsp of the dressing.
3. Pat scallops dry with a paper towel and season with remaining salt and ½ tsp ground fennel.
4. On medium fire, place a nonstick skillet and brush with 1 tsp oil. Once heated, add ½ of scallops and cook until lightly browned or for 5 minutes each side. Transfer to a plate and keep warm as you cook the second batch using the same process.
5. Mix together dressing, lettuce and fennel in a large salad bowl. Divide evenly onto 4 salad plates.
6. Evenly top each salad with scallops, grapefruit segments and almonds. Drizzle with reserved dressing, serve and enjoy.

NUTRITION:
Calories: 231.9; Protein: 25.3g; Carbs: 18.5g; Fat: 6.3g

107. Fruity Asparagus-Quinoa Salad

Servings: 8 | Cooking Time: 25 minutes

¼ cup chopped pecans, toasted	½ cup finely chopped white onion
½ jalapeno pepper, diced	½ lb. asparagus, sliced to 2-inch lengths, steamed and chilled
½ tsp kosher salt	1 cup fresh orange sections
1 cup uncooked quinoa	1 tsp olive oil
2 cups water	2 tbsp minced red onion
5 dates, pitted and chopped	**Dressing ingredients**
¼ tsp ground black pepper	¼ tsp kosher salt
1 garlic clove, minced	1 tbsp olive oil
2 tbsp chopped fresh mint	2 tbsp fresh lemon juice
Mint sprigs – optional	

1. Wash and rub with your hands the quinoa in a bowl at least three times, discarding water each and every time.
2. On medium high fire, place a large nonstick fry pan and heat 1 tsp olive oil. For two minutes, sauté onions before adding quinoa and sautéing for another five minutes.
3. Add ½ tsp salt and 2 cups water and bring to a boil. Lower fire to a simmer, cover and cook for 15 minutes. Turn off fire and let stand until water is absorbed.
4. Add pepper, asparagus, dates, pecans and orange sections into a salad bowl. Add cooked quinoa, toss to mix well.
5. In a small bowl, whisk mint, garlic, black pepper, salt, olive oil and lemon juice to create the dressing.
6. Pour dressing over salad, serve and enjoy.

NUTRITION:
Calories: 173; Fat: 6.3g; Protein: 4.3g; Carbohydrates: 24.7g

108. Garden Salad with Balsamic Vinegar

Servings: 1 | Cooking Time: 0 minutes

1 cup baby arugula
1 tbsp raisins
1 tbsp balsamic vinegar

1 cup spinach
1 tbsp almonds, shaved or chopped
½ tbsp extra virgin olive oil

1. In a plate, mix arugula and spinach.
2. Top with raisins and almonds.
3. Drizzle olive oil and balsamic vinegar.
4. Serve and enjoy.

NUTRITION:
Calories: 206; Fat: 15 g; Protein: 5g; Carbohydrates: 14g

109. Garden Salad with Oranges and Olives

Servings: 4 | Cooking Time: 15 minutes

½ cup red wine vinegar
1 tbsp finely chopped celery
16 large ripe black olives
2 navel oranges, peeled and segmented
4 garlic cloves, minced
Cracked black pepper to taste

1 tbsp extra virgin olive oil
1 tbsp finely chopped red onion
2 garlic cloves
4 boneless, skinless chicken breasts, 4-oz each
8 cups leaf lettuce, washed and dried

1. Prepare the dressing by mixing pepper, celery, onion, olive oil, garlic and vinegar in a small bowl. Whisk well to combine.
2. Lightly grease grate and preheat grill to high.
3. Rub chicken with the garlic cloves and discard garlic.
4. Grill chicken for 5 minutes per side or until cooked through.
5. Remove from grill and let it stand for 5 minutes before cutting into ½-inch strips.
6. In 4 serving plates, evenly arrange two cups lettuce, ¼ of the sliced oranges and 4 olives per plate.
7. Top each plate with ¼ serving of grilled chicken, evenly drizzle with dressing, serve and enjoy.

NUTRITION:
Calories: 259.8; Protein: 48.9g; Carbs: 12.9g; Fat: 1.4g

110. Garden Salad with Grapes

Servings: 6 | Cooking Time: 0 minutes

¼ tsp black pepper
½ tsp stone-ground mustard
1 tsp honey
2 cups red grapes, halved

2 tsp grapeseed oil
7 cups loosely packed baby arugula

¼ tsp salt
1 tsp chopped fresh thyme
1 tsp maple syrup
2 tbsp toasted sunflower seed kernels
3 tbsp red wine vinegar

1. In a small bowl whisk together mustard, syrup, honey and vinegar. Whisking continuously, slowly add oil.
2. In a large salad bowl, mix thyme, seeds, grapes and arugula.
3. Drizzle with the oil dressing, season with pepper and salt.
4. Gently toss to coat salad with the dressing.

NUTRITION:
Calories: 85.7; Protein: 1.6g; Carbs: 12.4g; Fat: 3.3g

111. Ginger Yogurt Dressed Citrus Salad

Servings: 6 | Cooking Time: minutes

2/3 cup minced crystallized ginger
¼ tsp ground cinnamon
½ cup dried cranberries
2 large tangerines, peeled

1 16-oz Greek yogurt
2 tbsp honey
3 navel oranges
1 pink grapefruit, peeled

1. Into sections, break tangerines and grapefruit.
2. Cut tangerine sections into half.
3. Into thirds, slice grapefruit sections.
4. Cut orange pith and peel in half and slice oranges into ¼ inch thick rounds, then quartered.
5. In a medium bowl, mix oranges, grapefruit, tangerines and its juices.
6. Add cinnamon, honey and ½ cup of cranberries.
7. Cover and place in the ref for an hour.
8. In a small bowl, mix ginger and yogurt.
9. To serve, add a dollop of yogurt dressing onto a serving of fruit and sprinkle with cranberries.

NUTRITION:
Calories: 190; Protein: 2.9g; Carbs: 16.7g; Fat: 12.4g

112. Goat Cheese and Oregano Dressing Salad

Servings: 4 | Cooking Time: 0 minutes

¾ cup crumbled soft fresh goat cheese
1 ½ large red bell peppers, diced
1/3 cup chopped red onion
2 tbsp fresh lemon juice

1 ½ cups diced celery
1 tbsp chopped fresh oregano
2 tbsp extra virgin olive oil
4 cups baby spinach leaves, coarsely chopped

1. In a large salad bowl, mix oregano, lemon juice and oil.
2. Add pepper and salt to taste.
3. Mix in red onion, goat cheese, celery, bell peppers and spinach.
4. Toss to coat well, serve and enjoy. Ingredients

NUTRITION:
Calories: 110.9; Protein: 6.9g; Carbs: 10.7g; Fat: 4.5g

113. Grape and Walnut Garden Salad

Servings: 2 | Cooking Time: 0 minutes

½ cup chopped walnuts, toasted
½ cup red grapes, halved lengthwise
1 tsp minced garlic
2 tbsp fresh lemon juice
6 cups baby spinach

1 ripe persimmon
1 shallot, minced
1 tsp whole grain mustard
3 tbsp extra virgin olive oil

1. Cut persimmon and red pear into ½-inch cubes. Discard seeds.
2. In a medium bowl, whisk garlic, shallot, olive oil, lemon juice and mustard to make the dressing.
3. In a medium salad bowl, toss to mix spinach, pear and persimmon.
4. Pour in dressing and toss to coat well.
5. Garnish with pecans.
6. Serve and enjoy.

NUTRITION:
Calories: 440; Protein: 6.1g; Carbs: 39.1g; Fat: 28.8g

114. Greek Antipasto Salad

Servings: 4 | Cooking Time: 0 minutes

½ cup artichoke hearts, chipped
½ cup sweet peppers, roasted

4 ounces cooked prosciutto, cut into thin strips
Italian dressing to taste

½ cup olives, sliced
1 large head romaine lettuce, chopped
4 ounces cooked salami, cubed

1. In a large mixing bowl, add all the ingredients except the Italian dressing. Mix everything until the vegetables are evenly distributed.
2. Add the Italian dressing and toss to combine.
3. Serve chilled.

NUTRITION:
Calories: 425.8; Fat: 38.9 g; Protein: 39.2 g; Carbs: 12.6 g

115. Grilled Halloumi Cheese Salad

Servings: 1 | Cooking Time: 10 minutes

0.5 oz chopped walnuts	1 handful baby arugula
1 Persian cucumber, sliced into circles about ½-inch thick	3 oz halloumi cheese
5 grape tomatoes, sliced in half	balsamic vinegar
olive oil	salt

1. Into 1/3 slices, cut the cheese. For 3 to 5 minutes each side, grill the kinds of cheese until you can see grill marks.
2. In a salad bowl, add arugula, cucumber, and tomatoes. Drizzle with olive oil and balsamic vinegar. Season with salt and toss well coat.
3. Sprinkle walnuts and add grilled halloumi.
4. Serve and enjoy.

NUTRITION:
Calories: 543; Protein: 21.0g; Carbs: 9.0g; Fat: 47.0g

116. Grilled Eggplant Salad

Servings: 4 | Cooking Time: 18 minutes

1 avocado, halved, pitted, peeled and cubed	1 Italian eggplant, cut into 1-inch thick slices
1 large red onion, cut into rounds	1 lemon, zested
1 tbsp coarsely chopped oregano leaves	1 tbsp red wine vinegar
1 tsp Dijon mustard	Canola oil
Freshly ground black pepper	Honey
Olive oil	Parsley sprigs for garnish
Salt	

1. With canola oil, brush onions and eggplant and place on grill.
2. Grill on high until onions are slightly charred and eggplants are soft around 5 minutes for onions and 8 to 12 minutes for eggplant.
3. Remove from grill and let cool for 5 minutes.
4. Roughly chop eggplants and onions and place in salad bowl.
5. Add avocado and toss to mix.
6. Whisk oregano, mustard and red wine vinegar in a small bowl.
7. Whisk in olive oil and honey to taste. Season with pepper and salt to taste.
8. Pour dressing to eggplant mixture, toss to mix well.
9. Garnish with parsley sprigs and lemon zest before serving.

NUTRITION:
Calories: 190; Protein: 2.9g; Carbs: 16.7g; Fat: 12.4g

117. Grilled Vegetable Salad

Servings: 3 | Cooking Time: 7 minutes

¼ cup extra virgin olive oil, for brushing	¼ cup fresh basil leaves
¼ lb. feta cheese	½ bunch asparagus, trimmed and cut into bite-size pieces
1 medium onion, cut into ½ inch rings	1-pint cherry tomatoes
1 red bell pepper, quartered, seeds and ribs removed	1 yellow bell pepper, quartered, seeds and ribs removed
Pepper and salt to taste	

1. Toss olive oil and vegetables in a big bowl. Season with salt and pepper.
2. Frill vegetables in a preheated griller for 5-7 minutes or until charred and tender.
3. Transfer veggies to a platter, add feta and basil.
4. In a separate small bowl, mix olive oil, balsamic vinegar, garlic seasoned with pepper and salt.
5. Drizzle dressing over vegetables and serve.

NUTRITION:
Calories: 147.6; Protein: 3.8g; Fat: 19.2g; Carbs: 13.9 g

118. Healthy Detox Salad

Servings: 4 | Cooking Time: 0 minutes

4 cups mixed greens	2 tbsp lemon juice
2 tbsp pumpkin seed oil	1 tbsp chia seeds
2 tbsp almonds, chopped	1 large apple, diced
1 large carrot, coarsely grated	1 large beet, coarsely grated

1. In a medium salad bowl, except for mixed greens, combine all ingredients thoroughly.
2. Into 4 salad plates, divide the mixed greens.
3. Evenly top mixed greens with the salad bowl mixture.
4. Serve and enjoy.

NUTRITION:
Calories: 141; Protein: 2.1g; Carbs: 14.7g; Fat: 8.2g

119. Herbed Calamari Salad

Servings: 6 | Cooking Time: 25 minutes

¼ cup finely chopped cilantro leaves	¼ cup finely chopped mint leaves
¼ tsp freshly ground black pepper	½ cup finely chopped flat leaf parsley leaves
¾ tsp kosher salt	2 ½ lbs. cleaned and trimmed uncooked calamari rings and tentacles, defrosted
3 medium garlic cloves, smashed and minced	3 tbsp extra virgin olive oil
A pinch of crushed red pepper flakes	Juice of 1 large lemon
Peel of 1 lemon, thinly sliced into strips	

1. On a nonstick large fry pan, heat 1 ½ tbsp olive oil. Once hot, sauté garlic until fragrant around a minute.
2. Add calamari, making sure that they are in one layer, if pan is too small then cook in batches.
3. Season with pepper and salt, after 2 to 4 minutes of searing, remove calamari from pan with a slotted spoon and transfer to a large bowl. Continue cooking remainder of calamari.
4. Season cooked calamari with herbs, lemon rind, lemon juice, red pepper flakes, pepper, salt, and remaining olive oil.
5. Toss well to coat, serve and enjoy.

NUTRITION:
Calories: 551.7; Protein: 7.3g; Carbs: 121.4g; Fat: 4.1g

120. Herbed Chicken Salad Greek Style

Servings: 6 | Cooking Time: 0 minutes

¼ cup or 1 oz crumbled feta cheese	½ tsp garlic powder
½ tsp salt	¾ tsp black pepper, divided
1 cup grape tomatoes, halved	1 cup peeled and chopped English cucumbers
1 cup plain fat-free yogurt	1 pound skinless, boneless chicken breast, cut into 1-inch cubes
1 tsp bottled minced garlic	1 tsp ground oregano
2 tsp sesame seed paste or tahini	5 tsp fresh lemon juice, divided
6 pitted kalamata olives, halved	8 cups chopped romaine lettuce
Cooking spray	

1. In a bowl, mix together ¼ tsp salt, ½ tsp pepper, garlic powder and oregano. Then on medium high heat place a skillet and coat with cooking spray and sauté together the spice mixture and chicken until chicken is cooked. Before transferring to bowl, drizzle with juice.
2. In a small bowl, mix thoroughly the following: garlic, tahini, yogurt, ¼ tsp pepper, ¼ tsp salt, and 2 tsp juice.
3. In another bowl, mix together olives, tomatoes, cucumber and lettuce.
4. To Serve salad, place 2 ½ cups of lettuce mixture on plate, topped with ½ cup chicken mixture, 3 tbsp yogurt mixture and 1 tbsp of cheese.

NUTRITION:
Calories: 170.1; Fat: 3.7g; Protein: 20.7g; Carbs: 13.5g

121. Kale Salad Recipe

Servings: 4 | Cooking Time: 7 minutes

¼ cup Kalamata olives
1 ½ tbsp flaxseeds
1 small cucumber, sliced thinly
2 tbsp green onion, chopped
6 cups dinosaur kale, chopped
a pinch of salt

½ of a lemon
1 garlic clove, minced
1 tbsp extra virgin olive oil
2 tbsp red onion, minced
a pinch of dried basil

1. Bring a medium pot, half-filled with water to a boil.
2. Rinse kale and cut into small strips. Place in a steamer and put on top of boiling water and steam for 5 – 7 minutes.
3. Transfer steamed kale to a salad bowl.
4. Season kale with oil, salt, basil and lemon. Toss to coat well.
5. Add remaining ingredients into salad bowl, toss to mix.
6. Serve and enjoy.

NUTRITION:
Calories: 92.7; Protein: 2.4g; Carbs: 6.6g; Fat: 6.3g

122. Cheesy Keto Zucchini Soup

Servings: 2 | Preparation time: 20 mins

½ medium onion, peeled and chopped
1 tablespoon coconut oil
½ tablespoon nutrition al yeast
½ tablespoon parsley, chopped, for garnish

1 cup bone broth
1½ zucchinis, cut into chunks
Dash of black pepper
½ tablespoon coconut cream, for garnish

1. Melt the coconut oil in a large pan over medium heat and add onions.
2. Sauté for about 3 minutes and add zucchinis and bone broth.
3. Reduce the heat to simmer for about 15 minutes and cover the pan.
4. Add nutrition al yeast and transfer to an immersion blender.
5. Blend until smooth and season with black pepper.
6. Top with coconut cream and parsley to serve.

NUTRITION:
Calories: 154 Carbs: 8.9g Fats: 8.1g Proteins: 13.4g Sodium: 93mg Sugar: 3.9g

123. Spring Soup with Poached Egg

Servings: 2 | Preparation time: 20 mins

32 oz vegetable broth
1 head romaine lettuce, chopped

2 eggs
Salt, to taste

1. Bring the vegetable broth to a boil and reduce the heat.
2. Poach the eggs for 5 minutes in the broth and remove them into 2 bowls.
3. Stir in romaine lettuce into the broth and cook for 4 minutes.
4. Dish out in a bowl and serve hot.

NUTRITION:
Calories: 158 Carbs: 6.9g Fats: 7.3g Proteins: 15.4g Sodium: 1513mg Sugar: 3.3g

124. Mint Avocado Chilled Soup

Servings: 2 | Preparation time: 15 mins

2 romaine lettuce leaves
1 medium ripe avocado
20 fresh mint leaves

1 Tablespoon lime juice
1 cup coconut milk, chilled
Salt to taste

1. Put all the ingredients in a blender and blend until smooth.
2. Refrigerate for about 10 minutes and serve chilled.

NUTRITION:
Calories: 432 Carbs: 16.1g Fats: 42.2g Proteins: 5.2g Sodium: 33mg Sugar: 4.5g

125. Easy Butternut Squash Soup

Servings: 4 | Preparation time: 1 hour 45 mins

1 small onion, chopped
4 cups chicken broth
1 butternut squash
3 tablespoons coconut oil
Salt, to taste
Nutmeg and pepper, to taste

1. Put oil and onions in a large pot and add onions.
2. Sauté for about 3 minutes and add chicken broth and butternut squash.
3. Simmer for about 1 hour on medium heat and transfer into an immersion blender.
4. Pulse until smooth and season with salt, pepper and nutmeg.
5. Return to the pot and cook for about 30 minutes.
6. Dish out and serve hot.

NUTRITION:
Calories: 149 Carbs: 6.6g Fats: 11.6g Proteins: 5.4g Sodium: 765mg Sugar: 2.2g

126. Spring Soup Recipe with Poached Egg

Servings: 2 | Preparation time: 20 mins

2 eggs
4 cups chicken broth
Salt, to taste

2 tablespoons butter
1 head of romaine lettuce, chopped

1. Boil the chicken broth and lower heat.
2. Poach the eggs in the broth for about 5 minutes and remove the eggs.
3. Place each egg into a bowl and add chopped romaine lettuce into the broth.
4. Cook for about 10 minutes and ladle the broth with the lettuce into the bowls.

NUTRITION:
Calories: 264 Carbs: 7g Fats: 18.9g Proteins: 16.1g Sodium: 1679mg Sugar: 3.4g

127. Cauliflower, leek & bacon soup

Servings: 4 | Preparation time: 10 mins

4 cups chicken broth
1 leek, chopped
5 bacon strips

½ cauliflower head, chopped
Salt and black pepper, to taste

1. Put the cauliflower, leek and chicken broth into the pot and cook for about 1 hour on medium heat.
2. Transfer into an immersion blender and pulse until smooth.
3. Return the soup into the pot and microwave the bacon strips for 1 minute.
4. Cut the bacon into small pieces and put into the soup.
5. Cook on for about 30 minutes on low heat.
6. Season with salt and pepper and serve.

NUTRITION:
Calories: 185 Carbs: 5.8g Fats: 12.7g Proteins: 10.8g Sodium: 1153mg Sugar: 2.4g

128. Swiss Chard Egg Drop Soup

Servings: 4 | Preparation time: 20 mins

3 cups bone broth
1 teaspoon ground oregano
2 cups Swiss chard, chopped
1 teaspoon ginger, grated

2 eggs, whisked
3 tablespoons butter
2 tablespoons coconut aminos
Salt and black pepper, to taste

1. Heat the bone broth in a saucepan and add whisked eggs while stirring slowly.

2. Add the swiss chard, butter, coconut aminos, ginger, oregano and salt and black pepper.
3. Cook for about 10 minutes and serve hot.

NUTRITION:
Calories: 185 Carbs: 2.9g Fats: 11g Proteins: 18.3g Sodium: 252mg Sugar: 0.4g

129. Mushroom Spinach Soup

Servings: 4 | Preparation time: 25 mins

1cup spinach, cleaned and chopped	100g mushrooms, chopped
1 onion	6 garlic cloves
½ teaspoon red chili powder	Salt and black pepper, to taste
3 tablespoons buttermilk	1 teaspoon almond flour
2 cups chicken broth	3 tablespoons butter
¼ cup fresh cream for garnish	

1. Heat butter in a pan and add onions and garlic.
2. Sauté for about 3 minutes and add spinach, salt and red chili powder.
3. Sauté for about 4 minutes and add mushrooms.
4. Transfer into a blender and blend to make a puree.
5. Return to the pan and add buttermilk and almond flour for creamy texture.
6. Mix well and simmer for about 2 minutes.
7. Garnish with fresh cream and serve hot.

NUTRITION:
Calories: 160 Carbs: 7g Fats: 13.3g Proteins: 4.7g Sodium: 462mg Sugar: 2.7g

130. Delicata Squash Soup

Servings: 5 | Preparation time: 45mins

1½ cups beef bone broth	1 small onion, peeled and grated.
½ teaspoon sea salt	¼ teaspoon poultry seasoning
2 small Delicata Squash, chopped	2 garlic cloves, minced
2 tablespoons olive oil	¼ teaspoon black pepper
1 small lemon, juiced	5 tablespoons sour cream

1. Put Delicata Squash and water in a medium pan and bring to a boil.
2. Reduce the heat and cook for about 20 minutes.
3. Drain and set aside.
4. Put olive oil, onions, garlic and poultry seasoning in a small sauce pan.
5. Cook for about 2 minutes and add broth.
6. Allow it to simmer for 5 minutes and remove from heat.
7. Whisk in the lemon juice and transfer the mixture in a blender.
8. Pulse until smooth and top with sour cream.

NUTRITION:
Calories: 109 Carbs: 4.9g Fats: 8.5g Proteins: 3g Sodium: 279mg Sugar: 2.4g

131. Broccoli Soup

Servings: 6 | Preparation time: 10 mins

3 tablespoons ghee	5 garlic cloves
1 teaspoon sage	¼ teaspoon ginger
2 cups broccoli	1 small onion
1 teaspoon oregano	½ teaspoon parsley
Salt and black pepper, to taste	6 cups vegetable broth
4 tablespoons butter	

1. Put ghee, onions, spices and garlic in a pot and cook for 3 minutes.
2. Add broccoli and cook for about 4 minutes.
3. Add vegetable broth, cover and allow it to simmer for about 30 minutes.
4. Transfer into a blender and blend until smooth.
5. Add the butter to give it a creamy delicious texture and flavor

NUTRITION:
Calories: 183 Carbs: 5.2g Fats: 15.6g Proteins: 6.1g Sodium: 829mg Sugar: 1.8g

132. Apple Pumpkin Soup

Servings: 8 | Preparation time: 10 mins

1 apple, chopped	1 whole kabocha pumpkin, peeled, seeded and cubed
1 cup almond flour	¼ cup ghee
1 pinch cardamom powder	2 quarts water
¼ cup coconut cream	1 pinch ground black pepper

1. Heat ghee in the bottom of a heavy pot and add apples.
2. Cook for about 5 minutes on a medium flame and add pumpkin.
3. Sauté for about 3 minutes and add almond flour.
4. Sauté for about 1 minute and add water.
5. Lower the flame and cook for about 30 minutes.
6. Transfer the soup into an immersion blender and blend until smooth.
7. Top with coconut cream and serve.

NUTRITION:
Calories: 186 Carbs: 10.4g Fats: 14.9g Proteins: 3.7g Sodium: 7mg Sugar: 5.4g

133. Keto French Onion Soup

Servings: 6 | Preparation time: 40 mins

5 tablespoons butter	500 g brown onion medium
4 drops liquid stevia	4 tablespoons olive oil
3 cups beef stock	

1. Put the butter and olive oil in a large pot over medium low heat and add onions and salt.
2. Cook for about 5 minutes and stir in stevia.
3. Cook for another 5 minutes and add beef stock.
4. Reduce the heat to low and simmer for about 25 minutes.
5. Dish out into soup bowls and serve hot.

NUTRITION:
Calories: 198 Carbs: 6g Fats: 20.6g Proteins: 2.9g Sodium: 883mg Sugar: 1.7g

134. Cauliflower and Thyme Soup

Servings: 6 | Preparation time: 30 mins

2 teaspoons thyme powder	1 head cauliflower
3 cups vegetable stock	½ teaspoon matcha green tea powder
3 tablespoons olive oil	Salt and black pepper, to taste
5 garlic cloves, chopped	

1. Put the vegetable stock, thyme and matcha powder to a large pot over medium-high heat and bring to a boil.
2. Add cauliflower and cook for about 10 minutes.
3. Meanwhile, put the olive oil and garlic in a small sauce pan and cook for about 1 minute.
4. Add the garlic, salt and black pepper and cook for about 2 minutes.
5. Transfer into an immersion blender and blend until smooth.
6. Dish out and serve immediately.

NUTRITION:
Calories: 79 Carbs: 3.8g Fats: 7.1g Proteins: 1.3g Sodium: 39mg Sugar: 1.5g

135. Homemade Thai Chicken Soup

Servings: 12 | Preparation time: 8 hours 25 mins

1 lemongrass stalk, cut into large chunks	5 thick slices of fresh ginger
1 whole chicken	20 fresh basil leaves
1 lime, juiced	1 tablespoon salt

1. Place the chicken, 10 basil leaves, lemongrass, ginger, salt and water into the slow cooker.
2. Cook for about 8 hours on low and dish out into a bowl.
3. Stir in fresh lime juice and basil leaves to serve.

NUTRITION:
Calories: 255 Carbs: 1.2g Fats: 17.6g Proteins: 25.2g Sodium: 582mg Sugar: 0.1g

136. Chicken Kale Soup

Servings: 6 | Preparation time: 6 hours 10 mins

2 pounds chicken breast, skinless	1/3 cup onion
1 tablespoon olive oil	14 ounces chicken bone broth
½ cup olive oil	4 cups chicken stock
¼ cup lemon juice	5 ounces baby kale leaves
Salt, to taste	

1. Season chicken with salt and black pepper.
2. Heat olive oil over medium heat in a large skillet and add seasoned chicken.
3. Reduce the temperature and cook for about 15 minutes.
4. Shred the chicken and place in the crock pot.
5. Process the chicken broth and onions in a blender and blend until smooth.
6. Pour into crock pot and stir in the remaining ingredients.
7. Cook on low for about 6 hours, stirring once while cooking.

NUTRITION:

Calories: 261 Carbs: 2g Fats: 21g Proteins: 14.1g Sodium: 264mg Sugar: 0.3g

137. Chicken Veggie Soup

Servings: 6 | Preparation time: 20 mins

5 chicken thighs	12 cups water
1 tablespoon adobo seasoning	4 celery ribs
1 yellow onion	1½ teaspoons whole black peppercorns
6 sprigs fresh parsley	2 teaspoons coarse sea salt
2 carrots	6 mushrooms, sliced
2 garlic cloves	1 bay leaf
3 sprigs fresh thyme	

1. Put water, chicken thighs, carrots, celery ribs, onion, garlic cloves and herbs in a large pot.
2. Bring to a boil and reduce the heat to low.
3. Cover the pot and simmer for about 30 minutes.
4. Dish out the chicken and shred it, removing the bones.
5. Put the bones back into the pot and simmer for about 20 minutes.
6. Strain the broth, discarding the chunks and put the liquid back into the pot.
7. Bring it to a boil and simmer for about 30 minutes.
8. Put the mushrooms in the broth and simmer for about 10 minutes.
9. Dish out to serve hot.

NUTRITION:

Calories: 250 Carbs: 6.4g Fats: 8.9g Proteins: 35.1g Sodium: 852mg Sugar: 2.5g

138. Chicken Mulligatawny Soup

Servings: 10 | Preparation time: 30 mins

1½ tablespoons curry powder	3 cups celery root, diced
2 tablespoons Swerve	10 cups chicken broth
5 cups chicken, chopped and cooked	¼ cup apple cider
½ cup sour cream	¼ cup fresh parsley, chopped
2 tablespoons butter	Salt and black pepper, to taste

1. Combine the broth, butter, chicken, curry powder, celery root and apple cider in a large soup pot.
2. Bring to a boil and simmer for about 30 minutes.
3. Stir in Swerve, sour cream, fresh parsley, salt and black pepper.
4. Dish out and serve hot.

NUTRITION:

Calories: 215 Carbs: 7.1g Fats: 8.5g Proteins: 26.4g Sodium: 878mg Sugar: 2.2g

139. Buffalo Ranch Chicken Soup

Servings: 4 | Preparation time: 40 mins

2 tablespoons parsley	2 celery stalks, chopped
6 tablespoons butter	1 cup heavy whipping cream
4 cups chicken, cooked and shredded	4 tablespoons ranch dressing
¼ cup yellow onions, chopped	8 oz cream cheese
8 cups chicken broth	7 hearty bacon slices, crumbled

1. Heat butter in a pan and add chicken.
2. Cook for about 5 minutes and add 1½ cups water.
3. Cover and cook for about 10 minutes.
4. Put the chicken and rest of the ingredients into the saucepan except parsley and cook for about 10 minutes.
5. Top with parsley and serve hot.

NUTRITION:

Calories: 444 Carbs: 4g Fats: 34g Proteins: 28g Sodium: 1572mg Sugar: 2g

140. Traditional Chicken Soup

Servings: 6 | Preparation time: 1 hour 45 mins

3 pounds chicken	4 quarts water
4 stalks celery	1/3 large red onion
1 large carrot	3 garlic cloves
2 thyme sprigs	2 rosemary sprigs
Salt and black pepper, to taste	

1. Put water and chicken in the stock pot on medium high heat.
2. Bring to a boil and allow it to simmer for about 10 minutes.
3. Add onion, garlic, celery, salt and pepper and simmer on medium low heat for 30 minutes.
4. Add thyme and carrots and simmer on low for another 30 minutes.
5. Dish out the chicken and shred the pieces, removing the bones.
6. Return the chicken pieces to the pot and add rosemary sprigs.
7. Simmer for about 20 minutes at low heat and dish out to serve.

NUTRITION:

Calories: 357 Carbs: 3.3g Fats: 7g Proteins: 66.2g Sodium: 175mg Sugar: 1.1g

141. Chicken Noodle Soup

Servings: 6 | Preparation time: 30 mins

1 onion, minced	1 rib celery, sliced
3 cups chicken, shredded	3 eggs, lightly beaten
1 green onion, for garnish	2 tablespoons coconut oil
1 carrot, peeled and thinly sliced	2 teaspoons dried thyme
2½ quarts homemade bone broth	¼ cup fresh parsley, minced
Salt and black pepper, to taste	

1. Heat coconut oil over medium-high heat in a large pot and add onions, carrots, and celery.
2. Cook for about 4 minutes and stir in the bone broth, thyme and chicken.
3. Simmer for about 15 minutes and stir in parsley.
4. Pour beaten eggs into the soup in a slow steady stream.
5. Remove soup from heat and let it stand for about 2 minutes.
6. Season with salt and black pepper and dish out to serve.

NUTRITION:

Calories: 226 Carbs: 3.5g Fats: 8.9g Proteins: 31.8g Sodium: 152mg Sugar: 1.6g

142. Chicken Cabbage Soup

Servings: 8 | Preparation time: 35 mins

2 celery stalks	2 garlic cloves, minced
4 oz. butter	6 oz. mushrooms, sliced
2 tablespoons onions, dried and minced	1 teaspoon salt
8 cups chicken broth	1 medium carrot
2 cups green cabbage, sliced into strips	2 teaspoons dried parsley
¼ teaspoon black pepper	1½ rotisserie chickens, shredded

1. Melt butter in a large pot and add celery, mushrooms, onions and garlic into the pot.
2. Cook for about 4 minutes and add broth, parsley, carrot, salt and black pepper.
3. Simmer for about 10 minutes and add cooked chicken and cabbage.
4. Simmer for an additional 12 minutes until the cabbage is tender.
5. Dish out and serve hot.

NUTRITION:
Calories: 184 Carbs: 4.2g Fats: 13.1g Proteins: 12.6g Sodium: 1244mg Sugar: 2.1g

143. Green Chicken Enchilada Soup

Servings: 5 | Preparation time: 20 mins

4 oz. cream cheese, softened
½ cup salsa verde
1 cup cheddar cheese, shredded
2 cups cooked chicken, shredded
2 cups chicken stock

1. Put salsa verde, cheddar cheese, cream cheese and chicken stock in an immersion blender and blend until smooth.
2. Pour this mixture into a medium saucepan and cook for about 5 minutes on medium heat.
3. Add the shredded chicken and cook for about 5 minutes.
4. Garnish with additional shredded cheddar and serve hot.

NUTRITION:
Calories: 265 Carbs: 2.2g Fats: 17.4g Proteins: 24.2g Sodium: 686mg Sugar: 0.8g

144. Keto BBQ Chicken Pizza Soup

Servings: 6 | Preparation time: 1 hour 30 mins

6 chicken legs	1 medium red onion, diced
4 garlic cloves	1 large tomato, unsweetened
4 cups green beans	¾ cup BBQ Sauce
1½ cups mozzarella cheese, shredded	¼ cup ghee
2 quarts water	2 quarts chicken stock
Salt and black pepper, to taste	Fresh cilantro, for garnishing

1. Put chicken, water and salt in a large pot and bring to a boil.
2. Reduce the heat to medium-low and cook for about 75 minutes.
3. Shred the meat off the bones using a fork and keep aside.
4. Put ghee, red onions and garlic in a large soup and cook over a medium heat.
5. Add chicken stock and bring to a boil over a high heat.
6. Add green beans and tomato to the pot and cook for about 15 minutes.
7. Add BBQ Sauce, shredded chicken, salt and black pepper to the pot.
8. Ladle the soup into serving bowls and top with shredded mozzarella cheese and cilantro to serve.

NUTRITION:
Calories: 449 Carbs: 7.1g Fats: 32.5g Proteins: 30.8g Sodium: 252mg Sugar: 4.7g

145. Salmon Stew Soup

Servings: 5 | Preparation time: 25 mins

4 cups chicken broth	3 salmon fillets, chunked
2 tablespoons butter	1 cup parsley, chopped
3 cups Swiss chard, roughly chopped	2 Italian squash, chopped
1 garlic clove, crushed	½ lemon, juiced
Salt and black pepper, to taste	2 eggs

1. Put the chicken broth and garlic into a pot and bring to a boil.
2. Add salmon, lemon juice and butter in the pot and cook for about 10 minutes on medium heat.
3. Add Swiss chard, Italian squash, salt and pepper and cook for about 10 minutes.
4. Whisk eggs and add to the pot, stirring continuously.
5. Garnish with parsley and serve.

NUTRITION:
Calories: 262 Carbs: 7.8g Fats: 14g Proteins: 27.5g Sodium: 1021mg Sugar: 1.2g

146. Spicy Halibut Tomato Soup

Servings: 8 | Preparation time: 1 hour 5mins

2 garlic cloves, minced	1 tablespoon olive oil
¼ cup fresh parsley, chopped	10 anchovies canned in oil, minced
6 cups vegetable broth	1 teaspoon black pepper
1 pound halibut fillets, chopped	3 tomatoes, peeled and diced
1 teaspoon salt	1 teaspoon red chili flakes

1. Heat olive oil in a large stockpot over medium heat and add garlic and half of the parsley.
2. Add anchovies, tomatoes, vegetable broth, red chili flakes, salt and black pepper and bring to a boil.
3. Reduce the heat to medium-low and simmer for about 20 minutes.
4. Add halibut fillets and cook for about 10 minutes.
5. Dish out the halibut and shred into small pieces.
6. Mix back with the soup and garnish with the remaining fresh parsley to serve.

NUTRITION:
Calories: 170 Carbs: 3g Fats: 6.7g Proteins: 23.4g Sodium: 2103mg Sugar: 1.8g

PASTA, RICE & GRAINS

147. Delicious Chicken Pasta

Preparation Time: 10 minutes | Cooking Time: 17 minutes | Servings: 4

3 chicken breasts, skinless, boneless, cut into pieces
1/2 cup olives, sliced
1 tbsp roasted red peppers, chopped
2 cups marinara sauce
Pepper

9 oz whole-grain pasta
1/2 cup sun-dried tomatoes
14 oz can tomatoes, diced
1 cup chicken broth
Salt

1. Add all ingredients except whole-grain pasta into the instant pot and stir well.
2. Seal pot with lid and cook on high for 12 minutes.
3. Once done, allow to release pressure naturally. Remove lid.
4. Add pasta and stir well. Seal pot again and select manual and set timer for 5 minutes.
5. Once done, allow to release pressure naturally for 5 minutes then release remaining using quick release. Remove lid.
6. Stir well and serve.

NUTRITION:
Calories 615 Fat 15.4 g Carbohydrates 71 g Sugar 17.6 g Protein 48 g Cholesterol 100 mg

148. Flavors Taco Rice Bowl

Preparation Time: 10 minutes | Cooking Time: 14 minutes | Servings: 8

1 lb ground beef
14 oz can red beans
16 oz salsa
2 cups brown rice
Salt

8 oz cheddar cheese, shredded
2 oz taco seasoning
2 cups of water
Pepper

1. Set instant pot on sauté mode.
2. Add meat to the pot and sauté until brown.
3. Add water, beans, rice, taco seasoning, pepper, and salt and stir well.
4. Top with salsa. Seal pot with lid and cook on high for 14 minutes.
5. Once done, release pressure using quick release. Remove lid.
6. Add cheddar cheese and stir until cheese is melted.
7. Serve and enjoy.

NUTRITION:
Calories 464 Fat 15.3 g Carbohydrates 48.9 g Sugar 2.8 g Protein 32.2 g Cholesterol 83 mg

149. Flavorful Mac & Cheese

Preparation Time: 10 minutes | Cooking Time: 10 minutes | Servings: 6

16 oz whole-grain elbow pasta
1 cup can tomatoes, diced
2 tbsp olive oil
1/2 cup parmesan cheese, grated
1 cup cheddar cheese, grated
1 cup unsweetened almond milk
1/2 cup sun-dried tomatoes, sliced
1 tsp salt

4 cups of water
1 tsp garlic, chopped
1/4 cup green onions, chopped
1/2 cup mozzarella cheese, grated
1/4 cup passata
1 cup marinated artichoke, diced
1/2 cup olives, sliced

1. Add pasta, water, tomatoes, garlic, oil, and salt into the instant pot and stir well.
2. Seal pot with lid and cook on high for 4 minutes.
3. Once done, allow to release pressure naturally for 5 minutes then release remaining using quick release. Remove lid.

4. Set pot on sauté mode. Add green onion, parmesan cheese, mozzarella cheese, cheddar cheese, passata, almond milk, artichoke, sun-dried tomatoes, and olive. Mix well.
5. Stir well and cook until cheese is melted.
6. Serve and enjoy.

NUTRITION:
Calories 519 Fat 17.1 g Carbohydrates 66.5 g Sugar 5.2 g Protein 25 g Cholesterol 26 mg

150. Cucumber Olive Rice

Preparation Time: 10 minutes | Cooking Time: 10 minutes | Servings: 8

2 cups rice, rinsed
1 cup cucumber, chopped
1 tsp lemon zest, grated
2 tbsp olive oil
1/2 tsp dried oregano
1/2 cup onion, chopped
Pepper

1/2 cup olives, pitted
1 tbsp red wine vinegar
1 tbsp fresh lemon juice
2 cups vegetable broth
1 red bell pepper, chopped
1 tbsp olive oil
Salt

1. Add oil into the inner pot of instant pot and set the pot on sauté mode.
2. Add onion and sauté for 3 minutes.
3. Add bell pepper and oregano and sauté for 1 minute.
4. Add rice and broth and stir well.
5. Seal pot with lid and cook on high for 6 minutes.
6. Once done, allow to release pressure naturally for 10 minutes then release remaining using quick release. Remove lid.
7. Add remaining ingredients and stir everything well to mix.
8. Serve immediately and enjoy it.

NUTRITION:
Calories 229 Fat 5.1 g Carbohydrates 40.2 g Sugar 1.6 g Protein 4.9 g Cholesterol 0 mg

151. Flavors Herb Risotto

Preparation Time: 10 minutes | Cooking Time: 15 minutes | Servings: 4

2 cups of rice
3.5 oz heavy cream
1 tbsp fresh basil, chopped
1 onion, chopped
1 tsp garlic, minced
Pepper

2 tbsp parmesan cheese, grated
1 tbsp fresh oregano, chopped
1/2 tbsp sage, chopped
2 tbsp olive oil
4 cups vegetable stock
Salt

1. Add oil into the inner pot of instant pot and set the pot on sauté mode.
2. Add garlic and onion and sauté for 2-3 minutes.
3. Add remaining ingredients except for parmesan cheese and heavy cream and stir well.
4. Seal pot with lid and cook on high for 12 minutes.
5. Once done, allow to release pressure naturally for 10 minutes then release remaining using quick release. Remove lid.
6. Stir in cream and cheese and serve.

NUTRITION:
Calories 514 Fat 17.6 g Carbohydrates 79.4 g Sugar 2.1 g Protein 8.8 g Cholesterol 36 mg

152. Delicious Pasta Primavera

Preparation Time: 10 minutes | Cooking Time: 4 minutes | Servings: 4

8 oz whole wheat penne pasta	1 tbsp fresh lemon juice
2 tbsp fresh parsley, chopped	1/4 cup almonds slivered
1/4 cup parmesan cheese, grated	14 oz can tomatoes, diced
1/2 cup prunes	1/2 cup zucchini, chopped
1/2 cup asparagus, cut into 1-inch pieces	1/2 cup carrots, chopped
1/2 cup broccoli, chopped	1 3/4 cups vegetable stock
Pepper	Salt

1. Add stock, pars, tomatoes, prunes, zucchini, asparagus, carrots, and broccoli into the instant pot and stir well.
2. Seal pot with lid and cook on high for 4 minutes.
3. Once done, release pressure using quick release. Remove lid.
4. Add remaining ingredients and stir well and serve.

NUTRITION:

Calories 303 Fat 2.6 g Carbohydrates 63.5 g Sugar 13.4 g Protein 12.8 g Cholesterol 1 mg

153. Roasted Pepper Pasta

Preparation Time: 10 minutes | Cooking Time: 13 minutes | Servings: 6

1 lb whole wheat penne pasta	1 tbsp Italian seasoning
4 cups vegetable broth	1 tbsp garlic, minced
1/2 onion, chopped	14 oz jar roasted red peppers
1 cup feta cheese, crumbled	1 tbsp olive oil
Pepper	Salt

1. Add roasted pepper into the blender and blend until smooth.
2. Add oil into the inner pot of instant pot and set the pot on sauté mode.
3. Add garlic and onion and sauté for 2-3 minutes.
4. Add blended roasted pepper and sauté for 2 minutes.
5. Add remaining ingredients except feta cheese and stir well.
6. Seal pot with lid and cook on high for 8 minutes.
7. Once done, allow to release pressure naturally for 5 minutes then release remaining using quick release. Remove lid.
8. Top with feta cheese and serve.

NUTRITION:

Calories 459 Fat 10.6 g Carbohydrates 68.1 g Sugar 2.1 g Protein 21.3 g Cholesterol 24 mg

154. Cheese Basil Tomato Rice

Preparation Time: 10 minutes | Cooking Time: 26 minutes | Servings: 8

1 1/2 cups brown rice	1 cup parmesan cheese, grated
1/4 cup fresh basil, chopped	2 cups grape tomatoes, halved
8 oz can tomato sauce	1 3/4 cup vegetable broth
1 tbsp garlic, minced	1/2 cup onion, diced
1 tbsp olive oil	Pepper
Salt	

1. Add oil into the inner pot of instant pot and set the pot on sauté mode.
2. Add garlic and onion and sauté for 4 minutes.
3. Add rice, tomato sauce, broth, pepper, and salt and stir well.
4. Seal pot with lid and cook on high for 22 minutes.
5. Once done, allow to release pressure naturally for 10 minutes then release remaining using quick release. Remove lid.
6. Add remaining ingredients and stir well.
7. Serve and enjoy.

NUTRITION:

Calories 208 Fat 5.6 g Carbohydrates 32.1 g Sugar 2.8 g Protein 8.3 g Cholesterol 8 mg

155. Mac & Cheese

Preparation Time: 10 minutes | Cooking Time: 4 minutes | Servings: 8

1 lb whole grain pasta	1/2 cup parmesan cheese, grated
4 cups cheddar cheese, shredded	1 cup milk
1/4 tsp garlic powder	1/2 tsp ground mustard
2 tbsp olive oil	4 cups of water
Pepper	Salt

1. Add pasta, garlic powder, mustard, oil, water, pepper, and salt into the instant pot.
2. Seal pot with lid and cook on high for 4 minutes.
3. Once done, release pressure using quick release. Remove lid.
4. Add remaining ingredients and stir well and serve.

NUTRITION:

Calories 509 Fat 25.7 g Carbohydrates 43.8 g Sugar 3.8 g Protein 27.3 g Cholesterol 66 mg

156. Tuna Pasta

Preparation Time: 10 minutes | Cooking Time: 8 minutes | Servings: 6

10 oz can tuna, drained	15 oz whole wheat rotini pasta
4 oz mozzarella cheese, cubed	1/2 cup parmesan cheese, grated
1 tsp dried basil	14 oz can tomatoes, diced
4 cups vegetable broth	1 tbsp garlic, minced
8 oz mushrooms, sliced	2 zucchini, sliced
1 onion, chopped	2 tbsp olive oil
Pepper	Salt

1. Add oil into the inner pot of instant pot and set the pot on sauté mode.
2. Add mushrooms, zucchini, and onion and sauté until onion is softened.
3. Add garlic and sauté for a minute.
4. Add pasta, basil, tuna, tomatoes, and broth and stir well.
5. Seal pot with lid and cook on high for 4 minutes.
6. Once done, allow to release pressure naturally for 5 minutes then release remaining using quick release. Remove lid.
7. Add remaining ingredients and stir well and serve.

NUTRITION:

Calories 346 Fat 11.9 g Carbohydrates 31.3 g Sugar 6.3 g Protein 6.3 g Cholesterol 30 mg

157. Vegan Olive Pasta

Preparation Time: 10 minutes | Cooking Time: 5 minutes | Servings: 4

4 cups whole grain penne pasta	1/2 cup olives, sliced
1 tbsp capers	1/4 tsp red pepper flakes
3 cups of water	4 cups pasta sauce, homemade
1 tbsp garlic, minced	Pepper
Salt	

1. Add all ingredients into the inner pot of instant pot and stir well.
2. Seal pot with lid and cook on high for 5 minutes.
3. Once done, release pressure using quick release. Remove lid.
4. Stir and serve.

NUTRITION:

Calories 441 Fat 10.1 g Carbohydrates 77.3 g Sugar 24.1 g Protein 11.8 g Cholesterol 5 mg

158. Italian Mac & Cheese

Preparation Time: 10 minutes | Cooking Time: 6 minutes | Servings: 4

1 lb whole grain pasta	2 tsp Italian seasoning
1 1/2 tsp garlic powder	1 1/2 tsp onion powder
1 cup sour cream	4 cups of water
4 oz parmesan cheese, shredded	12 oz ricotta cheese
Pepper	Salt

1. Add all ingredients except ricotta cheese into the inner pot of instant pot and stir well.
2. Seal pot with lid and cook on high for 6 minutes.
3. Once done, allow to release pressure naturally for 5 minutes then release remaining using quick release. Remove lid.
4. Add ricotta cheese and stir well and serve.

NUTRITION
Calories 388 Fat 25.8 g Carbohydrates 18.1 g Sugar 4 g Protein 22.8 g Cholesterol 74 mg

159. Italian Chicken Pasta

Preparation Time: 10 minutes | Cooking Time: 9 minutes | Servings: 8

1 lb chicken breast, skinless, boneless, and cut into chunks	1/2 cup cream cheese
1 cup mozzarella cheese, shredded	1 1/2 tsp Italian seasoning
1 tsp garlic, minced	1 cup mushrooms, diced
1/2 onion, diced	2 tomatoes, diced
2 cups of water	16 oz whole wheat penne pasta
Pepper	Salt

1. Add all ingredients except cheeses into the inner pot of instant pot and stir well.
2. Seal pot with lid and cook on high for 9 minutes.
3. Once done, allow to release pressure naturally for 5 minutes then release remaining using quick release. Remove lid.
4. Add cheeses and stir well and serve.

NUTRITION:
Calories 328 Fat 8.5 g Carbohydrates 42.7 g Sugar 1.4 g Protein 23.7 g Cholesterol 55 mg

160. Delicious Greek Chicken Pasta

Preparation Time: 10 minutes | Cooking Time: 10 minutes | Servings: 6

2 chicken breasts, skinless, boneless, and cut into chunks	1/2 cup olives, sliced
2 cups vegetable stock	12 oz Greek vinaigrette dressing
1 lb whole grain pasta	Pepper
Salt	

1. Add all ingredients into the inner pot of instant pot and stir well.
2. Seal pot with lid and cook on high for 10 minutes.
3. Once done, release pressure using quick release. Remove lid.
4. Stir well and serve.

NUTRITION:
Calories 325 Fat 25.8 g Carbohydrates 10.5 g Sugar 4 g Protein 15.6 g Cholesterol 43 mg

161. Pesto Chicken Pasta

Preparation Time: 10 minutes | Cooking Time: 10 minutes | Servings: 6

1 lb chicken breast, skinless, boneless, and diced	3 tbsp olive oil
1/2 cup parmesan cheese, shredded	1 tsp Italian seasoning
1/4 cup heavy cream	16 oz whole wheat pasta
6 oz basil pesto	3 1/2 cups water
Pepper	Salt

1. Season chicken with Italian seasoning, pepper, and salt.
2. Add oil into the inner pot of instant pot and set the pot on sauté mode.
3. Add chicken to the pot and sauté until brown.
4. Add remaining ingredients except for parmesan cheese, heavy cream, and pesto and stir well.
5. Seal pot with lid and cook on high for 5 minutes.
6. Once done, release pressure using quick release. Remove lid.
7. Stir in parmesan cheese, heavy cream, and pesto and serve.

NUTRITION:
Calories 475 Fat 14.7 g Carbohydrates 57 g Sugar 2.8 g Protein 28.7 g Cholesterol 61 mg

162. Spinach Pesto Pasta

Preparation Time: 10 minutes | Cooking Time: 10 minutes | Servings: 4

8 oz whole-grain pasta	1/3 cup mozzarella cheese, grated
1/2 cup pesto	5 oz fresh spinach
1 3/4 cup water	8 oz mushrooms, chopped
1 tbsp olive oil	Pepper
Salt	

1. Add oil into the inner pot of instant pot and set the pot on sauté mode.
2. Add mushrooms and sauté for 5 minutes.
3. Add water and pasta and stir well.
4. Seal pot with lid and cook on high for 5 minutes.
5. Once done, release pressure using quick release. Remove lid.
6. Stir in remaining ingredients and serve.

NUTRITION:
Calories 213 Fat 17.3 g Carbohydrates 9.5 g Sugar 4.5 g Protein 7.4 g Cholesterol 9 mg

163. Fiber Packed Chicken Rice

Preparation Time: 10 minutes | Cooking Time: 16 minutes | Servings: 6

1 lb chicken breast, skinless, boneless, and cut into chunks	14.5 oz can cannellini beans
4 cups chicken broth	2 cups wild rice
1 tbsp Italian seasoning	1 small onion, chopped
1 tbsp garlic, chopped	1 tbsp olive oil
Pepper	Salt

1. Add oil into the inner pot of instant pot and set the pot on sauté mode.
2. Add garlic and onion and sauté for 2 minutes.
3. Add chicken and cook for 2 minutes.
4. Add remaining ingredients and stir well.
5. Seal pot with lid and cook on high for 12 minutes.
6. Once done, release pressure using quick release. Remove lid.
7. Stir well and serve.

NUTRITION:
Calories 399 Fat 6.4 g Carbohydrates 53.4 g Sugar 3 g Protein 31.6 g Cholesterol 50 mg

164. Tasty Greek Rice

Preparation Time: 10 minutes | Cooking Time: 10 minutes | Servings: 6

1 3/4 cup brown rice, rinsed and drained	3/4 cup roasted red peppers, chopped
1 cup olives, chopped	1 tsp dried oregano
1 tsp Greek seasoning	1 3/4 cup vegetable broth
2 tbsp olive oil	Salt

1. Add oil into the inner pot of instant pot and set the pot on sauté mode.

2. Add rice and cook for 5 minutes.
3. Add remaining ingredients except for red peppers and olives and stir well.
4. Seal pot with lid and cook on high for 5 minutes.
5. Once done, allow to release pressure naturally for 10 minutes then release remaining using quick release. Remove lid.
6. Add red peppers and olives and stir well.
7. Serve and enjoy. Ingredients

NUTRITION:
Calories 285 Fat 9.1 g Carbohydrates 45.7 g Sugar 1.2 g Protein 6 g Cholesterol 0 mg

165. Bulgur Salad

Preparation Time: 10 minutes | Cooking Time: 1 minute | Servings: 2

1/2 cup bulgur wheat	1/4 cup fresh parsley, chopped
1 tbsp fresh mint, chopped	1/3 cup feta cheese, crumbled
2 tbsp fresh lemon juice	2 tbsp olives, chopped
1/4 cup olive oil	1/2 cup tomatoes, chopped
1/3 cup cucumber, chopped	1/2 cup water
Salt	

1. Add the bulgur wheat, water, and salt into the instant pot.
2. Seal pot with lid and cook on high for 1 minute.
3. Once done, release pressure using quick release. Remove lid.
4. Transfer bulgur wheat to the mixing bowl. Add remaining ingredients to the bowl and mix well.
5. Serve and enjoy.

NUTRITION:
Calories 430 Fat 32.2 g Carbohydrates 31.5 g Sugar 3 g Protein 8.9 g Cholesterol 22 mg

166. Perfect Herb Rice

Preparation Time: 10 minutes | Cooking Time: 4 minutes | Servings: 4

1 cup brown rice, rinsed	1 tbsp olive oil
1 1/2 cups water	1/2 cup fresh mix herbs, chopped
1 tsp salt	

1. Add all ingredients into the inner pot of instant pot and stir well.
2. Seal pot with lid and cook on high for 4 minutes.
3. Once done, allow to release pressure naturally for 10 minutes then release remaining using quick release. Remove lid.
4. Stir well and serve.

NUTRITION:
Calories 264 Fat 9.9 g Carbohydrates 36.7 g Sugar 0.4 g Protein 7.3 g Cholesterol 0 mg

167. Herb Polenta

Preparation Time: 10 minutes | Cooking Time: 12 minutes | Servings: 6

1/4 tsp nutmeg	
3 tbsp fresh parsley, chopped	1/4 cup milk
1/2 cup parmesan cheese, grated	4 cups vegetable broth
2 tsp thyme, chopped	2 tsp rosemary, chopped
2 tsp sage, chopped	1 small onion, chopped

1. Add oil into the inner pot of instant pot and set the pot on sauté mode.
2. Add onion and herbs and sauté for 4 minutes.
3. Add polenta, broth, and salt and stir well.
4. Seal pot with lid and cook on high for 8 minutes.
5. Once done, allow to release pressure naturally. Remove lid.
6. Stir in remaining ingredients and serve.

NUTRITION:

Calories 196 Fat 7.8 g Carbohydrates 23.5 g Sugar 1.7 g Protein 8.2 g Cholesterol 6 mg

168. Pecorino Pasta with Sausage and Fresh Tomato

Servings: 4 | Cooking Time: 20 minutes

¼ cup torn fresh basil leaves	1/8 tsp black pepper
¼ tsp salt	6 tbsp grated fresh pecorino Romano cheese, divided
1 ¼ lbs. tomatoes, chopped	2 tsp minced garlic
1 cup vertically sliced onions	2 tsp olive oil
8 oz sweet Italian sausage	8 oz uncooked penne, cooked and drained

1. On medium high fire, place a nonstick fry pan with oil and cook for five minutes onion and sausage. Stir constantly to break sausage into pieces.
2. Stir in garlic and continue cooking for two minutes more.
3. Add tomatoes and cook for another two minutes.
4. Remove pan from fire, season with pepper and salt. Mix well.
5. Stir in 2 tbsp cheese and pasta. Toss well.
6. Transfer to a serving dish, garnish with basil and remaining cheese before serving.

NUTRITION:
Calories: 376; Carbs: 50.8g; Protein: 17.8g; Fat: 11.6g

169. Pesto Pasta and Shrimps

Servings: 4 | Cooking Time: 15 minutes

¼ cup pesto, divided	¼ cup shaved Parmesan Cheese
1 ¼ lbs. large shrimp, peeled and deveined	1 cup halved grape tomatoes
4-oz angel hair pasta, cooked, rinsed and drained	

1. On medium high fire, place a nonstick large fry pan and grease with cooking spray.
2. Add tomatoes, pesto and shrimp. Cook for 15 minutes or until shrimps are opaque, while covered.
3. Stir in cooked pasta and cook until heated through.
4. Transfer to a serving plate and garnish with Parmesan cheese.

NUTRITION:
Calories: 319; Carbs: 23.6g; Protein: 31.4g; Fat: 11g

170. Prosciutto e Faggioli

Servings: 4 | Cooking Time: 15 minutes

12 oz pasta, cooked and drained	Pepper and salt to taste
3 tbsp snipped fresh chives	3 cups arugula or watercress leaves, loosely packed
½ cup chicken broth, warm	1 tbsp Herbed garlic butter
½ cup shredded pecorino Toscano	4 oz prosciutto, cut into bite sizes
2 cups cherry tomatoes, halved	1 can of 19oz white kidney beans, rinsed and drained

1. Heat over medium low fire herbed garlic butter, cheese, prosciutto, tomatoes and beans in a big saucepan for 2 minutes.
2. Once mixture is simmering, stir constantly to melt cheese while gradually stirring in the broth.
3. Once cheese is fully melted and incorporated, add chives, arugula, pepper and salt.
4. Turn off the fire and toss in the cooked pasta. Serve and enjoy.

NUTRITION:
Calories: 452; Carbs: 57.9g; Protein: 30.64g; Fat: 11.7g

171. Puttanesca Style Bucatini

Servings: 4 | Cooking Time: 40 minutes

1 tbsp capers, rinsed	1 tsp coarsely chopped fresh oregano
1 tsp finely chopped garlic	1/8 tsp salt
12-oz bucatini pasta	2 cups coarsely chopped canned no-salt-added whole peeled tomatoes with their juice
3 tbsp extra virgin olive oil, divided	4 anchovy fillets, chopped
8 black Kalamata olives, pitted and sliced into slivers	

1. Cook bucatini pasta according to package directions. Drain, keep warm, and set aside.
2. On medium fire, place a large nonstick saucepan and heat 2 tbsp oil.
3. Sauté anchovies until it starts to disintegrate.
4. Add garlic and sauté for 15 seconds.
5. Add tomatoes, sauté for 15 to 20 minutes or until no longer watery. Season with 1/8 tsp salt.
6. Add oregano, capers, and olives.
7. Add pasta, sautéing until heated through.
8. To serve, drizzle pasta with remaining olive oil and enjoy.

NUTRITION:
Calories: 207.4; Carbs: 31g; Protein: 5.1g; Fat: 7g

172. Quinoa & Black Bean Stuffed Sweet Potatoes

Servings: 8 | Cooking Time: 60 minutes

4 sweet potatoes	½ onion, diced
1 garlic glove, crushed and diced	½ large bell pepper diced (about 2/3 cups)
Handful of diced cilantro	½ cup cooked quinoa
½ cup black beans	1 tbsp olive oil
1 tbsp chili powder	½ tbsp cumin
½ tbsp paprika	½ tbsp oregano
2 tbsp lime juice	2 tbsp honey
Sprinkle salt	1 cup shredded cheddar cheese
Chopped spring onions, for garnish (optional)	

1. Preheat oven to 400oF.
2. Wash and scrub outside of potatoes. Poke with fork a few times and then place on parchment paper on cookie sheet. Bake for 40-45 minutes or until it is cooked.
3. While potatoes are baking, sauté onions, garlic, olive oil and spices in a pan on the stove until onions are translucent and soft.
4. In the last 10 minutes while the potatoes are cooking, in a large bowl combine the onion mixture with the beans, quinoa, honey, lime juice, cilantro and ½ cup cheese. Mix well.
5. When potatoes are cooked, remove from oven and let cool slightly. When cool to touch, cut in half (hot dog style) and scoop out most of the insides. Leave a thin ring of potato so that it will hold its shape. You can save the sweet potato guts for another recipe, such as my veggie burgers (recipe posted below).
6. Fill with bean and quinoa mixture. Top with remaining cheddar cheese.
7. (If making this a freezer meal, stop here. Individually wrap potato skins in plastic wrap and place on flat surface to freeze. Once frozen, place all potatoes in large zip lock container or Tupperware.)
8. Return to oven for an additional 10 minutes or until cheese is melted.

NUTRITION:
Calories: 243; Carbs: 37.6g; Protein: 8.5g; Fat: 7.3g

173. Quinoa and Three Beans Recipe

Servings: 8, | Cooking Time: 35 minutes

1 cup grape tomatoes, sliced in half	1 cup quinoa
1 cup seedless cucumber, chopped	1 red bell pepper, seeds removed and chopped

1 tablespoon balsamic vinegar	1 yellow bell pepper, seeds removed and chopped
1/2-pound green beans, trimmed and snapped into 2-inch pieces	1/3 cup pitted kalamata olives, cut in half
1/4 cup chopped fresh basil	1/4 cup diced red onion
1/4 cup feta cheese crumbles	1/4 cup olive oil
1/4 teaspoon dried basil	1/4 teaspoon dried oregano
15 ounces garbanzo beans, drained and rinsed	15 ounces white beans, drained and rinsed
2 cups water	2 garlic cloves, smashed
kosher salt and freshly ground black pepper to taste	

1. Bring water and quinoa to a boil in a medium saucepan. Cover, reduce heat to low, and cook until quinoa is tender, around 15 minutes.
2. Remove from heat and let stand for 5 minutes, covered.
3. Remove lid and fluff with a fork. Transfer to a large salad bowl.
4. Meanwhile, Bring a large pot of salted water to a boil and blanch the green beans for two minutes. Drain and place in a bowl of ice water. Drain well.
5. Add the fresh basil, olives, feta cheese, red onion, tomatoes, cucumbers, peppers, white beans, garbanzo beans, and green beans in bowl of quinoa.
6. In a small bowl, whisk together the pepper, salt, oregano, dried basil, balsamic, and olive oil. Pour dressing over the salad and gently toss salad until coated with dressing.
7. Season with additional salt and pepper if needed.
8. Serve and enjoy.

NUTRITION:
Calories: 249; Carbs: 31.0g; Protein: 8.0g; Fat: 10.0g

174. Quinoa Buffalo Bites

Servings: 4 | Cooking Time: 15 minutes

2 cups cooked quinoa	1 cup shredded mozzarella
1/2 cup buffalo sauce	1/4 cup +1 Tbsp flour
1 egg	1/4 cup chopped cilantro
1 small onion, diced	

1. Preheat oven to 350oF.
2. Mix all ingredients in large bowl.
3. Press mixture into greased mini muffin tins.
4. Bake for approximately 15 minutes or until bites are golden.
5. Enjoy on its own or with blue cheese or ranch dip.

NUTRITION:
Calories: 212; Carbs: 30.6g; Protein: 15.9g; Fat: 3.0g

175. Raisins, Nuts and Beef on Hashweh Rice

Servings: 8 | Cooking Time: 50 minutes

½ cup dark raisins, soaked in 2 cups water for an hour	1/3 cup slivered almonds, toasted and soaked in 2 cups water overnight
1/3 cup pine nuts, toasted and soaked in 2 cups water overnight	½ cup fresh parsley leaves, roughly chopped
Pepper and salt to taste	¾ tsp ground cinnamon, divided
¾ tsp cloves, divided	1 tsp garlic powder
1 ¾ tsp allspice, divided	1 lb. lean ground beef or lean ground lamb
1 small red onion, finely chopped	Olive oil
1 ½ cups medium grain rice	

1. For 15 to 20 minutes, soak rice in cold water. You will know that soaking is enough when you can snap a grain of rice easily between your thumb and index finger. Once soaking is done, drain rice well.
2. Meanwhile, drain pine nuts, almonds and raisins for at least a minute and transfer to one bowl. Set aside.
3. On a heavy cooking pot on medium high fire, heat 1 tbsp olive oil.
4. Once oil is hot, add red onions. Sauté for a minute before adding ground meat and sauté for another minute.
5. Season ground meat with pepper, salt, ½ tsp ground cinnamon, ½ tsp ground cloves, 1 tsp garlic powder, and 1 ¼ tsp allspice.

6. Sauté ground meat for 10 minutes or until browned and cooked fully. Drain fat.
7. In same pot with cooked ground meat, add rice on top of meat.
8. Season with a bit of pepper and salt. Add remaining cinnamon, ground cloves, and allspice. Do not mix.
9. Add 1 tbsp olive oil and 2 ½ cups of water. Bring to a boil and once boiling, lower fire to a simmer. Cook while covered until liquid is fully absorbed, around 20 to 25 minutes.
10. Turn of fire.
11. To serve, place a large serving platter that fully covers the mouth of the pot. Place platter upside down on mouth of pot, and invert pot. The inside of the pot should now rest on the platter with the rice on bottom of plate and ground meat on top of it.
12. Garnish the top of the meat with raisins, almonds, pine nuts, and parsley.
13. Serve and enjoy.

NUTRITION:
Calories: 357; Carbs: 39.0g; Protein: 16.7g; Fat: 15.9g

176. Raw Tomato Sauce & Brie on Linguine
Servings: 4, | Cooking Time: 12 minutes

¼ cup grated low-fat Parmesan cheese
12 oz whole wheat linguine
2 green onions, green parts only, sliced thinly
2 tbsp extra virgin olive oil
3 oz low-fat Brie cheese, cubed, rind removed and discarded
Pepper and salt to taste

½ cup loosely packed fresh basil leaves, torn
2 cups loosely packed baby arugula
2 tbsp balsamic vinegar

3 large vine-ripened tomatoes
3 tbsp toasted pine nuts

1. Toss together pepper, salt, vinegar, oil, onions, Parmesan, basil, arugula, Brie and tomatoes in a large bowl and set aside.
2. Cook linguine following package instructions. Reserve 1 cup of pasta cooking water after linguine is cooked. Drain and discard the rest of the pasta. Do not run under cold water, instead immediately add into bowl of salad. Let it stand for a minute without mixing.
3. Add ¼ cup of reserved pasta water into bowl to make a creamy sauce. Add more pasta water if desired. Toss to mix well.
4. Serve and enjoy.

NUTRITION:
Calories: 274.7; Carbs: 30.9g; Protein: 14.6g; Fat: 10.3g

177. Red Quinoa Peach Porridge
Servings: 1 | Cooking Time: 30 minutes

¼ cup old fashioned rolled oats
½ cup milk
2 peaches, peeled and sliced

¼ cup red quinoa
1 ½ cups water

1. On a small saucepan, place the peaches and quinoa. Add water and cook for 30 minutes.
2. Add the oatmeal and milk last and cook until the oats become tender.
3. Stir occasionally to avoid the porridge from sticking on the bottom of the pan.

NUTRITION:
Calories: 456.6; Carbs: 77.3g; Protein: 16.6g; Fat: 9g

178. Red Wine Risotto
Servings: 8 | Cooking Time: 25 minutes

Pepper to taste

2 tsp tomato paste
¼ tsp salt
2 cloves garlic, minced
2 tbsp extra-virgin olive oil

1 cup finely shredded Parmigian-Reggiano cheese, divided
1 ¾ cups dry red wine
1 ½ cups Italian 'risotto' rice
1 medium onion, freshly chopped
4 ½ cups reduced sodium beef broth

1. On medium high fire, bring to a simmer broth in a medium fry pan. Lower fire so broth is steaming but not simmering.
2. On medium low heat, place a Dutch oven and heat oil.
3. Sauté onions for 5 minutes. Add garlic and cook for 2 minutes.
4. Add rice, mix well, and season with salt.
5. Into rice, add a generous splash of wine and ½ cup of broth.
6. Lower fire to a gentle simmer, cook until liquid is fully absorbed while stirring rice every once in a while.
7. Add another splash of wine and ½ cup of broth. Stirring once in a while.
8. Add tomato paste and stir to mix well.
9. Continue cooking and adding wine and broth until broth is used up.
10. Once done cooking, turn off fire and stir in pepper and ¾ cup cheese.
11. To serve, sprinkle with remaining cheese and enjoy.

NUTRITION:
Calories: 231; Carbs: 33.9g; Protein: 7.9g; Fat: 5.7g

179. Rice & Currant Salad Mediterranean Style
Servings: 4 | Cooking Time: 50 minutes

1 cup basmati rice
2 1/2 Tablespoons lemon juice
2 Tablespoons fresh orange juice
1/2 teaspoon cinnamon
4 chopped green onions
3/4 cup shelled pistachios or almonds

salt
1 teaspoon grated orange zest
1/4 cup olive oil
Salt and pepper to taste
1/2 cup dried currants
1/4 cup chopped fresh parsley

1. Place a nonstick pot on medium high fire and add rice. Toast rice until opaque and starts to smell, around 10 minutes.
2. Add 4 quarts of boiling water to pot and 2 tsp salt. Boil until tender, around 8 minutes uncovered.
3. Drain the rice and spread out on a lined cookie sheet to cool completely.
4. In a large salad bowl, whisk well the oil, juices and spices. Add salt and pepper to taste.
5. Add half of the green onions, half of parsley, currants, and nuts.
6. Toss with the cooled rice and let stand for at least 20 minutes.
7. If needed adjust seasoning with pepper and salt.
8. Garnish with remaining parsley and green onions.

NUTRITION:
Calories: 450; Carbs: 50.0g; Protein: 9.0g; Fat: 24.0g

180. Ricotta and Spinach Ravioli
Servings: 2 | Cooking Time: 15 minutes

1 cup chicken stock
1 batch pasta dough
3 tbsp heavy cream
1 ¾ cups baby spinach
2 tbsp butter

1 cup frozen spinach, thawed
INGREDIENTS Filling
1 cup ricotta
1 small onion, finely chopped

1. Create the filling: In a fry pan, sauté onion and butter around five minutes. Add the baby spinach leaves and continue simmering for another four minutes. Remove from fire, drain liquid and mince the onion and leaves. Then combine with 2 tbsp cream and the ricotta ensuring that it is well combined. Add pepper and salt to taste.
2. With your pasta dough, divide it into four balls. Roll out one ball to ¼ inch thick rectangular spread. Cut a 1 ½ inch by 3-inch rectangles. Place filling on the middle of the rectangles, around 1 tablespoonful and brush filling with cold water. Fold the rectangles in half, ensuring that no air is trapped within and seal using a cookie cutter. Use up all the filling.
3. Create Pasta Sauce: Until smooth, puree chicken stock and spinach. Pour into heated fry pan and for two minutes cook it. Add 1 tbsp cream and season with pepper and salt. Continue cooking for a minute and turn of fire.
4. Cook the raviolis by submerging in a boiling pot of water with salt. Cook until al dente then drain. Then quickly transfer the cooked ravioli into the fry pan of pasta sauce, toss to mix and serve.

NUTRITION:
Calories: 443; Carbs: 12.3g; Protein: 18.8g; Fat: 36.8g

181. Roasted Red Peppers and Shrimp Pasta

Servings: 6 | Cooking Time: 10 minutes

12 oz pasta, cooked and drained	1 cup finely shredded Parmesan Cheese
¼ cup snipped fresh basil	½ cup whipping cream
½ cup dry white wine	1 12oz jar roasted red sweet peppers, drained and chopped
¼ tsp crushed red pepper	6 cloves garlic, minced
1/3 cup finely chopped onion	2 tbsp olive oil
¼ cup butter	1 ½ lbs. fresh, peeled, deveined, rinsed and drained medium shrimps

1. On medium high fire, heat butter in a big fry pan and add garlic and onions. Stir fry until onions are soft, around two minutes. Add crushed red pepper and shrimps, sauté for another two minutes before adding wine and roasted peppers.
2. Allow mixture to boil before lowering heat to low fire and for two minutes, let the mixture simmer uncovered. Stirring occasionally, add cream once shrimps are cooked and simmer for a minute.
3. Add basil and remove from fire. Toss in the pasta and mix gently. Transfer to serving plates and top with cheese.

NUTRITION:
Calories: 418; Carbs: 26.9g; Protein: 37.1g; Fat: 18.8g

182. Seafood and Veggie Pasta

Servings: 4 | Cooking Time: 20 minutes

¼ tsp pepper	¼ tsp salt
1 lb raw shelled shrimp	1 lemon, cut into wedges
1 tbsp butter	1 tbsp olive oil
2 5-oz cans chopped clams, drained (reserve 2 tbsp clam juice)	2 tbsp dry white wine
4 cloves garlic, minced	4 cups zucchini, spiraled (use a veggie spiralizer)
4 tbsp Parmesan Cheese	Chopped fresh parsley to garnish

1. Ready the zucchini and spiralize with a veggie spiralizer. Arrange 1 cup of zucchini noodle per bowl. Total of 4 bowls.
2. On medium fire, place a large nonstick saucepan and heat oil and butter.
3. For a minute, sauté garlic. Add shrimp and cook for 3 minutes until opaque or cooked.
4. Add white wine, reserved clam juice and clams. Bring to a simmer and continue simmering for 2 minutes or until half of liquid has evaporated. Stir constantly.
5. Season with pepper and salt. And if needed add more to taste.
6. Remove from fire and evenly distribute seafood sauce to 4 bowls.
7. Top with a tablespoonful of Parmesan cheese per bowl, serve and enjoy.

NUTRITION:
Calories: 324.9; Carbs: 12g; Protein: 43.8g; Fat: 11.3g

183. Seafood Paella with Couscous

Servings: 4 | Cooking Time: 15 minutes

½ cup whole wheat couscous	4 oz small shrimp, peeled and deveined
4 oz bay scallops, tough muscle removed	¼ cup vegetable broth
1 cup freshly diced tomatoes and juice	Pinch of crumbled saffron threads
¼ tsp freshly ground pepper	¼ tsp salt
½ tsp fennel seed	½ tsp dried thyme
1 clove garlic, minced	1 medium onion, chopped
2 tsp extra virgin olive oil	

DIRECTIONS
1. Put on medium fire a large saucepan and add oil. Stir in the onion and sauté for three minutes before adding: saffron, pepper, salt, fennel seed, thyme, and garlic. Continue to sauté for another minute.
2. Then add the broth and tomatoes and let boil. Once boiling, reduce the fire, cover and continue to cook for another 2 minutes.
3. Add the scallops and increase fire to medium and stir occasionally and cook for two minutes. Add the shrimp and wait for two minutes more

before adding the couscous. Then remove from fire, cover and set aside for five minutes before carefully mixing.

NUTRITION :
Calories: 117; Carbs: 11.7g; Protein: 11.5g; Fat: 3.1g

184. Shrimp Paella Made with Quinoa

Servings: 7 | Cooking Time: 40 minutes

1 lb. large shrimp, peeled, deveined and thawed	1 tsp seafood seasoning
1 cup frozen green peas	1 red bell pepper, cored, seeded & membrane removed, sliced into ½" strips
½ cup sliced sun-dried tomatoes, packed in olive oil	Salt to taste
½ tsp black pepper	½ tsp Spanish paprika
½ tsp saffron threads (optional turmeric)	1 bay leaf
¼ tsp crushed red pepper flakes	3 cups chicken broth, fat free, low sodium
1 ½ cups dry quinoa, rinse well	1 tbsp olive oil
2 cloves garlic, minced	1 yellow onion, diced

1. Season shrimps with seafood seasoning and a pinch of salt. Toss to mix well and refrigerate until ready to use.
2. Prepare and wash quinoa. Set aside.
3. On medium low fire, place a large nonstick skillet and heat oil. Add onions and for 5 minutes sauté until soft and tender.
4. Add paprika, saffron (or turmeric), bay leaves, red pepper flakes, chicken broth and quinoa. Season with salt and pepper.
5. Cover skillet and bring to a boil. Once boiling, lower fire to a simmer and cook until all liquid is absorbed, around ten minutes.
6. Add shrimp, peas and sun-dried tomatoes. For 5 minutes, cover and cook.
7. Once done, turn off fire and for ten minutes allow paella to set while still covered.
8. To serve, remove bay leaf and enjoy with a squeeze of lemon if desired.

NUTRITION:
Calories: 324.4; Protein: 22g; Carbs: 33g; Fat: 11.6g

185. Shrimp, Lemon and Basil Pasta

Servings: 4 | Cooking Time: 25 minutes

2 cups baby spinach	½ tsp salt
2 tbsp fresh lemon juice	2 tbsp extra virgin olive oil
3 tbsp drained capers	¼ cup chopped fresh basil
1 lb. peeled and deveined large shrimp	8 oz uncooked spaghetti
3 quarts water	

1. In a pot, bring to boil 3 quarts water. Add the pasta and allow to boil for another eight mins before adding the shrimp and boiling for another three mins or until pasta is cooked.
2. Drain the pasta and transfer to a bowl. Add salt, lemon juice, olive oil, capers and basil while mixing well.
3. To serve, place baby spinach on plate around ½ cup and topped with ½ cup of pasta.

NUTRITION:
Calories: 151; Carbs: 18.9g; Protein: 4.3g; Fat: 7.4g

186. Simple Penne Anti-Pasto

Servings: 4 | Cooking Time: 15 minutes

¼ cup pine nuts, toasted	½ cup grated Parmigiano-Reggiano cheese, divided
8oz penne pasta, cooked and drained	1 6oz jar drained, sliced, marinated and quartered artichoke hearts
1 7 oz jar drained and chopped sun-dried tomato halves packed in oil	3 oz chopped prosciutto
1/3 cup pesto	½ cup pitted and chopped Kalamata olives
1 medium red bell pepper	

1. Slice bell pepper, discard membranes, seeds and stem. On a foiled lined baking sheet, place bell pepper halves, press down by hand and broil in oven for eight minutes. Remove from oven, put in a sealed bag for 5 minutes before peeling and chopping.
2. Place chopped bell pepper in a bowl and mix in artichokes, tomatoes, prosciutto, pesto and olives.
3. Toss in ¼ cup cheese and pasta. Transfer to a serving dish and garnish with ¼ cup cheese and pine nuts. Serve and enjoy!

NUTRITION:
Calories: 606; Carbs: 70.3g; Protein: 27.2g; Fat: 27.6g

187. Spaghetti in Lemon Avocado White Sauce

Servings: 6 | Cooking Time: 30 minutes

Freshly ground black pepper	Zest and juice of 1 lemon
1 avocado, pitted and peeled	1-pound spaghetti
Salt	1 tbsp Olive oil
8 oz small shrimp, shelled and deveined	¼ cup dry white wine
1 large onion, finely sliced	

1. Let a big pot of water boil. Once boiling add the spaghetti or pasta and cook following manufacturer's instructions until al dente. Drain and set aside.
2. In a large fry pan, over medium fire sauté wine and onions for ten minutes or until onions are translucent and soft.
3. Add the shrimps into the fry pan and increase fire to high while constantly sautéing until shrimps are cooked around five minutes. Turn the fire off. Season with salt and add the oil right away. Then quickly toss in the cooked pasta, mix well.
4. In a blender, until smooth, puree the lemon juice and avocado. Pour into the fry pan of pasta, combine well. Garnish with pepper and lemon zest then serve.

NUTRITION:
Calories: 206; Carbs: 26.3g; Protein: 10.2g; Fat: 8.0g

188. Spanish Rice Casserole with Cheesy Beef

Servings: 2 | Cooking Time: 32 minutes

2 tablespoons chopped green bell pepper	1/4 teaspoon Worcestershire sauce
1/4 teaspoon ground cumin	1/4 cup shredded Cheddar cheese
1/4 cup finely chopped onion	1/4 cup chile sauce
1/3 cup uncooked long grain rice	1/2-pound lean ground beef
1/2 teaspoon salt	1/2 teaspoon brown sugar
1/2 pinch ground black pepper	1/2 cup water
1/2 (14.5 ounce) can canned tomatoes	1 tablespoon chopped fresh cilantro

1. Place a nonstick saucepan on medium fire and brown beef for 10 minutes while crumbling beef. Discard fat.
2. Stir in pepper, Worcestershire sauce, cumin, brown sugar, salt, chile sauce, rice, water, tomatoes, green bell pepper, and onion. Mix well and cook for 10 minutes until blended and a bit tender.
3. Transfer to an ovenproof casserole and press down firmly. Sprinkle cheese on top and cook for 7 minutes at 400oF preheated oven. Broil for 3 minutes until top is lightly browned.
4. Serve and enjoy with chopped cilantro.

NUTRITION:
Calories: 460; Carbohydrates: 35.8g; Protein: 37.8g; Fat: 17.9g

189. Squash and Eggplant Casserole

Servings: 2 | Cooking Time: 45 minutes

½ cup dry white wine	1 eggplant, halved and cut to 1-inch slices
1 large onion, cut into wedges	1 red bell pepper, seeded and cut to julienned strips
1 small butternut squash, cut into 1-inch slices	1 tbsp olive oil
12 baby corn	2 cups low sodium vegetable broth
Salt and pepper to taste	Polenta Ingredients
¼ cup parmesan cheese, grated	1 cup instant polenta
2 tbsp fresh oregano, chopped	Topping Ingredients
1 garlic clove, chopped	2 tbsp slivered almonds
5 tbsp parsley, chopped	Grated zest of 1 lemon

1. Preheat the oven to 350 degrees Fahrenheit.
2. In a casserole, heat the oil and add the onion wedges and baby corn. Sauté over medium high heat for five minutes. Stir occasionally to prevent the onions and baby corn from sticking at the bottom of the pan.
3. Add the butternut squash to the casserole and toss the vegetables. Add the eggplants and the red pepper.
4. Cover the vegetables and cook over low to medium heat.
5. Cook for about ten minutes before adding the wine. Let the wine sizzle before stirring in the broth. Bring to a boil and cook in the oven for 30 minutes.
6. While the casserole is cooking inside the oven, make the topping by spreading the slivered almonds on a baking tray and toasting under the grill until they are lightly browned.
7. Place the toasted almonds in a small bowl and mix the remaining ingredients for the toppings.
8. Prepare the polenta. In a large saucepan, bring 3 cups of water to boil over high heat.
9. Add the polenta and continue whisking until it absorbs all the water.
10. Reduce the heat to medium until the polenta is thick. Add the parmesan cheese and oregano.
11. Serve the polenta on plates and add the casserole on top. Sprinkle the toppings on top.

NUTRITION:
Calories: 579.3; Carbs: 79.2g; Protein: 22.2g; Fat: 19.3g

190. Stuffed Tomatoes with Green Chili

Servings: 6 | Cooking Time: 55 minutes

4 oz Colby-Jack shredded cheese	¼ cup water
1 cup uncooked quinoa	6 large ripe tomatoes
¼ tsp freshly ground black pepper	¾ tsp ground cumin
1 tsp salt, divided	1 tbsp fresh lime juice
1 tbsp olive oil	1 tbsp chopped fresh oregano
1 cup chopped onion	2 cups fresh corn kernels
2 poblano chilies	

1. Preheat broiler to high.
2. Slice lengthwise the chilies and press on a baking sheet lined with foil. Broil for 8 minutes. Remove from oven and let cool for 10 minutes. Peel the chilies and chop coarsely and place in medium sized bowl.
3. Place onion and corn in baking sheet and broil for ten minutes. Stir two times while broiling. Remove from oven and mix in with chopped chilies.
4. Add black pepper, cumin, ¼ tsp salt, lime juice, oil and oregano. Mix well.
5. Cut off the tops of tomatoes and set aside. Leave the tomato shell intact as you scoop out the tomato pulp.
6. Drain tomato pulp as you press down with a spoon. Reserve 1 ¼ cups of tomato pulp liquid and discard the rest. Invert the tomato shells on a wire rack for 30 mins and then wipe the insides dry with a paper towel.
7. Season with ½ tsp salt the tomato pulp.

8. On a sieve over a bowl, place quinoa. Add water until it covers quinoa. Rub quinoa grains for 30 seconds together with hands; rinse and drain. Repeat this procedure two times and drain well at the end.
9. In medium saucepan bring to a boil remaining salt, ¼ cup water, quinoa and tomato liquid.
10. Once boiling, reduce heat and simmer for 15 minutes or until liquid is fully absorbed. Remove from heat and fluff quinoa with fork. Transfer and mix well the quinoa with the corn mixture.
11. Spoon ¾ cup of the quinoa-corn mixture into the tomato shells, top with cheese and cover with the tomato top. Bake in a preheated 350oF oven for 15 minutes and then broil high for another 1.5 minutes.

NUTRITION:
Calories: 276; Carbs: 46.3g; Protein: 13.4g; Fat: 4.1g

191. Tasty Lasagna Rolls
Servings: 6, | Cooking Time: 20 minutes

¼ tsp crushed red pepper	¼ tsp salt
½ cup shredded mozzarella cheese	½ cups parmesan cheese, shredded
1 14-oz package tofu, cubed	1 25-oz can of low-sodium marinara sauce
1 tbsp extra virgin olive oil	12 whole wheat lasagna noodles
2 tbsp Kalamata olives, chopped	3 cloves minced garlic
3 cups spinach, chopped	

1. Put enough water on a large pot and cook the lasagna noodles according to package instructions. Drain, rinse and set aside until ready to use.
2. In a large skillet, sauté garlic over medium heat for 20 seconds. Add the tofu and spinach and cook until the spinach wilts. Transfer this mixture in a bowl and add parmesan olives, salt, red pepper and 2/3 cup of the marinara sauce.
3. In a pan, spread a cup of marinara sauce on the bottom. To make the rolls, place noodle on a surface and spread ¼ cup of the tofu filling. Roll up and place it on the pan with the marinara sauce. Do this procedure until all lasagna noodles are rolled.
4. Place the pan over high heat and bring to a simmer. Reduce the heat to medium and let it cook for three more minutes. Sprinkle mozzarella cheese and let the cheese melt for two minutes. Serve hot.

NUTRITION:
Calories: 304; Carbs: 39.2g; Protein: 23g; Fat: 19.2g

192. Tasty Mushroom Bolognese
Servings: 6 | Cooking Time: 65 minutes

¼ cup chopped fresh parsley	oz Parmigiano-Reggiano cheese, grated
1 tbsp kosher salt	10-oz whole wheat spaghetti, cooked and drained
¼ cup milk	1 14-oz can whole peeled tomatoes
½ cup white wine	2 tbsp tomato paste
1 tbsp minced garlic	8 cups finely chopped cremini mushrooms
½ lb. ground pork	½ tsp freshly ground black pepper, divided
¾ tsp kosher salt, divided	2 ½ cups chopped onion
1 tbsp olive oil	1 cup boiling water
½-oz dried porcini mushrooms	

1. Let porcini stand in a boiling bowl of water for twenty minutes, drain (reserve liquid), rinse and chop. Set aside.
2. On medium high fire, place a Dutch oven with olive oil and cook for ten minutes cook pork, ¼ tsp pepper, ¼ tsp salt and onions. Constantly mix to break ground pork pieces.
3. Stir in ¼ tsp pepper, ¼ tsp salt, garlic and cremini mushrooms. Continue cooking until liquid has evaporated, around fifteen minutes.
4. Stirring constantly, add porcini and sauté for a minute.
5. Stir in wine, porcini liquid, tomatoes and tomato paste. Let it simmer for forty minutes. Stir occasionally. Pour milk and cook for another two minutes before removing from fire.
6. Stir in pasta and transfer to a serving dish. Garnish with parsley and cheese before serving.

NUTRITION:
Calories: 358; Carbs: 32.8g; Protein: 21.1g; Fat: 15.4g

193. Tortellini Salad with Broccoli
Servings: 12 | Cooking Time: 20 minutes

1 red onion, chopped finely	1 cup sunflower seeds
1 cup raisins	3 heads fresh broccoli, cut into florets
2 tsp cider vinegar	½ cup white sugar
½ cup mayonnaise	20-oz fresh cheese filled tortellini

1. In a large pot of boiling water, cook tortellini according to manufacturer's instructions. Drain and rinse with cold water and set aside.
2. Whisk vinegar, sugar and mayonnaise to create your salad dressing.
3. Mix together in a large bowl red onion, sunflower seeds, raisins, tortellini and broccoli. Pour dressing and toss to coat.
4. Serve and enjoy.

NUTRITION:
Calories: 272; Carbs: 38.7g; Protein: 5.0g; Fat: 8.1g

194. Turkey and Quinoa Stuffed Peppers
Servings: 6 | Cooking Time: 55 minutes

3 large red bell peppers	2 tsp chopped fresh rosemary
2 tbsp chopped fresh parsley	3 tbsp chopped pecans, toasted
¼ cup extra virgin olive oil	½ cup chicken stock
½ lb. fully cooked smoked turkey sausage, diced	½ tsp salt
2 cups water	1 cup uncooked quinoa

1. On high fire, place a large saucepan and add salt, water and quinoa. Bring to a boil.
2. Once boiling, reduce fire to a simmer, cover and cook until all water is absorbed around 15 minutes.
3. Uncover quinoa, turn off fire and let it stand for another 5 minutes.
4. Add rosemary, parsley, pecans, olive oil, chicken stock and turkey sausage into pan of quinoa. Mix well.
5. Slice peppers lengthwise in half and discard membranes and seeds. In another boiling pot of water, add peppers, boil for 5 minutes, drain and discard water.
6. Grease a 13 x 9 baking dish and preheat oven to 350oF.
7. Place boiled bell pepper onto prepared baking dish, evenly fill with the quinoa mixture and pop into oven.
8. Bake for 15 minutes.

NUTRITION :
Calories: 255.6; Carbs: 21.6g; Protein: 14.4g; Fat: 12.4g

195. Veggie Pasta with Shrimp, Basil and Lemon
Servings: 4 | Cooking Time: 5 minutes

2 cups baby spinach	½ tsp salt
2 tbsp fresh lemon juice	2 tbsp extra virgin olive oil
3 tbsp drained capers	¼ cup chopped fresh basil
1 lb. peeled and deveined large shrimp	4 cups zucchini, spirals

1. divide into 4 serving plates, top with ¼ cup of spinach, serve and enjoy.

NUTRITION:
Calories: 51; Carbs: 4.4g; Protein: 1.8g; Fat: 3.4g

196. Veggies and Sun-Dried Tomato Alfredo

Servings: 4 | Cooking Time: 30 minutes

2 tsp finely shredded lemon peel	½ cup finely shredded Parmesan cheese
1 ¼ cups milk	2 tbsp all-purpose flour
8 fresh mushrooms, sliced	1 ½ cups fresh broccoli florets
4 oz fresh trimmed and quartered Brussels sprouts	4 oz trimmed fresh asparagus spears
1 tbsp olive oil	4 tbsp butter
½ cup chopped dried tomatoes	8 oz dried fettuccine

1. In a boiling pot of water, add fettuccine and cook following manufacturer's instructions. Two minutes before the pasta is cooked, add the dried tomatoes. Drain pasta and tomatoes and return to pot to keep warm. Set aside.
2. On medium high fire, in a big fry pan with 1 tbsp butter, fry mushrooms, broccoli, Brussels sprouts and asparagus. Cook for eight minutes while covered, transfer to a plate and put aside.
3. Using same fry pan, add remaining butter and flour. Stirring vigorously, cook for a minute or until thickened. Add Parmesan cheese, milk and mix until cheese is melted around five minutes.
4. Toss in the pasta and mix. Transfer to serving dish. Garnish with Parmesan cheese and lemon peel before serving.

NUTRITION:
Calories: 439; Carbs: 52.0g; Protein: 16.3g; Fat: 19.5g

197. Yangchow Chinese Style Fried Rice

Servings: 4 | Cooking Time: 20 minutes

4 cups cold cooked rice	1/2 cup peas
1 medium yellow onion, diced	5 tbsp olive oil
4 oz frozen medium shrimp, thawed, shelled, deveined and chopped finely	6 oz roast pork
3 large eggs	Salt and freshly ground black pepper
1/2 tsp cornstarch	

1. Combine the salt and ground black pepper and 1/2 tsp cornstarch, coat the shrimp with it. Chop the roasted pork. Beat the eggs and set aside.
2. Stir-fry the shrimp in a wok on high fire with 1 tbsp heated oil until pink, around 3 minutes. Set the shrimp aside and stir fry the roasted pork briefly. Remove both from the pan.
3. In the same pan, stir-fry the onion until soft, Stir the peas and cook until bright green. Remove both from pan.
4. Add 2 tbsp oil in the same pan, add the cooked rice. Stir and separate the individual grains. Add the beaten eggs, toss the rice. Add the roasted pork, shrimp, vegetables and onion. Toss everything together. Season with salt and pepper to taste.

NUTRITION:
Calories: 556; Carbs: 60.2g; Protein: 20.2g; Fat: 25.2g

SEAFOOD & FISH RECIPES

198. Mediterranean Fish Fillets

Preparation Time: 10 minutes | Cooking Time: 3 minutes | Servings: 4

4 cod fillets	1 lb grape tomatoes, halved
1 cup olives, pitted and sliced	2 tbsp capers
1 tsp dried thyme	2 tbsp olive oil
1 tsp garlic, minced	Pepper
Salt	

1. Pour 1 cup water into the instant pot then place steamer rack in the pot.
2. Spray heat-safe baking dish with cooking spray.
3. Add half grape tomatoes into the dish and season with pepper and salt.
4. Arrange fish fillets on top of cherry tomatoes. Drizzle with oil and season with garlic, thyme, capers, pepper, and salt.
5. Spread olives and remaining grape tomatoes on top of fish fillets.
6. Place dish on top of steamer rack in the pot.
7. Seal pot with a lid and select manual and cook on high for 3 minutes.
8. Once done, release pressure using quick release. Remove lid.
9. Serve and enjoy.

NUTRITION:

Calories 212 Fat 11.9 g Carbohydrates 7.1 g Sugar 3 g Protein 21.4 g Cholesterol 55 mg

199. Flavors Cioppino

Preparation Time: 10 minutes | Cooking Time: 5 minutes | Servings: 6

1 lb codfish, cut into chunks	1 1/2 lbs shrimp
28 oz can tomatoes, diced	1 cup dry white wine
1 bay leaf	1 tsp cayenne
1 tsp oregano	1 shallot, chopped
1 tsp garlic, minced	1 tbsp olive oil
1/2 tsp salt	

1. Add oil into the inner pot of instant pot and set the pot on sauté mode.
2. Add shallot and garlic and sauté for 2 minutes.
3. Add wine, bay leaf, cayenne, oregano, and salt and cook for 3 minutes.
4. Add remaining ingredients and stir well.
5. Seal pot with a lid and select manual and cook on low for 0 minutes.
6. Once done, release pressure using quick release. Remove lid.
7. Serve and enjoy.

NUTRITION:

Calories 281 Fat 5 g Carbohydrates 10.5 g Sugar 4.9 g Protein 40.7 g Cholesterol 266 mg

200. Delicious Shrimp Alfredo

Preparation Time: 10 minutes | Cooking Time: 3 minutes | Servings: 4

12 shrimp, remove shells	1 tbsp garlic, minced
1/4 cup parmesan cheese	2 cups whole wheat rotini noodles
1 cup fish broth	15 oz alfredo sauce
1 onion, chopped	Salt

1. Add all ingredients except parmesan cheese into the instant pot and stir well.
2. Seal pot with lid and cook on high for 3 minutes.
3. Once done, release pressure using quick release. Remove lid.
4. Stir in cheese and serve.

NUTRITION:

Calories 669 Fat 23.1 g Carbohydrates 76 g Sugar 2.4 g Protein 37.8 g Cholesterol 190 mg

201. Tomato Olive Fish Fillets

Preparation Time: 10 minutes | Cooking Time: 8 minutes | Servings: 4

2 lbs halibut fish fillets	2 oregano sprigs
2 rosemary sprigs	2 tbsp fresh lime juice
1 cup olives, pitted	28 oz can tomatoes, diced
1 tbsp garlic, minced	1 onion, chopped
2 tbsp olive oil	

1. Add oil into the inner pot of instant pot and set the pot on sauté mode.
2. Add onion and sauté for 3 minutes.
3. Add garlic and sauté for a minute.
4. Add lime juice, olives, herb sprigs, and tomatoes and stir well.
5. Seal pot with lid and cook on high for 3 minutes.
6. Once done, release pressure using quick release. Remove lid.
7. Add fish fillets and seal pot again with lid and cook on high for 2 minutes.
8. Once done, release pressure using quick release. Remove lid.
9. Serve and enjoy.

NUTRITION:

Calories 333 Fat 19.1 g Carbohydrates 31.8 g Sugar 8.4 g Protein 13.4 g Cholesterol 5 mg

202. Shrimp Scampi

Preparation Time: 10 minutes | Cooking Time: 8 minutes | Servings: 6

1 lb whole wheat penne pasta	1 lb frozen shrimp
2 tbsp garlic, minced	1/4 tsp cayenne
1/2 tbsp Italian seasoning	1/4 cup olive oil
3 1/2 cups fish stock	Pepper
Salt	

1. Add all ingredients into the inner pot of instant pot and stir well.
2. Seal pot with lid and cook on high for 6 minutes.
3. Once done, release pressure using quick release. Remove lid.
4. Stir well and serve.

NUTRITION:

Calories 435 Fat 12.6 g Carbohydrates 54.9 g Sugar 0.1 g Protein 30.6 g Cholesterol 116 mg

203. Easy Salmon Stew

Preparation Time: 10 minutes | Cooking Time: 8 minutes | Servings: 6

2 lbs salmon fillet, cubed	1 onion, chopped
2 cups fish broth	1 tbsp olive oil
Pepper	salt

1. Add oil into the inner pot of instant pot and set the pot on sauté mode.
2. Add onion and sauté for 2 minutes.
3. Add remaining ingredients and stir well.
4. Seal pot with lid and cook on high for 6 minutes.
5. Once done, release pressure using quick release. Remove lid.
6. Stir and serve.

NUTRITION:

Calories 243 Fat 12.6 g Carbohydrates 0.8 g Sugar 0.3 g Protein 31 g Cholesterol 78 mg

204.   Italian Tuna Pasta

Preparation Time: 10 minutes | Cooking Time: 5 minutes | Servings: 6

15 oz whole wheat pasta	2 tbsp capers
3 oz tuna	2 cups can tomatoes, crushed
2 anchovies	1 tsp garlic, minced
1 tbsp olive oil	Salt

1. Add oil into the inner pot of instant pot and set the pot on sauté mode.
2. Add anchovies and garlic and sauté for 1 minute.
3. Add remaining ingredients and stir well. Pour enough water into the pot to cover the pasta.
4. Seal pot with a lid and select manual and cook on low for 4 minutes.
5. Once done, release pressure using quick release. Remove lid.
6. Stir and serve.

NUTRITION:
Calories 339 Fat 6 g Carbohydrates 56.5 g Sugar 5.2 g Protein 15.2 g Cholesterol 10 mg

205.   Garlicky Clams

Preparation Time: 10 minutes | Cooking Time: 5 minutes | Servings: 4

3 lbs clams, clean	4 garlic cloves
1/4 cup olive oil	1/2 cup fresh lemon juice
1 cup white wine	Pepper
Salt	

1. Add oil into the inner pot of instant pot and set the pot on sauté mode.
2. Add garlic and sauté for 1 minute.
3. Add wine and cook for 2 minutes.
4. Add remaining ingredients and stir well.
5. Seal pot with lid and cook on high for 2 minutes.
6. Once done, allow to release pressure naturally. Remove lid.
7. Serve and enjoy.

NUTRITION:
Calories 332 Fat 13.5 g Carbohydrates 40.5 g Sugar 12.4 g Protein 2.5 g Cholesterol 0 mg

206.   Delicious Fish Tacos

Preparation Time: 10 minutes | Cooking Time: 8 minutes | Servings: 8

4 tilapia fillets	1/4 cup fresh cilantro, chopped
1/4 cup fresh lime juice	2 tbsp paprika
1 tbsp olive oil	Pepper
Salt	

1. Pour 2 cups of water into the instant pot then place steamer rack in the pot.
2. Place fish fillets on parchment paper.
3. Season fish fillets with paprika, pepper, and salt and drizzle with oil and lime juice.
4. Fold parchment paper around the fish fillets and place them on a steamer rack in the pot.
5. Seal pot with lid and cook on high for 8 minutes.
6. Once done, release pressure using quick release. Remove lid.
7. Remove fish packet from pot and open it.
8. Shred the fish with a fork and serve.

NUTRITION:
Calories 67 Fat 2.5 g Carbohydrates 1.1 g Sugar 0.2 g Protein 10.8 g Cholesterol 28 mg

207.   Pesto Fish Fillet

Preparation Time: 10 minutes | Cooking Time: 8 minutes | Servings: 4

4 halibut fillets	1/2 cup water
1 tbsp lemon zest, grated	1 tbsp capers
1/2 cup basil, chopped	1 tbsp garlic, chopped
1 avocado, peeled and chopped	Pepper
Salt	

1. Add lemon zest, capers, basil, garlic, avocado, pepper, and salt into the blender blend until smooth.
2. Place fish fillets on aluminum foil and spread a blended mixture on fish fillets.
3. Fold foil around the fish fillets.
4. Pour water into the instant pot and place trivet in the pot.
5. Place foil fish packet on the trivet.
6. Seal pot with lid and cook on high for 8 minutes.
7. Once done, allow to release pressure naturally. Remove lid.
8. Serve and enjoy.

NUTRITION:
Calories 426 Fat 16.6 g Carbohydrates 5.5 g Sugar 0.4 g Protein 61.8 g Cholesterol 93 mg

208.   Tuna Risotto

Preparation Time: 10 minutes | Cooking Time: 23 minutes | Servings: 6

1 cup of rice	1/3 cup parmesan cheese, grated
1 1/2 cups fish broth	1 lemon juice
1 tbsp garlic, minced	1 onion, chopped
2 tbsp olive oil	2 cups can tuna, cut into chunks
Pepper	Salt

1. Add oil into the inner pot of instant pot and set the pot on sauté mode.
2. Add garlic, onion, and tuna and cook for 3 minutes.
3. Add remaining ingredients except for parmesan cheese and stir well.
4. Seal pot with lid and cook on high for 20 minutes.
5. Once done, release pressure using quick release. Remove lid.
6. Stir in parmesan cheese and serve.

NUTRITION:
Calories 228 Fat 7 g Carbohydrates 27.7 g Sugar 1.2 g Protein 12.6 g Cholesterol 21 mg

209.   Salsa Fish Fillets

Preparation Time: 10 minutes | Cooking Time: 2 minutes | Servings: 4

1 lb tilapia fillets	1/2 cup salsa
1 cup of water	Pepper
Salt	

1. Place fish fillets on aluminum foil and top with salsa and season with pepper and salt.
2. Fold foil around the fish fillets.
3. Pour water into the instant pot and place trivet in the pot.
4. Place foil fish packet on the trivet.
5. Seal pot with lid and cook on high for 2 minutes.
6. Once done, release pressure using quick release. Remove lid.
7. Serve and enjoy.

NUTRITION:
Calories 342 Fat 10.5 g Carbohydrates 41.5 g Sugar 1.9 g Protein 18.9 g Cholesterol 31 mg

211. Coconut Clam Chowder

Preparation Time: 10 minutes | Cooking Time: 7 minutes | Servings: 6

6 oz clams, chopped	1 cup heavy cream
1/4 onion, sliced	1 cup celery, chopped
1 lb cauliflower, chopped	1 cup fish broth
1 bay leaf	2 cups of coconut milk
Salt	

1. Add all ingredients except clams and heavy cream and stir well.
2. Seal pot with lid and cook on high for 5 minutes.
3. Once done, release pressure using quick release. Remove lid.
4. Add heavy cream and clams and stir well and cook on sauté mode for 2 minutes.
5. Stir well and serve.

NUTRITION:

Calories 301 Fat 27.2 g Carbohydrates 13.6 g Sugar 6 g Protein 4.9 g Cholesterol 33 mg

212. Feta Tomato Sea Bass

Preparation Time: 10 minutes | Cooking Time: 8 minutes | Servings: 4

4 sea bass fillets	1 1/2 cups water
1 tbsp olive oil	1 tsp garlic, minced
1 tsp basil, chopped	1 tsp parsley, chopped
1/2 cup feta cheese, crumbled	1 cup can tomatoes, diced
Pepper	Salt

1. Season fish fillets with pepper and salt.
2. Pour 2 cups of water into the instant pot then place steamer rack in the pot.
3. Place fish fillets on steamer rack in the pot.
4. Seal pot with lid and cook on high for 5 minutes.
5. Once done, release pressure using quick release. Remove lid.
6. Remove fish fillets from the pot and clean the pot.
7. Add oil into the inner pot of instant pot and set the pot on sauté mode.
8. Add garlic and sauté for 1 minute.
9. Add tomatoes, parsley, and basil and stir well and cook for 1 minute.
10. Add fish fillets and top with crumbled cheese and cook for a minute.
11. Serve and enjoy.

NUTRITION:

Calories 219 Fat 10.1 g Carbohydrates 4 g Sugar 2.8 g Protein 27.1 g Cholesterol 70 mg

213. Stewed Mussels & Scallops

Preparation Time: 10 minutes | Cooking Time: 11 minutes | Servings: 4

2 cups mussels	1 cup scallops
2 cups fish stock	2 bell peppers, diced
2 cups cauliflower rice	1 onion, chopped
1 tbsp olive oil	Pepper
Salt	

1. Add oil into the inner pot of instant pot and set the pot on sauté mode.
2. Add onion and peppers and sauté for 3 minutes.
3. Add scallops and cook for 2 minutes.
4. Add remaining ingredients and stir well.
5. Seal pot with lid and cook on high for 6 minutes.
6. Once done, allow to release pressure naturally. Remove lid.
7. Stir and serve.

NUTRITION:

Calories 191 Fat 7.4 g Carbohydrates 13.7 g Sugar 6.2 g Protein 18 g Cholesterol 29 mg

214. Healthy Halibut Soup

Preparation Time: 10 minutes | Cooking Time: 13 minutes | Servings: 4

1 lb halibut, skinless, boneless, & cut into chunks	2 tbsp ginger, minced
2 celery stalks, chopped	1 carrot, sliced
1 onion, chopped	1 cup of water
2 cups fish stock	1 tbsp olive oil
Pepper	Salt

1. Add oil into the inner pot of instant pot and set the pot on sauté mode.
2. Add onion and sauté for 3-4 minutes.
3. Add water, celery, carrot, ginger, and stock and stir well.
4. Seal pot with lid and cook on high for 5 minutes.
5. Once done, release pressure using quick release. Remove lid.
6. Add fish and stir well. Seal pot again and cook on high for 4 minutes.
7. Once done, release pressure using quick release. Remove lid.
8. Stir and serve.

NUTRITION:

Calories 4586 Fat 99.6 g Carbohydrates 6.3 g Sugar 2.1 g Protein 861 g Cholesterol 1319 mg

215. Creamy Fish Stew

Preparation Time: 10 minutes | Cooking Time: 8 minutes | Servings: 6

1 lb white fish fillets, cut into chunks	2 tbsp olive oil
1 cup kale, chopped	1 cup cauliflower, chopped
1 cup broccoli, chopped	3 cups fish broth
1 cup heavy cream	2 celery stalks, diced
1 carrot, sliced	1 onion, diced
Pepper	Salt

1. Add oil into the inner pot of instant pot and set the pot on sauté mode.
2. Add onion and sauté for 3 minutes.
3. Add remaining ingredients except for heavy cream and stir well.
4. Seal pot with lid and cook on high for 5 minutes.
5. Once done, allow to release pressure naturally. Remove lid.
6. Stir in heavy cream and serve.

NUTRITION:

Calories 296 Fat 19.3 g Carbohydrates 7.5 g Sugar 2.6 g Protein 22.8 g Cholesterol 103 mg

216. Nutritious Broccoli Salmon

Preparation Time: 10 minutes | Cooking Time: 4 minutes | Servings: 4

4 salmon fillets	10 oz broccoli florets
1 1/2 cups water	1 tbsp olive oil
Pepper	Salt

1. Pour water into the instant pot then place steamer basket in the pot.
2. Place salmon in the steamer basket and season with pepper and salt and drizzle with oil.
3. Add broccoli on top of salmon in the steamer basket.
4. Seal pot with lid and cook on high for 4 minutes.
5. Once done, release pressure using quick release. Remove lid.
6. Serve and enjoy.

NUTRITION:

Calories 290 Fat 14.7 g Carbohydrates 4.7 g Sugar 1.2 g Protein 36.5 g Cholesterol 78 mg

218. Shrimp Zoodles

Preparation Time: 10 minutes | Cooking Time: 5 minutes | Servings: 4

2 zucchini, spiralized
1/2 tsp paprika
1/2 lemon juice
2 tbsp olive oil
Pepper

1 lb shrimp, peeled and deveined
1 tbsp basil, chopped
1 tsp garlic, minced
1 cup vegetable stock
Salt

1. Add oil into the inner pot of instant pot and set the pot on sauté mode.
2. Add garlic and sauté for a minute.
3. Add shrimp and lemon juice and stir well and cook for 1 minute.
4. Add remaining ingredients and stir well.
5. Seal pot with lid and cook on high for 3 minutes.
6. Once done, release pressure using quick release. Remove lid.
7. Serve and enjoy.

NUTRITION:
Calories 215 Fat 9.2 g Carbohydrates 5.8 g Sugar 2 g Protein 27.3 g Cholesterol 239 mg

219. Healthy Carrot & Shrimp

Preparation Time: 10 minutes | Cooking Time: 6 minutes | Servings: 4

1 lb shrimp, peeled and deveined
1 onion, chopped
1 cup fish stock
Pepper and Salt

1 tbsp chives, chopped
1 tbsp olive oil
1 cup carrots, sliced

1. Add oil into the inner pot of instant pot and set the pot on sauté mode.
2. Add onion and sauté for 2 minutes.
3. Add shrimp and stir well.
4. Add remaining ingredients and stir well.
5. Seal pot with lid and cook on high for 4 minutes.
6. Once done, release pressure using quick release. Remove lid.
7. Serve and enjoy.

NUTRITION:
Calories 197 Fat 5.9 g Carbohydrates 7 g Sugar 2.5 g Protein 27.7 g Cholesterol 239 mg

220. Salmon with Potatoes

Preparation Time: 10 minutes | Cooking Time: 15 minutes | Servings: 4

1 1/2 lbs Salmon fillets, boneless and cubed
1 cup fish stock
1 tsp garlic, minced
Pepper

2 tbsp olive oil

2 tbsp parsley, chopped
1 lb baby potatoes, halved
Salt

1. Add oil into the inner pot of instant pot and set the pot on sauté mode.
2. Add garlic and sauté for 2 minutes.
3. Add remaining ingredients and stir well.
4. Seal pot with lid and cook on high for 13 minutes.
5. Once done, release pressure using quick release. Remove lid.
6. Serve and enjoy.

NUTRITION:
Calories 362 Fat 18.1 g Carbohydrates 14.5 g Sugar 0 g Protein 37.3 g Cholesterol 76 mg

221. Honey Garlic Shrimp

Preparation Time: 10 minutes | Cooking Time: 5 minutes | Servings: 4

1 lb shrimp, peeled and deveined   1/4 cup honey

1 tbsp garlic, minced
1 tbsp olive oil
Pepper

1 tbsp ginger, minced
1/4 cup fish stock
Salt

1. Add shrimp into the large bowl. Add remaining ingredients over shrimp and toss well.
2. Transfer shrimp into the instant pot and stir well.
3. Seal pot with lid and cook on high for 5 minutes.
4. Once done, release pressure using quick release. Remove lid.
5. Serve and enjoy.

NUTRITION:
Calories 240 Fat 5.6 g Carbohydrates 20.9 g Sugar 17.5 g Protein 26.5 g Cholesterol 239 mg

222. Simple Lemon Clams

Preparation Time: 10 minutes | Cooking Time: 10 minutes | Servings: 4

1 lb clams, clean
1 lemon zest, grated
1/2 cup fish stock
Salt

1 tbsp fresh lemon juice
1 onion, chopped
Pepper

1. Add all ingredients into the inner pot of instant pot and stir well.
2. Seal pot with lid and cook on high for 10 minutes.
3. Once done, release pressure using quick release. Remove lid.
4. Serve and enjoy.

NUTRITION:
Calories 76 Fat 0.6 g Carbohydrates 16.4 g Sugar 5.4 g Protein 1.8 g Cholesterol 0 mg

223. Crab Stew

Preparation Time: 10 minutes | Cooking Time: 13 minutes | Servings: 2

1/2 lb lump crab meat
1 tbsp olive oil
1/2 lb shrimp, shelled and chopped
1/2 tsp garlic, chopped
Pepper

2 tbsp heavy cream
2 cups fish stock
1 celery stalk, chopped
1/4 onion, chopped
Salt

1. Add oil into the inner pot of instant pot and set the pot on sauté mode.
2. Add onion and sauté for 3 minutes.
3. Add garlic and sauté for 30 seconds.
4. Add remaining ingredients except for heavy cream and stir well.
5. Seal pot with lid and cook on high for 10 minutes.
6. Once done, release pressure using quick release. Remove lid.
7. Stir in heavy cream and serve.

NUTRITION:
Calories 376 Fat 25.5 g Carbohydrates 5.8 g Sugar 0.7 g Protein 48.1 g Cholesterol 326 mg

224. Honey Balsamic Salmon

Preparation Time: 10 minutes \ Cooking Time: 3 minutes | Servings: 2

2 salmon fillets
2 tbsp honey
1 cup of water
Salt

1/4 tsp red pepper flakes
2 tbsp balsamic vinegar
Pepper

1. Pour water into the instant pot and place trivet in the pot.
2. In a small bowl, mix together honey, red pepper flakes, and vinegar.
3. Brush fish fillets with honey mixture and place on top of the trivet.
4. Seal pot with lid and cook on high for 3 minutes.
5. Once done, release pressure using quick release. Remove lid.
6. Serve and enjoy.

NUTRITION:
Calories 303 Fat 11 g Carbohydrates 17.6 g Sugar 17.3 g Protein 34.6 g Cholesterol 78 mg

225. Spicy Tomato Crab Mix

Preparation Time: 10 minutes | Cooking Time: 12 minutes | Servings: 4

1 lb crab meat	1 tsp paprika
1 cup grape tomatoes, cut into half	2 tbsp green onion, chopped
1 tbsp olive oil	Pepper
Salt	

1. Add oil into the inner pot of instant pot and set the pot on sauté mode.
2. Add paprika and onion and sauté for 2 minutes.
3. Add the rest of the ingredients and stir well.
4. Seal pot with lid and cook on high for 10 minutes.
5. Once done, release pressure using quick release. Remove lid.
6. Serve and enjoy.

NUTRITION:
Calories 142 Fat 5.7 g Carbohydrates 4.3 g Sugar 1.3 g Protein 14.7 g Cholesterol 61 mg

226. Dijon Fish Fillets

Preparation Time: 10 minutes | Cooking Time: 3 minutes | Servings: 2

2 white fish fillets	1 tbsp Dijon mustard
1 cup of water	Pepper
Salt	

1. Pour water into the instant pot and place trivet in the pot.
2. Brush fish fillets with mustard and season with pepper and salt and place on top of the trivet.
3. Seal pot with lid and cook on high for 3 minutes.
4. Once done, release pressure using quick release. Remove lid.
5. Serve and enjoy.

NUTRITION:
Calories 270 Fat 11.9 g Carbohydrates 0.5 g Sugar 0.1 g Protein 38 g Cholesterol 119 mg

227. Lemoney Prawns

Preparation Time: 10 minutes | Cooking Time: 3 minutes | Servings: 2

1/2 lb prawns	1/2 cup fish stock
1 tbsp fresh lemon juice	1 tbsp lemon zest, grated
1 tbsp olive oil	1 tbsp garlic, minced
Pepper	Salt

1. Add all ingredients into the inner pot of instant pot and stir well.
2. Seal pot with lid and cook on high for 3 minutes.
3. Once done, release pressure using quick release. Remove lid.
4. Drain prawns and serve.

NUTRITION:
Calories 215 Fat 9.5 g Carbohydrates 3.9 g Sugar 0.4 g Protein 27.6 g Cholesterol 239 mg

228. Lemon Cod Peas

Preparation Time: 10 minutes | Cooking Time: 10 minutes | Servings: 4

1 lb cod fillets, skinless, boneless and cut into chunks	1 cup fish stock
1 tbsp fresh parsley, chopped	1/2 tbsp lemon juice
1 green chili, chopped	3/4 cup fresh peas
2 tbsp onion, chopped	Pepper
Salt	

1. Add all ingredients into the inner pot of instant pot and stir well.
2. Seal pot with lid and cook on high for 10 minutes.
3. Once done, release pressure using quick release. Remove lid.

4. Stir and serve.

NUTRITION:
Calories 128 Fat 1.6 g Carbohydrates 5 g Sugar 2.1 g Protein 23.2 g Cholesterol 41 mg

229. Quick & Easy Shrimp

Preparation Time: 10 minutes | Cooking Time: 1 minute | Servings: 6

1 3/4 lbs shrimp, frozen and deveined	1/2 cup fish stock
1/2 cup apple cider vinegar	Pepper
Salt	

1. Add all ingredients into the inner pot of instant pot and stir well.
2. Seal pot with lid and cook on high for 1 minute.
3. Once done, release pressure using quick release. Remove lid.
4. Stir and serve.

NUTRITION:
Calories 165 Fat 2.4 g Carbohydrates 2.2 g Sugar 0.1 g Protein 30.6 g Cholesterol 279 mg

230. Creamy Curry Salmon

Preparation time: 10 minutes | Cooking time: 20 minutes | Servings: 2

2 salmon fillets, boneless and cubed	1 tablespoon olive oil
1 tablespoon basil, chopped	Sea salt and black pepper to the taste
1 cup Greek yogurt	2 teaspoons curry powder
1 garlic clove, minced	½ teaspoon mint, chopped

1. Heat up a pan with the oil over medium-high heat, add the salmon and cook for 3 minutes.
2. Add the rest of the ingredients, toss, cook for 15 minutes more, divide between plates and serve.

NUTRITION:
Calories 284, fat 14.1, fiber 8.5, carbs 26.7, protein 31.4

231. Mahi Mahi and Pomegranate Sauce

Preparation time: 10 minutes | Cooking time: 10 minutes | Servings: 4

1 and ½ cups chicken stock	1 tablespoon olive oil
4 mahi mahi fillets, boneless	4 tablespoons tahini paste
Juice of 1 lime	Seeds from 1 pomegranate
1 tablespoon parsley, chopped	

1. Heat up a pan with the oil over medium-high heat, add the fish and cook for 3 minutes on each side.
2. Add the rest of the ingredients, flip the fish again, cook for 4 minutes more, divide everything between plates and serve.

NUTRITION:
Calories 224, fat 11.1, fiber 5.5, carbs 16.7, protein 11.4

232. Smoked Salmon and Veggies Mix

Preparation time: 10 minutes | Cooking time: 20 minutes | Servings: 4

3 red onions, cut into wedges	¾ cup green olives, pitted and halved
3 red bell peppers, roughly chopped	½ teaspoon smoked paprika
Salt and black pepper to the taste	3 tablespoons olive oil
4 salmon fillets, skinless and boneless	2 tablespoons chives, chopped

1. In a roasting pan, combine the salmon with the onions and the rest of the ingredients, introduce in the oven and bake at 390 degrees F for 20 minutes.
2. Divide the mix between plates and serve.

NUTRITION:
Calories 301, fat 5.9, fiber 11.9, carbs 26.4, protein 22.4

233. Salmon and Mango Mix

Preparation time: 10 minutes | Cooking time: 25 minutes | Servings: 2

2 salmon fillets, skinless and boneless
2 tablespoons olive oil
2 mangos, peeled and cubed
1 small piece ginger, grated
1 tablespoon cilantro, chopped

Salt and pepper to the taste
2 garlic cloves, minced
1 red chili, chopped
Juice of 1 lime

1. In a roasting pan, combine the salmon with the oil, garlic and the rest of the ingredients except the cilantro, toss, introduce in the oven at 350 degrees F and bake for 25 minutes.
2. Divide everything between plates and serve with the cilantro sprinkled on top.

NUTRITION:
Calories 251, fat 15.9, fiber 5.9, carbs 26.4, protein 12.4

234. Salmon and Creamy Endives

Preparation time: 10 minutes | Cooking time: 15 minutes | Servings: 4

4 salmon fillets, boneless
Juice of 1 lime
¼ cup chicken stock
¼ cup green olives pitted and chopped
3 tablespoons olive oil

2 endives, shredded
Salt and black pepper to the taste
1 cup Greek yogurt
¼ cup fresh chives, chopped

1. Heat up a pan with half of the oil over medium heat, add the endives and the rest of the ingredients except the chives and the salmon, toss, cook for 6 minutes and divide between plates.
2. Heat up another pan with the rest of the oil, add the salmon, season with salt and pepper, cook for 4 minutes on each side, add next to the creamy endives mix, sprinkle the chives on top and serve.

NUTRITION:
Calories 266, fat 13.9, fiber 11.1, carbs 23.8, protein 17.5

235. Trout and Tzatziki Sauce

Preparation time: 10 minutes | Cooking time: 10 minutes | Servings: 4

Juice of ½ lime
1 and ½ teaspoon coriander, ground
4 trout fillets, boneless
2 tablespoons avocado oil
1 cucumber, chopped
1 tablespoon olive oil
1 and ½ cups Greek yogurt

Salt and black pepper to the taste
1 teaspoon garlic, minced
1 teaspoon sweet paprika
For the sauce:
4 garlic cloves, minced
1 teaspoon white vinegar
A pinch of salt and white pepper

1. Heat up a pan with the avocado oil over medium-high heat, add the fish, salt, pepper, lime juice, 1 teaspoon garlic and the paprika, rub the fish gently and cook for 4 minutes on each side.
2. In a bowl, combine the cucumber with 4 garlic cloves and the rest of the ingredients for the sauce and whisk well.
3. Divide the fish between plates, drizzle the sauce all over and serve with a side salad.

NUTRITION:
Calories 393, fat 18.5, fiber 6.5, carbs 18.3, protein 39.6

236. Parsley Trout and Capers

Preparation time: 10 minutes | Cooking time: 10 minutes | Servings: 4

4 trout fillets, boneless
A handful parsley, chopped
Salt and black pepper to the taste

3 ounces tomato sauce
2 tablespoons olive oil

1. Heat up a pan with the oil over medium-high heat, add the fish, salt and pepper and cook for 3 minutes on each side.
2. Add the rest of the ingredients, cook everything for 4 minutes more.
3. Divide everything between plates and serve.

NUTRITION:
Calories 308, fat 17, fiber 1, carbs 3, protein 16

237. Baked Trout and Fennel

Preparation time: 10 minutes | Cooking time: 22 minutes | Servings: 4

1 fennel bulb, sliced
1 yellow onion, sliced
4 rainbow trout fillets, boneless
½ cup kalamata olives, pitted and halved

2 tablespoons olive oil
3 teaspoons Italian seasoning
¼ cup panko breadcrumbs
Juice of 1 lemon

1. Spread the fennel the onion and the rest of the ingredients except the trout and the breadcrumbs on a baking sheet lined with parchment paper, toss them and cook at 400 degrees F for 10 minutes.
2. Add the fish dredged in breadcrumbs and seasoned with salt and pepper and cook it at 400 degrees F for 6 minutes on each side.
3. Divide the mix between plates and serve.

NUTRITION:
Calories 306, fat 8.9, fiber 11.1, carbs 23.8, protein 14.5

238. Lemon Rainbow Trout

Preparation time: 10 minutes | Cooking time: 15 minutes | Servings: 2

2 rainbow trout
3 tablespoons olive oil
A pinch of salt and black pepper

Juice of 1 lemon
4 garlic cloves, minced

1. Line a baking sheet with parchment paper, add the fish and the rest of the ingredients and rub.
2. Bake at 400 degrees F for 15 minutes, divide between plates and serve with a side salad.

NUTRITION:
Calories 521, fat 29, fiber 5, carbs 14, protein 52

239. Trout and Peppers Mix

Preparation: 10 minutes | Cooking: 20 minutes Servings: 4

4 trout fillets, boneless

1 tablespoon capers, drained
A pinch of salt and black pepper
1 yellow bell pepper, chopped
1 green bell pepper, chopped

2 tablespoons kalamata olives, pitted and chopped
2 tablespoons olive oil
1 and ½ teaspoons chili powder
1 red bell pepper, chopped

1. Heat up a pan with the oil over medium-high heat, add the trout, salt and pepper and cook for 10 minutes.
2. Flip the fish, add the peppers and the rest of the ingredients, cook for 10 minutes more, divide the whole mix between plates and serve.

NUTRITION:
Calories 572, fat 17.4, fiber 6, carbs 71, protein 33.7

240. Cod and Cabbage

Preparation time: 10 minutes | Cooking time: 15 minutes | Servings: 4

3 cups green cabbage, shredded
A pinch of salt and black pepper
4 teaspoons olive oil
¼ cup green olives, pitted and chopped

1 sweet onion, sliced
½ cup feta cheese, crumbled
4 cod fillets, boneless

1. Grease a roasting pan with the oil, add the fish, the cabbage and the rest of the ingredients, introduce in the pan and cook at 450 degrees F for 15 minutes.
2. Divide the mix between plates and serve.

NUTRITION:
Calories 270, fat 10, fiber 3, carbs 12, protein 31

241. Mediterranean Mussels

Preparation time: 10 minutes | Cooking time: 10 minutes | Servings: 4

1 white onion, sliced
2 teaspoons fennel seeds
1 teaspoon red pepper, crushed
1 cup chicken stock
2 and ½ pounds mussels, scrubbed
½ cup tomatoes, cubed

3 tablespoons olive oil
4 garlic cloves, minced
A pinch of salt and black pepper
1 tablespoon lemon juice
½ cup parsley, chopped

1. Heat up a pan with the oil over medium-high heat, add the onion and the garlic and sauté for 2 minutes.
2. Add the rest of the ingredients except the mussels, stir and cook for 3 minutes more.
3. Add the mussels, cook everything for 6 minutes more, divide everything into bowls and serve.

NUTRITION:
Calories 276, fat 9.8, fiber 4.8, carbs 6.5, protein 20.5

242. Mussels Bowls

Preparation time: 10 minutes | Cooking time: 10 minutes | Servings: 4

2 pounds mussels, scrubbed
1 tablespoon basil, chopped
6 tomatoes, cubed
2 tablespoons olive oil

1 tablespoon garlic, minced
1 yellow onion, chopped
1 cup heavy cream
1 tablespoon parsley, chopped

1. Heat up a pan with the oil over medium-high heat, add the garlic and the onion and sauté for 2 minutes.
2. Add the mussels and the rest of the ingredients, toss, cook for 7 minutes more, divide into bowls and serve.

NUTRITION:
Calories 266, fat 11.8, fiber 5.8, carbs 16.5, protein 10.5

243. Calamari and Dill Sauce

Preparation time: 10 minutes | Cooking time: 15 minutes | Servings: 4

1 and ½ pound calamari, sliced into rings
2 tablespoons olive oil
2 tablespoons balsamic vinegar
A pinch of salt and black pepper

10 garlic cloves, minced
Juice of 1 and ½ lime
3 tablespoons dill, chopped

1. Heat up a pan with the oil over medium-high heat, add the garlic, lime juice and the other ingredients except the calamari and cook for 5 minutes.
2. Add the calamari rings, cook everything for 10 minutes more, divide between plates and serve.

NUTRITION:
Calories 282, fat 18.6, fiber 4, carbs 9.2, protein 18.5

244. Chili Calamari and Veggie Mix

Preparation time: 10 minutes | Cooking time: 40 minutes | Servings: 4

1 pound calamari rings
2 tablespoons olive oil
14 ounces canned tomatoes, chopped
1 tablespoon thyme, chopped
2 tablespoons capers, drained

2 red chili peppers, chopped
3 garlic cloves, minced
2 tablespoons tomato paste
Salt and black pepper to the taste
12 black olives, pitted and halved

1. Heat up a pan with the oil over medium-high heat, add the garlic and the chili peppers and sauté for 2 minutes.
2. Add the rest of the ingredients except the olives and capers, stir, bring to a simmer and cook for 22 minutes.
3. Add the olives and capers, cook everything for 15 minutes more, divide everything into bowls and serve.

NUTRITION:
Calories 274, fat 11.6, fiber 2.8, carbs 13.5, protein 15.4

245. Cheesy Crab and Lime Spread

Preparation time: 10 minutes | Cooking time: 25 minutes | Servings: 8

1 pound crab meat, flaked
1 tablespoon chives, chopped
1 teaspoon lime zest, grated

4 ounces cream cheese, soft
1 teaspoon lime juice

1. 350 degrees F, bake for 25 minutes, divide into bowls and serve.

NUTRITION:
Calories 284, fat 14.6, fiber 5.8, carbs 16.5, protein 15.4

246. Horseradish Cheesy Salmon Mix

Preparation time: 1 hour | Servings: 8

2 ounces feta cheese, crumbled
3 tablespoons already prepared horseradish
2 teaspoons lime zest, grated
3 tablespoons chives, chopped

4 ounces cream cheese, soft
1 pound smoked salmon, skinless, boneless and flaked
1 red onion, chopped

DIRECTIONS
1. In your food processor, mix cream cheese with horseradish, goat cheese and lime zest and blend very well.
2. In a bowl, combine the salmon with the rest of the ingredients, toss and serve cold.

NUTRITION:
Calories 281, fat 17.9, fiber 1, carbs 4.2, protein 25.3

247. Greek Trout Spread

Preparation time: 5 minutes | Servings: 8

4 ounces smoked trout, skinless, boneless and flaked
1 cup Greek yogurt
Salt and black pepper to the taste

1 tablespoon lemon juice
tablespoon dill, chopped
A drizzle of olive oil

1. In a bowl, combine the trout with the lemon juice and the rest of the ingredients and whisk really well.
2. Divide the spread into bowls and serve.

NUTRITION:
Calories 258, fat 4,5, fiber 2, carbs 5.5, protein 7.6

248.   Scallions and Salmon Tartar

Preparation time: 5 minutes | Servings: 4

4 tablespoons scallions, chopped
1 tablespoon chives, minced
1 pound salmon, skinless, boneless and minced
1 tablespoon parsley, chopped

2 teaspoons lemon juice
1 tablespoon olive oil
Salt and black pepper to the taste

1.   In a bowl, combine the scallions with the salmon and the rest of the ingredients, stir well, divide into small moulds between plates and serve.

NUTRITION:
Calories 224, fat 14.5, fiber 5.2, carbs 12.7, protein 5.3

249.   Salmon and Green Beans

Preparation time: 10 minutes | Cooking time: 15 minutes | Servings: 4

3 tablespoons balsamic vinegar
1 garlic clove, minced

½ teaspoon lime zest, grated

Salt and black pepper to the taste
4 salmon fillets, boneless

2 tablespoons olive oil
½ teaspoons red pepper flakes, crushed
1 and ½ pounds green beans, chopped
1 red onion, sliced

1.   Heat up a pan with half of the oil, add the vinegar, onion, garlic and the other ingredients except the salmon, toss, cook for 6 minutes and divide between plates.
2.   Heat up the same pan with the rest of the oil over medium-high heat, add the salmon, salt and pepper, cook for 4 minutes on each side, add next to the green beans and serve.

NUTRITION:
Calories 224, fat 15.5, fiber 8.2, carbs 22.7, protein 16.3

250.   Cayenne Cod and Tomatoes

Preparation time: 10 minutes | Cooking time: 25 minutes | Servings: 4

1 teaspoon lime juice
1 teaspoon sweet paprika
2 tablespoons olive oil
2 garlic cloves, minced
A pinch of cloves, ground
½ pound cherry tomatoes, cubed

Salt and black pepper to the taste
1 teaspoon cayenne pepper
1 yellow onion, chopped
4 cod fillets, boneless
½ cup chicken stock

1.   Heat up a pan with the oil over medium-high heat add the cod, salt, pepper and the cayenne, cook for 4 minutes on each side and divide between plates.
2.   Heat up the same pan over medium-high heat, add the onion and garlic and sauté for 5 minutes.
3.   Add the rest of the ingredients, stir, bring to a simmer and cook for 10 minutes more.
4.   Divide the mix next to the fish and serve.

NUTRITION:
Calories 232, fat 16.5, fiber 11.1, carbs 24.8, protein 16.5

251. Salmon and Watermelon Gazpacho

Preparation time: 4 hours | Servings: 4

¼ cup basil, chopped
1 pound watermelon, cubed
1/3 cup avocado oil
1 cup smoked salmon, skinless, boneless and cubed

1 pound tomatoes, cubed
¼ cup red wine vinegar
2 garlic cloves, minced
A pinch of salt and black pepper

1.   In your blender, combine the basil with the watermelon and the rest of the ingredients except the salmon, pulse well and divide into bowls.
2.   Top each serving with the salmon and serve cold.

NUTRITION:
Calories 252, fat 16.5, fiber 9.1, carbs 24.8, protein 15.5

252.   Shrimp and Calamari Mix

Preparation time: 10 minutes | Cooking time: 12 minutes | Servings: 4

1 pound shrimp, peeled and deveined
3 garlic cloves, minced
½ pound calamari rings
1 teaspoon rosemary, dried
1 cup chicken stock
1 tablespoon parsley, chopped

Salt and black pepper to the taste

1 tablespoon avocado oil
½ teaspoon basil, dried
1 red onion, chopped
Juice of 1 lemon

1.   Heat up a pan with the oil over medium-high heat, add the onion and the garlic and sauté for 4 minutes.
2.   Add the shrimp, the calamari and the rest of the ingredients except the parsley, stir, bring to a simmer and cook for 8 minutes.
3.   Add the parsley, divide everything into bowls and serve.

NUTRITION:
Calories 288, fat 12.8, fiber 10.2, carbs 22.2, protein 6.8

253.   Shrimp and Dill Mix

Preparation time: 10 minutes | Cooking time: 10 minutes | Servings: 4

1 pound shrimp, cooked, peeled and deveined
1 cup spring onion, chopped
2 tablespoons capers, chopped
Salt and black pepper to the taste

½ cup raisins

2 tablespoons olive oil
2 tablespoons dill, chopped

1.   Heat up a pan with the oil over medium-high heat, add the onions and raisins and sauté for 2-3 minutes.
2.   Add the shrimp and the rest of the ingredients, toss, cook for 6 minutes more, divide between plates and serve with a side salad.

NUTRITION:
Calories 218, fat 12.8, fiber 6.2, carbs 22.2, protein 4.8

254.   Minty Sardines Salad

Preparation time: 10 minutes | Servings: 4

4 ounces canned sardines in olive oil, skinless, boneless and flaked
2 tablespoons mint, chopped
1 avocado, peeled, pitted and cubed
2 tomatoes, cubed

2 teaspoons avocado oil

A pinch of salt and black pepper
1 cucumber, cubed
2 spring onions, chopped

1.   In a bowl, combine the sardines with the oil and the rest of the ingredients, toss, divide into small cups and keep in the fridge for 10 minutes before serving.

NUTRITION:
Calories 261, fat 7.6, fiber 2.2, carbs 22.8, protein 12.5

VEGETABLES

255. Potato Salad

Preparation Time: 10 minutes | Cooking Time: 10 minutes | Servings: 8

5 cups potato, cubed
1/4 tsp red pepper flakes
1/3 cup mayonnaise
2 tbsp capers
1 cup olives, halved
3/4 cup onion, chopped
Salt
1/4 cup fresh parsley, chopped
1 tbsp olive oil
1/2 tbsp oregano
3/4 cup feta cheese, crumbled
3 cups of water
Pepper

1. Add potatoes, onion, and salt into the instant pot.
2. Seal pot with lid and cook on high for 3 minutes.
3. Once done, release pressure using quick release. Remove lid.
4. Remove potatoes from pot and place in a large mixing bowl.
5. Add remaining ingredients and stir everything well.
6. Serve and enjoy.

NUTRITION:
Calories 152 Fat 9.9 g Carbohydrates 13.6 g Sugar 2.1 g Protein 3.5 g Cholesterol 15 mg

256. Greek Green Beans

Preparation Time: 10 minutes | Cooking Time: 15 minutes | Servings: 4

1 lb green beans, remove stems
1 1/2 onion, sliced
1/4 cup dill, chopped
1 zucchini, quartered
1 cup of water
Pepper
2 potatoes, quartered
1 tsp dried oregano
1/4 cup fresh parsley, chopped
1/2 cup olive oil
k14.5 oz can tomatoes, diced
Salt

1. Add all ingredients into the inner pot of instant pot and stir everything well.
2. Seal pot with lid and cook on high for 15 minutes.
3. Once done, release pressure using quick release. Remove lid.
4. Stir well and serve.

NUTRITION:
Calories 381 Fat 25.8 g Carbohydrates 37.7 g Sugar 9 g Protein 6.6 g Cholesterol 0 mg

257. Healthy Vegetable Medley

Preparation Time: 10 minutes | Cooking Time: 17 minutes | Servings: 6

3 cups broccoli florets
1 tsp garlic, minced
28 oz can tomatoes, chopped

1 onion, chopped
1 tsp Italian seasoning
Salt
1 sweet potato, chopped
14 oz coconut milk
14 oz can chickpeas, drained and rinsed
1 tbsp olive oil
Pepper

1. Add oil into the inner pot of instant pot and set the pot on sauté mode.
2. Add garlic and onion and sauté until onion is softened.
3. Add remaining ingredients and stir everything well.
4. Seal pot with lid and cook on high for 12 minutes.
5. Once done, allow to release pressure naturally for 10 minutes then release remaining using quick release. Remove lid.
6. Stir well and serve.

NUTRITION:

Calories 322 Fat 19.3 g Carbohydrates 34.3 g Sugar 9.6 g Protein 7.9 g Cholesterol 1 mg

258. Spicy Zucchini

Preparation Time: 10 minutes | Cooking Time: 5 minutes | Servings: 4

4 zucchini, cut into 1/2-inch pieces
1/2 tsp Italian seasoning
1 tsp garlic, minced
1/2 cup can tomato, crushed
1 cup of water
1/2 tsp red pepper flakes
1 tbsp olive oil
Salt

1. Add water and zucchini into the instant pot.
2. Seal pot with lid and cook on high for 2 minutes.
3. Once done, release pressure using quick release. Remove lid.
4. Drain zucchini well and clean the instant pot.
5. Add oil into the inner pot of instant pot and set the pot on sauté mode.
6. Add garlic and sauté for 30 seconds.
7. Add remaining ingredients and stir well and cook for 2-3 minutes.
8. Serve and enjoy.

NUTRITION:
Calories 69 Fat 4.1 g Carbohydrates 7.9 g Sugar 3.5 g Protein 2.7 g Cholesterol 0 mg

259. Healthy Garlic Eggplant

Preparation Time: 10 minutes | Cooking Time: 10 minutes | Servings: 4

1 eggplant, cut into 1-inch pieces
1/4 cup can tomato, crushed
1 tsp paprika
1 tsp garlic powder
Salt
1/2 cup water
1/2 tsp Italian seasoning
1/2 tsp chili powder
2 tbsp olive oil

1. Add water and eggplant into the instant pot.
2. Seal pot with lid and cook on high for 5 minutes.
3. Once done, release pressure using quick release. Remove lid.
4. Drain eggplant well and clean the instant pot.
5. Add oil into the inner pot of instant pot and set the pot on sauté mode.
6. Add eggplant along with remaining ingredients and stir well and cook for 5 minutes.
7. Serve and enjoy.

NUTRITION:
Calories 97 Fat 7.5 g Carbohydrates 8.2 g Sugar 3.7 g Protein 1.5 g Cholesterol 0 mg

260. Carrot Potato Medley

Preparation Time: 10 minutes | Cooking Time: 15 minutes | Servings: 6

4 lbs baby potatoes, clean and cut in half
1 tsp Italian seasoning
1 tbsp garlic, chopped
2 tbsp olive oil
Salt
1 1/2 lbs carrots, cut into chunks
1 1/2 cups vegetable broth
1 onion, chopped
Pepper

1. Add oil into the inner pot of instant pot and set the pot on sauté mode.
2. Add onion and sauté for 5 minutes.
3. Add carrots and cook for 5 minutes.
4. Add remaining ingredients and stir well.
5. Seal pot with lid and cook on high for 5 minutes.

6. Once done, allow to release pressure naturally for 10 minutes then release remaining using quick release. Remove lid.
7. Stir and serve.

NUTRITION:
Calories 283 Fat 5.6 g Carbohydrates 51.3 g Sugar 6.6 g Protein 10.2 g Cholesterol 1 mg

261. Lemon Herb Potatoes

Preparation Time: 10 minutes | **Cooking Time:** 11 minutes |
Servings: 6

1 1/2 lbs baby potatoes, rinsed and pat dry	1/2 fresh lemon juice
1 tsp dried oregano	1/2 tsp garlic, minced
1 tbsp olive oil	1 cup vegetable broth
1/2 tsp sea salt	

1. Add broth and potatoes into the instant pot.
2. Seal pot with lid and cook on high for 8 minutes.
3. Once done, release pressure using quick release. Remove lid.
4. Drain potatoes well and clean the instant pot.
5. Add oil into the inner pot of instant pot and set the pot on sauté mode.
6. Add potatoes, garlic, oregano, lemon juice, and salt and cook for 3 minutes.
7. Serve and enjoy.

NUTRITION:
Calories 94 Fat 2.7 g Carbohydrates 14.6 g Sugar 0.2 g Protein 3.8 g Cholesterol 0 mg

262. Flavors Basil Lemon Ratatouille

Preparation Time: 10 minutes | **Cooking Time:** 10 minutes |
Servings: 8

1 small eggplant, cut into cubes	1 cup fresh basil
2 cups grape tomatoes	1 onion, chopped
2 summer squash, sliced	2 zucchini, sliced
2 tbsp vinegar	2 tbsp tomato paste
1 tbsp garlic, minced	1 fresh lemon juice
1/4 cup olive oil	Salt

1. Add basil, vinegar, tomato paste, garlic, lemon juice, oil, and salt into the blender and blend until smooth.
2. Add eggplant, tomatoes, onion, squash, and zucchini into the instant pot.
3. Pour blended basil mixture over vegetables and stir well.
4. Seal pot with lid and cook on high for 10 minutes.
5. Once done, allow to release pressure naturally. Remove lid.
6. Stir well and serve.

NUTRITION:
Calories 103 Fat 6.8 g Carbohydrates 10.6 g Sugar 6.1 g Protein 2.4 g Cholesterol 0 mg

263. Garlic Basil Zucchini

Preparation Time: 10 minutes | **Cooking Time:** 8 minutes | **Servings:** 4

14 oz zucchini, sliced	1/4 cup fresh basil, chopped
1/2 tsp red pepper flakes	14 oz can tomatoes, chopped
1 tsp garlic, minced	1/2 onion, chopped
1/4 cup feta cheese, crumbled	1 tbsp olive oil
Salt	

1. Add oil into the inner pot of instant pot and set the pot on sauté mode.
2. Add onion and garlic and sauté for 2 minutes.
3. Add remaining ingredients except feta cheese and stir well.
4. Seal pot with lid and cook on high for 6 minutes.
5. Once done, allow to release pressure naturally. Remove lid.
6. Top with feta cheese and serve.

NUTRITION:
Calories 99 Fat 5.7 g Carbohydrates 10.4 g Sugar 6.1 g Protein 3.7 g Cholesterol 8 mg

264. Feta Green Beans

Preparation Time: 10 minutes | **Cooking Time:** 15 minutes |
Servings: 4

1 1/2 lbs green beans, trimmed	1/4 cup feta cheese, crumbled
28 oz can tomatoes, crushed	2 tsp oregano
1 tsp cumin	1/2 cup water
1 tbsp olive oil	1 tbsp garlic, minced
1 onion, chopped	1 lb baby potatoes, clean and cut into chunks
Pepper	Salt

1. Add oil into the inner pot of instant pot and set the pot on sauté mode.
2. Add onion and garlic and sauté for 3-5 minutes.
3. Add remaining ingredients except feta cheese and stir well.
4. Seal pot with lid and cook on high for 10 minutes.
5. Once done, allow to release pressure naturally for 5 minutes then release remaining using quick release. Remove lid.
6. Top with feta cheese and serve.

NUTRITION:
Calories 234 Fat 6.1 g Carbohydrates 40.7 g Sugar 10.7 g Protein 9.7 g Cholesterol 8 mg

265. Garlic Parmesan Artichokes

Preparation Time: 10 minutes | **Cooking Time:** 10 minutes | **Servings:** 4

4 artichokes, wash, trim, and cut top	1/2 cup vegetable broth
1/4 cup parmesan cheese, grated	1 tbsp olive oil
2 tsp garlic, minced	

1. Pour broth into the instant pot then place steamer rack in the pot.
2. Place artichoke steam side down on steamer rack into the pot.
3. Sprinkle garlic and grated cheese on top of artichokes and season with salt. Drizzle oil over artichokes.
4. Seal pot with lid and cook on high for 10 minutes.
5. Once done, release pressure using quick release. Remove lid.
6. Serve and enjoy.

NUTRITION:
Calories 132 Fat 5.2 g Carbohydrates 17.8 g Sugar 1.7 g Protein 7.9 g Cholesterol 4 mg

266. Delicious Pepper Zucchini

Preparation Time: 10 minutes | **Cooking Time:** 10 minutes |
Servings: 6

1 zucchini, sliced	2 poblano peppers, sliced
1 tbsp sour cream	1/2 tsp ground cumin
1 yellow squash, sliced	1 tbsp garlic, minced
1/2 onion, sliced	1 tbsp olive oil
Salt	

1. Add oil into the inner pot of instant pot and set the pot on sauté mode.
2. Add poblano peppers and sauté for 5 minutes.
3. Add onion and garlic and sauté for 3 minutes.
4. Add remaining ingredients except for sour cream and stir well.
5. Seal pot with lid and cook on high for 2 minutes.
6. Once done, release pressure using quick release. Remove lid.
7. Add sour cream and stir well and serve.

NUTRITION:
Calories 42 Fat 2.9 g Carbohydrates 4 g Sugar 1.7 g Protein 1 g Cholesterol 1 mg

267. Celery Carrot Brown Lentils

Preparation Time: 10 minutes | Cooking Time: 25 minutes | Servings: 6

2 cups dry brown lentils, rinsed and drained
2 tomatoes, chopped
1/2 tsp ground cinnamon
1 tbsp tomato paste
2 carrots, grated
2 onions, chopped
Pepper

2 1/2 cups vegetable stock
1/2 tsp red pepper flakes
1 bay leaf
2 celery stalks, diced
1 tbsp garlic, minced
1/4 cup olive oil
Salt

1. Add oil into the inner pot of instant pot and set the pot on sauté mode.
2. Add celery, carrot, garlic, onion, pepper, and salt and sauté for 3 minutes.
3. Add remaining ingredients and stir everything well.
4. Seal pot with lid and cook on high for 22 minutes.
5. Once done, release pressure using quick release. Remove lid.
6. Stir well and serve.

NUTRITION:
Calories 137 Fat 8.8 g Carbohydrates 12.3 g Sugar 4.7 g Protein 3.1 g Cholesterol 0 mg

268. Lemon Artichokes

Preparation Time: 10 minutes | Cooking Time: 20 minutes | Servings: 4

4 artichokes, trim and cut the top
2 cups vegetable stock
Pepper

1/4 cup fresh lemon juice
1 tsp lemon zest, grated
Salt

1. Pour the stock into the instant pot then place steamer rack in the pot.
2. Place artichoke steam side down on steamer rack into the pot.
3. Sprinkle lemon zest over artichokes. Season with pepper and salt.
4. Pour lemon juice over artichokes.
5. Seal pot with lid and cook on high for 20 minutes.
6. Once done, allow to release pressure naturally for 5 minutes then release remaining using quick release. Remove lid.
7. Serve and enjoy.

NUTRITION:
Calories 83 Fat 0.4 g Carbohydrates 17.9 g Sugar 2.3 g Protein 5.6 g Cholesterol 0 mg

269. Easy Chili Pepper Zucchinis

Preparation Time: 10 minutes | Cooking Time: 10 minutes | Servings: 4

4 zucchinis, cut into cubes
1/2 tsp cayenne
1/4 cup vegetable stock

1/2 tsp red pepper flakes
1 tbsp chili powder
Salt

1. Add all ingredients into the inner pot of instant pot and stir well.
2. Seal pot with lid and cook on high for 10 minutes.
3. Once done, allow to release pressure naturally for 10 minutes then release remaining using quick release. Remove lid.
4. Stir and serve.

NUTRITION:
Calories 38 Fat 0.7 g Carbohydrates 8.8 g Sugar 3.6 g Protein 2.7 g Cholesterol 0 mg

270. Delicious Okra

Preparation Time: 10 minutes | Cooking Time: 10 minutes | Servings: 4

2 cups okra, chopped
1 tbsp paprika
Pepper

2 tbsp fresh dill, chopped
1 cup can tomato, crushed
Salt

1. Add all ingredients into the inner pot of instant pot and stir well.
2. Seal pot with lid and cook on high for 10 minutes.
3. Once done, allow to release pressure naturally for 5 minutes then release remaining using quick release. Remove lid.
4. Stir well and serve.

NUTRITION:
Calories 37 Fat 0.5 g Carbohydrates 7.4 g Sugar 0.9 g Protein 2 g Cholesterol 0 mg

271. Tomato Dill Cauliflower

Preparation Time: 10 minutes | Cooking Time: 12 minutes | Servings: 4

1 lb cauliflower florets, chopped
1/4 tsp Italian seasoning
1 cup can tomatoes, crushed
1 tsp garlic, minced
Salt

1 tbsp fresh dill, chopped
1 tbsp vinegar
1 cup vegetable stock
Pepper

1. Add all ingredients except dill into the instant pot and stir well.
2. Seal pot with lid and cook on high for 12 minutes.
3. Once done, allow to release pressure naturally for 10 minutes then release remaining using quick release. Remove lid.
4. Garnish with dill and serve.

NUTRITION:
Calories 47 Fat 0.3 g Carbohydrates 10 g Sugar 5 g Protein 3.1 g Cholesterol 0 mg

272. Parsnips with Eggplant

Preparation Time: 10 minutes | Cooking Time: 12 minutes | Servings: 4

2 parsnips, sliced
1/2 tsp ground cumin
1 tsp garlic, minced
1/4 tsp dried basil
Salt

1 cup can tomatoes, crushed
1 tbsp paprika
1 eggplant, cut into chunks
Pepper

1. Add all ingredients into the instant pot and stir well.
2. Seal pot with lid and cook on high for 12 minutes.
3. Once done, release pressure using quick release. Remove lid.
4. Stir and serve.

NUTRITION:
Calories 98 0.7 g Carbohydrates 23 g Sugar 8.8 g Protein 2.8 g Cholesterol 0 mg

273. Easy Garlic Beans

Preparation Time: 10 minutes | Cooking Time: 5 minutes | Servings: 4

1 lb green beans, trimmed
1 tsp garlic, minced
Pepper

1 1/2 cup vegetable stock
1 tbsp olive oil
Salt

1. Add all ingredients into the instant pot and stir well.
2. Seal pot with lid and cook on high for 5 minutes.
3. Once done, release pressure using quick release. Remove lid.
4. Stir and serve.

NUTRITION:
Calories 69 Fat 3.7 g Carbohydrates 8.7 g Sugar 1.9 g Protein 2.3 g Cholesterol 0 mg

274. Eggplant with Olives

Preparation Time: 10 minutes | Cooking Time: 12 minutes | Servings: 4

4 cups eggplants, cut into cubes
1 tsp chili powder
1 onion, chopped
1/4 cup grape tomatoes
Salt

1/2 cup vegetable stock
1 cup olives, pitted and sliced
1 tbsp olive oil
Pepper

1. Add oil into the inner pot of instant pot and set the pot on sauté mode.
2. Add onion and sauté for 2 minutes.
3. Add remaining ingredients and stir everything well.
4. Seal pot with lid and cook on high for 12 minutes.
5. Once done, allow to release pressure naturally for 10 minutes then release remaining using quick release. Remove lid.
6. Stir and serve.

NUTRITION:
Calories 105 Fat 7.4 g Carbohydrates 10.4 g Sugar 4.1 g Protein 1.6 g Cholesterol 0 mg

275. Vegan Carrots & Broccoli

Preparation Time: 10 minutes | Cooking Time: 5 minutes | Servings: 6

4 cups broccoli florets
1/4 cup water
1 tsp garlic, minced
1/4 cup vegetable stock
Salt

2 carrots, peeled and sliced
1/2 lemon juice
1 tbsp olive oil
1/4 tsp Italian seasoning

1. Add oil into the inner pot of instant pot and set the pot on sauté mode.
2. Add garlic and sauté for 30 seconds.
3. Add carrots and broccoli and cook for 2 minutes.
4. Add remaining ingredients and stir everything well.
5. Seal pot with lid and cook on high for 3 minutes.
6. Once done, release pressure using quick release. Remove lid.
7. Stir well and serve.

NUTRITION:
Calories 51 Fat 2.6 g Carbohydrates 6.3 g Sugar 2.2 g Protein 2 g Cholesterol 0 mg

276. Zucchini Tomato Potato Ratatouille

Preparation Time: 10 minutes | Cooking Time: 10 minutes | Servings: 6

1 1/2 lbs potatoes, cut into cubes
28 oz fire-roasted tomatoes, chopped
4 mushrooms, sliced
12 oz eggplant, diced
8 oz yellow squash, diced
Salt

1/2 cup fresh basil
1 onion, chopped

1 bell pepper, diced
8 oz zucchini, diced
Pepper

1. Add all ingredients except basil into the instant pot and stir well.
2. Seal pot with lid and cook on high for 10 minutes.
3. Once done, release pressure using quick release. Remove lid.
4. Add basil and stir well and serve.

NUTRITION:
Calories 175 Fat 1.9 g

POULTRY

277. Duck and Blackberries

Preparation time: 10 minutes | Cooking time: 25 minutes | Servings: 4

4 duck breasts, boneless and skin scored
Salt and black pepper to the taste
4 ounces blackberries
2 tablespoons avocado oil

2 tablespoons balsamic vinegar
1 cup chicken stock
¼ cup chicken stock

1. between plates and serve.

NUTRITION:
Calories 239, fat 10.5, fiber 10.2, carbs 21.1, protein 33.3

278. Ginger Ducated

Preparation time: 10 minutes | Cooking time: 40 minutes | Servings: 4

2 big duck breasts, boneless and skin scored
Salt and black pepper to the taste
1 tablespoon lime juice
1 Serrano chili, chopped
1 cucumber, sliced
¼ cup oregano, chopped

2 tablespoons olive oil
1 tablespoon fish sauce
1 garlic clove, minced
1 small shallot, sliced
2 mangos, peeled and sliced

DIRECTIONS
1. Heat up a pan with the oil over medium-high heat, add the duck breasts skin side down and cook for 5 minutes.
2. Add the orange zest, salt, pepper, fish sauce and the rest of the ingredients, bring to a simmer and cook over medium-low heat for 45 minutes.
3. Divide everything between plates and serve.

NUTRITION:
Calories 297, fat 9.1, fiber 10.2, carbs 20.8, protein 16.5

279. Turkey and Cranberry Sauce

Preparation time: 10 minutes | Cooking time: 50 minutes | Servings: 4

1 cup chicken stock
½ cup cranberry sauce

1 yellow onion, roughly chopped

2 tablespoons avocado oil
1 big turkey breast, skinless, boneless and sliced
Salt and black pepper to the taste

1. Heat up a pan with the avocado oil over medium-high heat, add the onion and sauté for 5 minutes.
2. Add the turkey and brown for 5 minutes more.
3. Add the rest of the ingredients, toss, introduce in the oven at 350 degrees F and cook for 40 minutes

NUTRITION:
Calories 382, fat 12.6, fiber 9.6, carbs 26.6, protein 17.6

280. Sage Turkey Mix

Preparation time: 10 minutes | Cooking time: 40 minutes | Servings: 4

1 big turkey breast, skinless, boneless and roughly cubed
2 tablespoons avocado oil
2 tablespoons sage, chopped
1 cup chicken stock

Juice of 1 lemon

1 red onion, chopped
1 garlic clove, minced

1. Heat up a pan with the avocado oil over medium-high heat, add the turkey and brown for 3 minutes on each side.

2. Add the rest of the ingredients, bring to a simmer and cook over medium heat for 35 minutes.
3. Divide the mix between plates and serve with a side dish.

NUTRITION:
Calories 382, fat 12.6, fiber 9.6, carbs 16.6, protein 33.2

281. Turkey and Asparagus Mix

Preparation time: 10 minutes | Cooking time: 30 minutes | Servings: 4

1 bunch asparagus, trimmed and halved
1 teaspoon basil, dried
A pinch of salt and black pepper
1 tablespoon chives, chopped

1 big turkey breast, skinless, boneless and cut into strips
2 tablespoons olive oil
½ cup tomato sauce

1. Heat up a pan with the oil over medium-high heat, add the turkey and brown for 4 minutes.
2. Add the asparagus and the rest of the ingredients except the chives, bring to a simmer and cook over medium heat for 25 minutes.
3. Add the chives, divide the mix between plates and serve.

NUTRITION:
Calories 337, fat 21.2, fiber 10.2, carbs 21.4, protein 17.6

282. Herbed Almond Turkey

Preparation time: 10 minutes | Cooking time: 40 minutes | Servings: 4

1 big turkey breast, skinless, boneless and cubed
½ cup chicken stock
1 tablespoon rosemary, chopped
1 tablespoon parsley, chopped
½ cup almonds, toasted and chopped

1 tablespoon olive oil
1 tablespoon basil, chopped
1 tablespoon oregano, chopped
3 garlic cloves, minced
3 cups tomatoes, chopped

1. Heat up a pan with the oil over medium-high heat, add the turkey and the garlic and brown for 5 minutes.
2. Add the stock and the rest of the ingredients, bring to a simmer over medium heat and cook for 35 minutes.
3. Divide the mix between plates and serve.

NUTRITION:
Calories 297, fat 11.2, fiber 9.2, carbs 19.4, protein 23.6

283. Thyme Chicken and Potatoes

Preparation time: 10 minutes | Cooking time: 50 minutes | Servings: 4

1 tablespoon olive oil
A pinch of salt and black pepper
12 small red potatoes, halved

1 cup red onion, sliced
2 tablespoons basil, chopped

4 garlic cloves, minced
2 teaspoons thyme, dried
2 pounds chicken breast, skinless, boneless and cubed
¾ cup chicken stock

1. In a baking dish greased with the oil, add the potatoes, chicken and the rest of the ingredients, toss a bit, introduce in the oven and bake at 400 degrees F for 50 minutes.
2. Divide between plates and serve.

NUTRITION:
Calories 281, fat 9.2, fiber 10.9, carbs 21.6, protein 13.6

284. Turkey, Artichokes and Asparagus

Preparation time: 10 minutes | Cooking time: 30 minutes | Servings: 4

2 turkey breasts, boneless, skinless and halved	3 tablespoons olive oil
1 and ½ pounds asparagus, trimmed and halved	1 cup chicken stock
A pinch of salt and black pepper	1 cup canned artichoke hearts, drained
¼ cup kalamata olives, pitted and sliced	1 shallot, chopped
3 garlic cloves, minced	3 tablespoons dill, chopped

1. Heat up a pan with the oil over medium-high heat, add the turkey and the garlic and brown for 4 minutes on each side.
2. Add the asparagus, the stock and the rest of the ingredients except the dill, bring to a simmer and cook over medium heat for 20 minutes.
3. Add the dill, divide the mix between plates and serve.

NUTRITION:
Calories 291, fat 16, fiber 10.3, carbs 22.8, protein 34.5

285. Lemony Turkey and Pine Nuts

Preparation time: 10 minutes | Cooking time: 30 minutes | Servings: 4

2 turkey breasts, boneless, skinless and halved	A pinch of salt and black pepper
2 tablespoons avocado oil	Juice of 2 lemons
1 tablespoon rosemary, chopped	3 garlic cloves, minced
¼ cup pine nuts, chopped	1 cup chicken stock

1. Heat up a pan with the oil over medium-high heat, add the garlic and the turkey and brown for 4 minutes on each side.
2. Add the rest of the ingredients, bring to a simmer and cook over medium heat for 20 minutes.
3. Divide the mix between plates and serve with a side salad.

NUTRITION:
Calories 293, fat 12.4, fiber 9.3, carbs 17.8, protein 24.5

286. Yogurt Chicken and Red Onion Mix

Preparation time: 10 minutes | Cooking time: 30 minutes | Servings: 4

2 pounds chicken breast, skinless, boneless and sliced	3 tablespoons olive oil
¼ cup Greek yogurt	2 garlic cloves, minced
½ teaspoon onion powder	A pinch of salt and black pepper
4 red onions, sliced	

1. In a roasting pan, combine the chicken with the oil, the yogurt and the other ingredients, introduce in the oven at 375 degrees F and bake for 30 minutes.
2. Divide chicken mix between plates and serve hot.

NUTRITION:
Calories 278, fat 15, fiber 9.2, carbs 15.1, protein 23.3

287. Chicken and Mint Sauce

Preparation time: 10 minutes | Cooking time: 30 minutes | Servings: 4

2 and ½ tablespoons olive oil	2 pounds chicken breasts, skinless, boneless and halved
3 tablespoons garlic, minced	2 tablespoons lemon juice
1 tablespoon red wine vinegar	1/3 cup Greek yogurt
2 tablespoons mint, chopped	A pinch of salt and black pepper

1. In a blender, combine the garlic with the lemon juice and the other ingredients except the oil and the chicken and pulse well.
2. Heat up a pan with the oil over medium-high heat, add the chicken and brown for 3 minutes on each side.

3. Add the mint sauce, introduce in the oven and bake everything at 370 degrees F for 25 minutes.
4. Divide the mix between plates and serve.

NUTRITION:
Calories 278, fat 12, fiber 11.2, carbs 18.1, protein 13.3

288. Oregano Turkey and Peppers

Preparation time: 10 minutes | Cooking time: 1 hour | Servings: 4

2 red bell peppers, cut into strips	2 green bell peppers, cut into strips
1 red onion, chopped	4 garlic cloves, minced
½ cup black olives, pitted and sliced	2 cups chicken stock
1 big turkey breast, skinless, boneless and cut into strips	1 tablespoon oregano, chopped
½ cup cilantro, chopped	

1. In a baking pan, combine the peppers with the turkey and the rest of the ingredients, toss, introduce in the oven at 400 degrees F and roast for 1 hour.
2. Divide everything between plates and serve.

NUTRITION:
Calories 229, fat 8.9, fiber 8.2, carbs 17.8, protein 33.6

289. Chicken and Mustard Sauce

Preparation time: 10 minutes | Cooking time: 26 minutes | Servings: 4

1/3 cup mustard	Salt and black pepper to the taste
1 red onion, chopped	1 tablespoon olive oil
1 and ½ cups chicken stock	4 chicken breasts, skinless, boneless and halved
¼ teaspoon oregano, dried	

1. Heat up a pan with the stock over medium heat, add the mustard, onion, salt, pepper and the oregano, whisk, bring to a simmer and cook for 8 minutes.
2. Heat up a pan with the oil over medium-high heat, add the chicken and brown for 3 minutes on each side.
3. Add the chicken to the pan with the sauce, toss, simmer everything for 12 minutes more, divide between plates and serve.

NUTRITION:
Calories 247, fat 15.1, fiber 9.1, carbs 16.6, protein 26.1

290. Chicken and Sausage Mix

Preparation time: 10 minutes | Cooking time: 50 minutes | Servings: 4

2 zucchinis, cubed	1 pound Italian sausage, cubed
2 tablespoons olive oil	1 red bell pepper, chopped
1 red onion, sliced	2 tablespoons garlic, minced
2 chicken breasts, boneless, skinless and halved	Salt and black pepper to the taste
½ cup chicken stock	1 tablespoon balsamic vinegar

1. Heat up a pan with half of the oil over medium-high heat, add the sausages, brown for 3 minutes on each side and transfer to a bowl.
2. Heat up the pan again with the rest of the oil over medium-high heat, add the chicken and brown for 4 minutes on each side.
3. Return the sausage, add the rest of the ingredients as well, bring to a simmer, introduce in the oven and bake at 400 degrees F for 30 minutes.
4. Divide everything between plates and serve.

NUTRITION:
Calories 293, fat 13.1, fiber 8.1, carbs 16.6, protein 26.1

291. Coriander and Coconut Chicken

Preparation time: 10 minutes | Cooking time: 30 minutes | Servings: 4

2 pounds chicken thighs, skinless, boneless and cubed	2 tablespoons olive oil
Salt and black pepper to the taste	3 tablespoons coconut flesh, shredded
1 and ½ teaspoons orange extract	1 tablespoon ginger, grated
¼ cup orange juice	2 tablespoons coriander, chopped
1 cup chicken stock	¼ teaspoon red pepper flakes

1. Heat up a pan with the oil over medium-high heat, add the chicken and brown for 4 minutes on each side.
2. Add salt, pepper and the rest of the ingredients, bring to a simmer and cook over medium heat for 20 minutes.
3. Divide the mix between plates and serve hot.

NUTRITION:
Calories 297, fat 14.4, fiber 9.6, carbs 22, protein 25

292. Saffron Chicken Thighs and Green Beans

Preparation time: 10 minutes | Cooking time: 25 minutes | Servings: 4

2 pounds chicken thighs, boneless and skinless	2 teaspoons saffron powder
1 pound green beans, trimmed and halved	½ cup Greek yogurt
Salt and black pepper to the taste	1 tablespoon lime juice
1 tablespoon dill, chopped	

1. In a roasting pan, combine the chicken with the saffron, green beans and the rest of the ingredients, toss a bit, introduce in the oven and bake at 400 degrees F for 25 minutes.
2. Divide everything between plates and serve.

NUTRITION:
Calories 274, fat 12.3, fiber 5.3, carbs 20.4, protein 14.3

293. Chicken and Olives Salsa

Preparation time: 10 minutes | Cooking time: 25 minutes | Servings: 4

2 tablespoon avocado oil	4 chicken breast halves, skinless and boneless
Salt and black pepper to the taste	1 tablespoon sweet paprika
1 red onion, chopped	1 tablespoon balsamic vinegar
2 tablespoons parsley, chopped	1 avocado, peeled, pitted and cubed
2 tablespoons black olives, pitted and chopped	

1. Heat up your grill over medium-high heat, add the chicken brushed with half of the oil and seasoned with paprika, salt and pepper, cook for 7 minutes on each side and divide between plates.
2. Meanwhile, in a bowl, mix the onion with the rest of the ingredients and the remaining oil, toss, add on top of the chicken and serve.

NUTRITION:
Calories 289, fat 12.4, fiber 9.1, carbs 23.8, protein 14.3

294. Carrots and Tomatoes Chicken

Preparation: 10 minutes | Cooking time: 1 hour , 10 minutes | Servings: 4

2 pounds chicken breasts, skinless, boneless and halved	Salt and black pepper to the taste
3 garlic cloves, minced	3 tablespoons avocado oil
2 shallots, chopped	4 carrots, sliced
3 tomatoes, chopped	¼ cup chicken stock
1 tablespoon Italian seasoning	1 tablespoon parsley, chopped

1. Heat up a pan with the oil over medium-high heat, add the chicken, garlic, salt and pepper and brown for 3 minutes on each side.

2. Add the rest of the ingredients except the parsley, bring to a simmer and cook over medium-low heat for 40 minutes.
3. Add the parsley, divide the mix between plates and serve.

NUTRITION:
Calories 309, fat 12.4, fiber 11.1, carbs 23.8, protein 15.3

295. Smoked and Hot Turkey Mix

Preparation time: 10 minutes | Cooking time: 40 minutes | Servings: 4

1 red onion, sliced	1 big turkey breast, skinless, boneless and roughly cubed
1 tablespoon smoked paprika	2 chili peppers, chopped
Salt and black pepper to the taste	2 tablespoons olive oil
½ cup chicken stock	1 tablespoon parsley, chopped
1 tablespoon cilantro, chopped	

1. Grease a roasting pan with the oil, add the turkey, onion, paprika and the rest of the ingredients, toss, introduce in the oven and bake at 425 degrees F for 40 minutes.
2. Divide the mix between plates and serve right away.

NUTRITION:
Calories 310, fat 18.4, fiber 10.4, carbs 22.3, protein 33.4

296. Spicy Cumin Chicken

Preparation time: 10 minutes | Cooking time: 25 minutes | Servings: 4

2 teaspoons chili powder	2 and ½ tablespoons olive oil
Salt and black pepper to the taste	1 and ½ teaspoons garlic powder
1 tablespoon smoked paprika	½ cup chicken stock
1 pound chicken breasts, skinless, boneless and halved	2 teaspoons sherry vinegar
2 teaspoons hot sauce	2 teaspoons cumin, ground
½ cup black olives, pitted and sliced	

1. Heat up a pan with the oil over medium-high heat, add the chicken and brown for 3 minutes on each side.
2. Add the chili powder, salt, pepper, garlic powder and paprika, toss and cook for 4 minutes more.
3. Add the rest of the ingredients, toss, bring to a simmer and cook over medium heat for 15 minutes more.
4. Divide the mix between plates and serve.

NUTRITION:
Calories 230, fat 18.4, fiber 9.4, carbs 15.3, protein 13.4

297. Chicken with Artichokes and Beans

Preparation time: 10 minutes | Cooking time: 40 minutes | Servings: 4

2 tablespoons olive oil	2 chicken breasts, skinless, boneless and halved
Zest of 1 lemon, grated	3 garlic cloves, crushed
Juice of 1 lemon	Salt and black pepper to the taste
1 tablespoon thyme, chopped	6 ounces canned artichokes hearts, drained
1 cup canned fava beans, drained and rinsed	1 cup chicken stock
A pinch of cayenne pepper	Salt and black pepper to the taste

DIRECTIONS
1. Heat up a pan with the oil over medium-high heat, add chicken and brown for 5 minutes.
2. Add lemon juice, lemon zest, salt, pepper and the rest of the ingredients, bring to a simmer and cook over medium heat for 35 minutes.
3. Divide the mix between plates and serve right away.

NUTRITION:
Calories 291, fat 14.9, fiber 10.5, carbs 23.8, protein 24.2

298. Chicken and Olives Tapenade

Preparation time: 10 minutes | Cooking time: 25 minutes | Servings: 4

2 chicken breasts, boneless, skinless and halved
½ cup olive oil
½ cup mixed parsley, chopped
Salt and black pepper to the taste
Juice of ½ lime

1 cup black olives, pitted

Salt and black pepper to the taste
½ cup rosemary, chopped
4 garlic cloves, minced

1. In a blender, combine the olives with half of the oil and the rest of the ingredients except the chicken and pulse well.
2. Heat up a pan with the rest of the oil over medium-high heat, add the chicken and brown for 4 minutes on each side.
3. Add the olives mix, and cook for 20 minutes more tossing often.

NUTRITION: Calories 291, fat 12.9, fiber 8.5, carbs 15.8, protein 34.2

299. Spiced Chicken Meatballs

Preparation time: 10 minutes | Cooking time: 20 minutes | Servings: 4

1 pound chicken meat, ground

1 egg, whisked
2 garlic cloves, minced
1 and ¼ cups heavy cream
¼ cup parsley, chopped

1 tablespoon pine nuts, toasted and chopped
2 teaspoons turmeric powder
Salt and black pepper to the taste
2 tablespoons olive oil
1 tablespoon chives, chopped

1. In a bowl, combine the chicken with the pine nuts and the rest of the ingredients except the oil and the cream, stir well and shape medium meatballs out of this mix.
2. Heat up a pan with the oil over medium-high heat, add the meatballs and cook them for 4 minutes on each side.
3. Add the cream, toss gently, cook everything over medium heat for 10 minutes more, divide between plates and serve.

NUTRITION:
Calories 283, fat 9.2, fiber 12.8, carbs 24.4, protein 34.5

300. Sesame Turkey Mix

Preparation time: 10 minutes | Cooking time: 25 minutes | Servings: 4

2 tablespoons avocado oil
1 tablespoons sesame seeds, toasted
1 big turkey breast, skinless, boneless and sliced
4 ounces feta cheese, crumbled
1 tablespoon lemon juice

1 and ¼ cups chicken stock
Salt and black pepper to the taste
¼ cup parsley, chopped

¼ cup red onion, chopped

1. Heat up a pan with the oil over medium-high heat, add the meat and brown for 4 minutes on each side.
2. Add the rest of the ingredients except the cheese and the sesame seeds, bring everything to a simmer and cook over medium heat for 15 minutes.
3. Add the cheese, toss, divide the mix between plates, sprinkle the sesame seeds on top and serve.

NUTRITION:
Calories 283, fat 13.2, fiber 6.8, carbs 19.4, protein 24.5

301. Cardamom Chicken and Apricot Sauce

Preparation time: 10 minutes | Cooking time: 7 hours | Servings: 4

Juice of ½ lemon
2 teaspoons cardamom, ground
2 chicken breasts, skinless, boneless and halved
2 spring onions, chopped
2 garlic cloves, minced
½ cup chicken stock

Zest of ½ lemon, grated
Salt and black pepper to the taste
2 tablespoons olive oil

2 tablespoons tomato paste
1 cup apricot juice
¼ cup cilantro, chopped

1. In your slow cooker, combine the chicken with the lemon juice, lemon zest and the other ingredients except the cilantro, toss, put the lid on and cook on Low for 7 hours.
2. Divide the mix between plates, sprinkle the cilantro on top and serve.

NUTRITION: C
alories 323, fat 12, fiber 11, carbs 23.8, protein 16.4

MEAT

302. Moist Shredded Beef

Preparation Time: 10 minutes | Cooking Time: 20 minutes | Servings: 8

2 lbs beef chuck roast, cut into chunks	1/2 tbsp dried red pepper
1 tbsp Italian seasoning	1 tbsp garlic, minced
2 tbsp vinegar	14 oz can fire-roasted tomatoes
1/2 cup bell pepper, chopped	1/2 cup carrots, chopped
1 cup onion, chopped	1 tsp salt

1. Add all ingredients into the inner pot of instant pot and set the pot on sauté mode.
2. Seal pot with lid and cook on high for 20 minutes.
3. Once done, release pressure using quick release. Remove lid.
4. Shred the meat using a fork.
5. Stir well and serve.

NUTRITION:
Calories 456 Fat 32.7 g Carbohydrates 7.7 g Sugar 4.1 g Protein 31 g Cholesterol 118 mg

303. Hearty Beef Ragu

Preparation Time: 10 minutes | Cooking Time: 50 minutes | Servings: 4

1 1/2 lbs beef steak, diced	1 1/2 cup beef stock
1 tbsp coconut amino	14 oz can tomatoes, chopped
1/2 tsp ground cinnamon	1 tsp dried oregano
1 tsp dried thyme	1 tsp dried basil
1 tsp paprika	1 bay leaf
1 tbsp garlic, chopped	1/2 tsp cayenne pepper
1 celery stick, diced	1 carrot, diced
1 onion, diced	2 tbsp olive oil
1/4 tsp pepper	1 1/2 tsp sea salt

DIRECTIONS
1. Add oil into the instant pot and set the pot on sauté mode.
2. Add celery, carrots, onion, and salt and sauté for 5 minutes.
3. Add meat and remaining ingredients and stir everything well.
4. Seal pot with lid and cook on high for 30 minutes.
5. Once done, allow to release pressure naturally for 10 minutes then release remaining using quick release. Remove lid.
6. Shred meat using a fork. Set pot on sauté mode and cook for 10 minutes. Stir every 2-3 minutes.
7. Serve and enjoy.

NUTRITION:
Calories 435 Fat 18.1 g Carbohydrates 12.3 g Sugar 5.5 g Protein 54.4 g Cholesterol 152 mg

304. Dill Beef Brisket

Preparation Time: 10 minutes | Cooking Time: 50 minutes | Servings: 4

INGREDIENTS

2 1/2 lbs beef brisket, cut into cubes	2 1/2 cups beef stock
2 tbsp dill, chopped	1 celery stalk, chopped
1 onion, sliced	1 tbsp garlic, minced
Pepper	Salt

1. Add all ingredients into the inner pot of instant pot and stir well.
2. Seal pot with lid and cook on high for 50 minutes.
3. Once done, allow to release pressure naturally for 10 minutes then release remaining using quick release. Remove lid.
4. Serve and enjoy.

NUTRITION:
Calories 556 Fat 18.1 g Carbohydrates 4.3 g Sugar 1.3 g Protein 88.5 g Cholesterol 253 mg

305. Tasty Beef Stew

Preparation Time: 10 minutes | Cooking Time: 30 minutes | Servings: 4

2 1/2 lbs beef roast, cut into chunks	1 cup beef broth
1/2 cup balsamic vinegar	1 tbsp honey
1/2 tsp red pepper flakes	1 tbsp garlic, minced
Pepper	Salt

1. Add all ingredients into the inner pot of instant pot and stir well.
2. Seal pot with lid and cook on high for 30 minutes.
3. Once done, allow to release pressure naturally. Remove lid.
4. Stir well and serve.

NUTRITION:
Calories 562 Fat 18.1 g Carbohydrates 5.7 g Sugar 4.6 g Protein 87.4 g Cholesterol 253 mg Meatloaf Preparation Time: 10 minutes Cooking Time: 35 minutes Servings: 6

306. Italian Style Ground Beef

Preparation time: 10 minutes | Cooking time: 20 minutes | Servings: 4

2 lbs ground beef	2 eggs, lightly beaten
1/4 tsp dried basil	3 tbsp olive oil
1/2 tsp dried sage	1 1/2 tsp dried parsley
1 tsp oregano	2 tsp thyme
1 tsp rosemary	Pepper
Salt	

1. Pour 1 1/2 cups of water into the instant pot then place the trivet in the pot.
2. Spray loaf pan with cooking spray.
3. Add all ingredients into the mixing bowl and mix until well combined.
4. Transfer meat mixture into the prepared loaf pan and place loaf pan on top of the trivet in the pot.
5. Seal pot with lid and cook on high for 35 minutes.
6. Once done, allow to release pressure naturally for 10 minutes then release remaining using quick release. Remove lid.
7. Serve and enjoy.

NUTRITION:
Calories 365 Fat 18 g Carbohydrates 0.7 g Sugar 0.1 g Protein 47.8 g Cholesterol 190 mg

307. Flavorful Beef Bourguignon

Preparation Time: 10 minutes | Cooking Time: 20 minutes | Servings: 4

1 1/2 lbs beef chuck roast, cut into chunks	2/3 cup beef stock
2 tbsp fresh thyme	1 bay leaf
1 tsp garlic, minced	8 oz mushrooms, sliced
2 tbsp tomato paste	2/3 cup dry red wine
1 onion, sliced	4 carrots, cut into chunks
1 tbsp olive oil	Pepper
Salt	

1. Add oil into the instant pot and set the pot on sauté mode.
2. Add meat and sauté until brown. Add onion and sauté until softened.
3. Add remaining ingredients and stir well.
4. Seal pot with lid and cook on high for 12 minutes.
5. Once done, allow to release pressure naturally. Remove lid.

6. Stir well and serve.

NUTRITION:
Calories 744 Fat 51.3 g Carbohydrates 14.5 g Sugar 6.5 g Protein 48.1 g Cholesterol 175 mg

308. Delicious Beef Chili
Preparation Time: 10 minutes | Cooking Time: 35 minutes | Servings: 8

2 lbs ground beef	1 tsp olive oil
1 tsp garlic, minced	1 small onion, chopped
2 tbsp chili powder	1 tsp oregano
1/2 tsp thyme	28 oz can tomatoes, crushed
2 cups beef stock	2 carrots, chopped
3 sweet potatoes, peeled and cubed	Pepper
Salt	

1. Add oil into the instant pot and set the pot on sauté mode.
2. Add meat and cook until brown.
3. Add remaining ingredients and stir well.
4. Seal pot with lid and cook on high for 35 minutes.
5. Once done, allow to release pressure naturally. Remove lid.
6. Stir well and serve.

NUTRITION:
Calories 302 Fat 8.2 g Carbohydrates 19.2 g Sugar 4.8 g Protein 37.1 g Cholesterol 101 mg

309. Rosemary Creamy Beef
Preparation Time: 10 minutes | Cooking Time: 40 minutes | Servings: 4

2 lbs beef stew meat, cubed	2 tbsp fresh parsley, chopped
1 tsp garlic, minced	1/2 tsp dried rosemary
1 tsp chili powder	1 cup beef stock
1 cup heavy cream	1 onion, chopped
1 tbsp olive oil	Pepper
Salt	

1. Add oil into the instant pot and set the pot on sauté mode.
2. Add rosemary, garlic, onion, and chili powder and sauté for 5 minutes.
3. Add meat and cook for 5 minutes.
4. Add remaining ingredients and stir well.
5. Seal pot with lid and cook on high for 30 minutes.
6. Once done, allow to release pressure naturally for 10 minutes then release remaining using quick release. Remove lid.
7. Serve and enjoy.

NUTRITION:
Calories 574 Fat 29 g Carbohydrates 4.3 g Sugar 1.3 g Protein 70.6 g Cholesterol 244 mg

310. Spicy Beef Chili Verde
Preparation Time: 10 minutes | Cooking Time: 23 minutes | Servings: 2

1/2 lb beef stew meat, cut into cubes	1/4 tsp chili powder
1 tbsp olive oil	1 cup chicken broth
1 Serrano pepper, chopped	1 tsp garlic, minced
1 small onion, chopped	1/4 cup grape tomatoes, chopped
1/4 cup tomatillos, chopped	Pepper
Salt	

1. Add oil into the instant pot and set the pot on sauté mode.
2. Add garlic and onion and sauté for 3 minutes.
3. Add remaining ingredients and stir well.
4. Seal pot with lid and cook on high for 20 minutes.
5. Once done, allow to release pressure naturally. Remove lid.
6. Stir well and serve.

NUTRITION:

Calories 317 Fat 15.1 g Carbohydrates 6.4 g Sugar 2.6 g Protein 37.8 g Cholesterol 101 mg

311. Carrot Mushroom Beef Roast
Preparation Time: 10 minutes | Cooking Time: 40 minutes | Servings: 4

1 1/2 lbs beef roast	1 tsp paprika
1/4 tsp dried rosemary	1 tsp garlic, minced
1/2 lb mushrooms, sliced	1/2 cup chicken stock
2 carrots, sliced	Pepper
Salt	

1. Add all ingredients into the inner pot of instant pot and stir well.
2. Seal pot with lid and cook on high for 40 minutes.
3. Once done, allow to release pressure naturally for 10 minutes then release remaining using quick release. Remove lid.
4. Slice and serve.

NUTRITION:
Calories 345 Fat 10.9 g Carbohydrates 5.6 g Sugar 2.6 g Protein 53.8 g Cholesterol 152 mg

312. Italian Beef Roast
Preparation Time: 10 minutes | Cooking Time: 50 minutes | Servings: 6

2 1/2 lbs beef roast, cut into chunks	1 cup chicken broth
1 cup red wine	2 tbsp Italian seasoning
2 tbsp olive oil	1 bell pepper, chopped
2 celery stalks, chopped	1 tsp garlic, minced
1 onion, sliced	Pepper
Salt	

1. Add oil into the instant pot and set the pot on sauté mode.
2. Add the meat into the pot and sauté until brown.
3. Add onion, bell pepper, and celery and sauté for 5 minutes.
4. Add remaining ingredients and stir well.
5. Seal pot with lid and cook on high for 40 minutes.
6. Once done, allow to release pressure naturally. Remove lid.
7. Stir well and serve.

NUTRITION:
Calories 460 Fat 18.2 g Carbohydrates 5.3 g Sugar 2.7 g Protein 58.7 g Cholesterol 172 mg

313. Thyme Beef Round Roast
Preparation Time: 10 minutes | Cooking Time: 55 minutes | Servings: 8

4 lbs beef bottom round roast, cut into pieces	2 tbsp honey
5 fresh thyme sprigs	2 cups red wine
1 lb carrots, cut into chunks	2 cups chicken broth
6 garlic cloves, smashed	1 onion, diced
1/4 cup olive oil	2 lbs potatoes, peeled and cut into chunks
Pepper	Salt

1. Add all ingredients except carrots and potatoes into the instant pot.
2. Seal pot with lid and cook on high for 45 minutes.
3. Once done, release pressure using quick release. Remove lid.
4. Add carrots and potatoes and stir well.
5. Seal pot again with lid and cook on high for 10 minutes.
6. Once done, allow to release pressure naturally. Remove lid.
7. Stir well and serve.

NUTRITION:
Calories 648 Fat 21.7 g Carbohydrates 33.3 g Sugar 9.7 g Protein 67.1 g Cholesterol 200 mg

314. Jalapeno Beef Chili

Preparation Time: 10 minutes | Cooking Time: 40 minutes | Servings: 8

1 lb ground beef	1 tsp garlic powder
1 jalapeno pepper, chopped	1 tbsp ground cumin
1 tbsp chili powder	1 lb ground pork
4 tomatillos, chopped	1/2 onion, chopped
5 oz tomato paste	Pepper
Salt	

1. Add oil into the instant pot and set the pot on sauté mode.
2. Add beef and pork and cook until brown.
3. Add remaining ingredients and stir well.
4. Seal pot with lid and cook on high for 35 minutes.
5. Once done, allow to release pressure naturally. Remove lid.
6. Stir well and serve.

NUTRITION:

Calories 217 Fat 6.1 g Carbohydrates 6.2 g Sugar 2.7 g Protein 33.4 g Cholesterol 92 mg

315. Beef with Tomatoes

Preparation Time: 10 minutes | Cooking Time: 40 minutes | Servings: 4

2 lb beef roast, sliced	1 tbsp chives, chopped
1 tsp garlic, minced	1/2 tsp chili powder
2 tbsp olive oil	1 onion, chopped
1 cup beef stock	1 tbsp oregano, chopped
1 cup tomatoes, chopped	Pepper
Salt	

1. Add oil into the instant pot and set the pot on sauté mode.
2. Add garlic, onion, and chili powder and sauté for 5 minutes.
3. Add meat and cook for 5 minutes.
4. Add remaining ingredients and stir well.
5. Seal pot with lid and cook on high for 30 minutes.
6. Once done, allow to release pressure naturally for 10 minutes then release remaining using quick release. Remove lid.
7. Stir well and serve.

NUTRITION:

Calories 511 Fat 21.6 g Carbohydrates 5.6 g Sugar 2.5 g Protein 70.4 g Cholesterol 203 mg

316. Tasty Beef Goulash

Preparation Time: 10 minutes | Cooking Time: 30 minutes | Servings: 2

1/2 lb beef stew meat, cubed	1 tbsp olive oil
1/2 onion, chopped	1/2 cup sun-dried tomatoes, chopped
1/4 zucchini, chopped	1/2 cabbage, sliced
1 1/2 tbsp olive oil	2 cups chicken broth
Pepper	Salt

1. Add oil into the instant pot and set the pot on sauté mode.
2. Add onion and sauté for 3-5 minutes.
3. Add tomatoes and cook for 5 minutes.
4. Add remaining ingredients and stir well.
5. Seal pot with lid and cook on high for 20 minutes.
6. Once done, allow to release pressure naturally for 10 minutes then release remaining using quick release. Remove lid.
7. Stir well and serve.

NUTRITION:

Calories 389 Fat 15.8 g Carbohydrates 19.3 g Sugar 10.7 g Protein 43.2 g Cholesterol 101 mg

317. Beef & Beans

Preparation Time: 10 minutes | Cooking Time: 30 minutes | Servings: 4

1 1/2 lbs beef, cubed	8 oz can tomatoes, chopped
8 oz red beans, soaked overnight and rinsed	1 tsp garlic, minced
1 1/2 cups beef stock	1/2 tsp chili powder
1 tbsp paprika	2 tbsp olive oil
1 onion, chopped	Pepper
Salt	

1. Add oil into the instant pot and set the pot on sauté mode.
2. Add meat and cook for 5 minutes.
3. Add garlic and onion and sauté for 5 minutes.
4. Add remaining ingredients and stir well.
5. Seal pot with lid and cook on high for 25 minutes.
6. Once done, allow to release pressure naturally. Remove lid.
7. Stir well and serve.

NUTRITION:

Calories 604 Fat 18.7 g Carbohydrates 41.6 g Sugar 4.5 g Protein 66.6 g Cholesterol 152 mg

318. Delicious Ground Beef

Preparation Time: 10 minutes | Cooking Time: 10 minutes | Servings: 4

1 lb ground beef	1 tbsp olive oil
2 tbsp tomato paste	1 cup chicken broth
12 oz cheddar cheese, shredded	1 tbsp Italian seasoning
Pepper	Salt

1. Add oil into the instant pot and set the pot on sauté mode.
2. Add meat and cook until browned.
3. Add remaining ingredients except for cheese and stir well.
4. Seal pot with lid and cook on high for 7 minutes.
5. Once done, release pressure using quick release. Remove lid.
6. Add cheese and stir well and cook on sauté mode until cheese is melted.
7. Serve and enjoy.

NUTRITION:

Calories 610 Fat 40.2 g Carbohydrates 3.2 g Sugar 1.9 g Protein 57.2 g Cholesterol 193 mg

319. Bean Beef Chili

Preparation Time: 10 minutes | Cooking Time: 40 minutes | Servings: 4

1 lb ground beef	1/2 onion, diced
1/2 jalapeno pepper, minced	1 tsp chili powder
1/2 bell pepper, chopped	1 tsp garlic, chopped
1 cup chicken broth	14 oz can black beans, rinsed and drained
14 oz can red beans, rinsed and drained	Pepper
Salt	

1. Set instant pot on sauté mode.
2. Add meat and sauté until brown.
3. Add remaining ingredients and stir well.
4. Seal pot with lid and cook on high for 35 minutes.
5. Once done, release pressure using quick release. Remove lid.
6. Stir well and serve.

NUTRITION:

Calories 409 Fat 8.3 g Carbohydrates 36.3 g Sugar 4.2 g Protein 46.6 g Cholesterol 101 mg

320. Garlic Caper Beef Roast

Preparation Time: 10 minutes | Cooking Time: 40 minutes | Servings: 4

2 lbs beef roast, cubed
1 tbsp capers, chopped
1 cup chicken stock
1/2 tsp ground cumin
1 tbsp olive oil
Salt

1 tbsp fresh parsley, chopped
1 tbsp garlic, minced
1/2 tsp dried rosemary
1 onion, chopped
Pepper

1. Add oil into the instant pot and set the pot on sauté mode.
2. Add garlic and onion and sauté for 5 minutes.
3. Add meat and cook until brown.
4. Add remaining ingredients and stir well.
5. Seal pot with lid and cook on high for 30 minutes.
6. Once done, allow to release pressure naturally. Remove lid.
7. Stir well and serve.

NUTRITION:
Calories 470 Fat 17.9 g Carbohydrates 3.9 g Sugar 1.4 g Protein 69.5 g Cholesterol 203 mg

321. Cauliflower Tomato Beef

Preparation Time: 10 minutes | Cooking Time: 25 minutes | Servings: 2

1/2 lb beef stew meat, chopped
1 tbsp balsamic vinegar
1/4 cup grape tomatoes, chopped
1 tbsp olive oil
Pepper

1 tsp paprika
1 celery stalk, chopped
1 onion, chopped
1/4 cup cauliflower, chopped
Salt

1. Add oil into the instant pot and set the pot on sauté mode.
2. Add meat and sauté for 5 minutes.
3. Add remaining ingredients and stir well.
4. Seal pot with lid and cook on high for 20 minutes.
5. Once done, allow to release pressure naturally. Remove lid.
6. Stir and serve.

NUTRITION:
Calories 306 Fat 14.3 g Carbohydrates 7.6 g Sugar 3.5 g Protein 35.7 g Cholesterol 101 mg

322. Artichoke Beef Roast

Preparation Time: 10 minutes | Cooking Time: 45 minutes | Servings: 6

2 lbs beef roast, cubed
1 onion, chopped
1 tbsp parsley, chopped
1 tbsp capers, chopped

2 cups chicken stock
Pepper

1 tbsp garlic, minced
1/2 tsp paprika
2 tomatoes, chopped
10 oz can artichokes, drained and chopped
1 tbsp olive oil
Salt

1. Add oil into the instant pot and set the pot on sauté mode.
2. Add garlic and onion and sauté for 5 minutes.
3. Add meat and cook until brown.
4. Add remaining ingredients and stir well.
5. Seal pot with lid and cook on high for 35 minutes.
6. Once done, allow to release pressure naturally. Remove lid.
7. Serve and enjoy.

NUTRITION:
Calories 344 Fat 12.2 g Carbohydrates 9.2 g Sugar 2.6 g Protein 48.4 g Cholesterol 135 mg

323. Italian Beef

Preparation Time: 10 minutes | Cooking Time: 35 minutes | Servings: 4

1 lb ground beef
1/2 cup mozzarella cheese, shredded
1 tsp basil
1/2 onion, chopped
14 oz can tomatoes, diced
Salt

1 tbsp olive oil
1/2 cup tomato puree
1 tsp oregano
1 carrot, chopped
Pepper

1. Add oil into the instant pot and set the pot on sauté mode.
2. Add onion and sauté for 2 minutes.
3. Add meat and sauté until browned.
4. Add remaining ingredients except for cheese and stir well.
5. Seal pot with lid and cook on high for 35 minutes.
6. Once done, release pressure using quick release. Remove lid.
7. Add cheese and stir well and cook on sauté mode until cheese is melted.
8. Serve and enjoy.

NUTRITION:
Calories 297 Fat 11.3 g Carbohydrates 11.1 g Sugar 6.2 g Protein 37.1 g Cholesterol 103 mg

324. Greek Chuck Roast

Preparation Time: 10 minutes | Cooking Time: 35 minutes | Servings: 6

3 lbs beef chuck roast, boneless and cut into chunks
1 tsp oregano, chopped
1 cup tomatoes, diced
1 tbsp olive oil
Pepper

1/2 tsp dried basil
1 small onion, chopped
2 cups chicken broth
1 tbsp garlic, minced
Salt

1. Add oil into the instant pot and set the pot on sauté mode.
2. Add onion and garlic and sauté for 3-5 minutes.
3. Add meat and sauté for 5 minutes.
4. Add remaining ingredients and stir well.
5. Seal pot with lid and cook on high for 25 minutes.
6. Once done, allow to release pressure naturally. Remove lid.
7. Serve and enjoy.

NUTRITION:
Calories 869 Fat 66 g Carbohydrates 3.2 g Sugar 1.5 g Protein 61.5 g Cholesterol 234 mg

325. Beanless Beef Chili

Preparation Time: 10 minutes | Cooking Time: 20 minutes | Servings: 4

1 lb ground beef
1/2 tsp paprika
1/2 tsp chili powder
1 cup heavy cream
1 tsp garlic, minced
1 bell pepper, chopped
Pepper

1/2 tsp dried rosemary
1 tsp garlic powder
1/2 cup chicken broth
1 tbsp olive oil
1 small onion, chopped
2 cups tomatoes, diced
Salt

1. Add oil into the instant pot and set the pot on sauté mode.
2. Add meat, bell pepper, and onion and sauté for 5 minutes.
3. Add remaining ingredients except for heavy cream and stir well.
4. Seal pot with lid and cook on high for 5 minutes.
5. Once done, release pressure using quick release. Remove lid.
6. Add heavy cream and stir well and cook on sauté mode for 10 minutes.
7. Serve and enjoy.

NUTRITION:
Calories 387 Fat 22.2 g Carbohydrates 9.5 g Sugar 5 g Protein 37.2 g Cholesterol 142 mg

326.   Sage Tomato Beef

Preparation Time: 10 minutes | Cooking Time: 40 minutes | Servings: 4

2 lbs beef stew meat, cubed
1 tsp garlic, minced
1 onion, chopped
1 tbsp sage, chopped
Salt

1/4 cup tomato paste
2 cups chicken stock
2 tbsp olive oil
Pepper

1. Add oil into the instant pot and set the pot on sauté mode.
2. Add garlic and onion and sauté for 5 minutes.
3. Add meat and sauté for 5 minutes.
4. Add remaining ingredients and stir well.
5. Seal pot with lid and cook on high for 30 minutes.
6. Once done, allow to release pressure naturally. Remove lid.
7. Serve and enjoy.

NUTRITION:

Calories 515 Fat 21.5 g Carbohydrates 7 g Sugar 3.6 g Protein 70 g Cholesterol 203 mg

327.   Rosemary Beef Eggplant

Preparation Time: 10 minutes | Cooking Time: 30 minutes | Servings: 4

1 lb beef stew meat, cubed
1/4 tsp red pepper flakes
1/2 tsp paprika
1 onion, chopped
2 tbsp olive oil
Salt

2 tbsp green onion, chopped
1/2 tsp dried rosemary
1 cup chicken stock
1 eggplant, cubed
Pepper

1. Add oil into the instant pot and set the pot on sauté mode.
2. Add meat and onion and sauté for 5 minutes.
3. Add remaining ingredients and stir well.
4. Seal pot with lid and cook on high for 25 minutes.
5. Once done, allow to release pressure naturally. Remove lid.
6. Serve and enjoy.

NUTRITION:

Calories 315 Fat 14.5 g Carbohydrates 10 g Sugar 4.9 g Protein 36.1 g Cholesterol 101 mg

328.   Lemon Basil Beef

Preparation Time: 10 minutes | Cooking Time: 35 minutes | Servings: 4

1 1/2 lb beef stew meat, cut into cubes
1/2 tsp dried thyme
1 tsp garlic, minced
1 onion, chopped
Pepper

1/2 cup fresh basil, chopped
2 cups chicken stock
2 tbsp lemon juice
2 tbsp olive oil
Salt

1. Add oil into the instant pot and set the pot on sauté mode.
2. Add meat, garlic, and onion and sauté for 5 minutes.
3. Add remaining ingredients and stir well.
4. Seal pot with lid and cook on high for 30 minutes.
5. Once done, allow to release pressure naturally. Remove lid.
6. Serve and enjoy.

NUTRITION:

Calories 396 Fat 18 g Carbohydrates 3.5 g Sugar 1.7 g Protein 52.4 g Cholesterol 152 mg

329.   Thyme Ginger Garlic Beef

Preparation Time: 10 minutes | Cooking Time: 45 minutes | Servings: 2

1 lb beef roast
1/2 tsp ginger, grated
1/2 tsp garlic powder
1/4 tsp pepper

2 whole cloves
1/2 cup beef stock
1/2 tsp thyme
1/4 tsp salt

1. Mix together ginger, cloves, thyme, garlic powder, pepper, and salt and rub over beef.
2. Place meat into the instant pot. Pour stock around the meat.
3. Seal pot with lid and cook on high for 45 minutes.
4. Once done, release pressure using quick release. Remove lid.
5. Shred meat using a fork and serve.

NUTRITION:

Calories 452 Fat 15.7 g Carbohydrates 5.2 g Sugar 0.4 g Protein 70.1 g Cholesterol 203 mg

330.   Beef Shawarma

Preparation Time: 10 minutes | Cooking Time: 10 minutes | Servings: 2

1/2 lb ground beef
1/2 tsp dried oregano
1/2 cup bell pepper, sliced
1/4 tsp cumin
1/4 tsp ground allspice
1/2 tsp salt

1/4 tsp cinnamon
1 cup cabbage, cut into strips
1/4 tsp ground coriander
1/4 tsp cayenne pepper
1/2 cup onion, chopped

1. Set instant pot on sauté mode.
2. Add meat to the pot and sauté until brown.
3. Add remaining ingredients and stir well.
4. Seal pot with lid and cook on high for 5 minutes.
5. Once done, release pressure using quick release. Remove lid.
6. Stir and serve.

NUTRITION:

Calories 245 Fat 7.4 g Carbohydrates 7.9 g Sugar 3.9 g Protein 35.6 g Cholesterol 101 mg

331. Beef Curry

Preparation Time: 10 minutes | Cooking Time: 30 minutes | Servings: 2

1/2 lb beef stew meat, cubed
1 cup beef stock
1/2 tsp ground cumin
1/2 tsp cayenne pepper
2 tbsp olive oil
1 green chili peppers, chopped

1 bell peppers, sliced
1 tbsp fresh ginger, grated
1 tsp ground coriander
1/2 cup sun-roasted tomatoes, diced
1 tsp garlic, crushed

1. Add all ingredients into the instant pot and stir well.
2. Seal pot with lid and cook on high for 30 minutes.
3. Once done, allow to release pressure naturally. Remove lid.
4. Serve and enjoy.

NUTRITION:

Calories 391 Fat 21.9 g Carbohydrates 11.6 g Sugar 5.8 g Protein 37.4 g Cholesterol 101 mg

332. Breakfast Egg on Avocado

Servings: 6 | Cooking Time: 15 minutes

1 tsp garlic powder	1/2 tsp sea salt
1/4 cup Parmesan cheese (grated or shredded)	1/4 tsp black pepper
3 medium avocados (cut in half, pitted, skin on)	6 medium eggs

1. Prepare muffin tins and preheat the oven to 350oF.
2. To ensure that the egg would fit inside the cavity of the avocado, lightly scrape off 1/3 of the meat.
3. Place avocado on muffin tin to ensure that it faces with the top up.
4. Evenly season each avocado with pepper, salt, and garlic powder.
5. Add one egg on each avocado cavity and garnish tops with cheese.
6. Pop in the oven and bake until the egg white is set, about 15 minutes.
7. Serve and enjoy.

NUTRITION:
Calories: 252; Protein: 14.0g; Carbs: 4.0g; Fat: 20.0g

333. Breakfast Egg-Artichoke Casserole

Servings: 8 | Cooking Time: 35 minutes

16 large eggs	14 ounce can artichoke hearts, drained
10-ounce box frozen chopped spinach, thawed and drained well	1 cup shredded white cheddar
1 garlic clove, minced	1 teaspoon salt
1/2 cup parmesan cheese	1/2 cup ricotta cheese
1/2 teaspoon dried thyme	1/2 teaspoon crushed red pepper
1/4 cup milk	1/4 cup shaved onion

1. Lightly grease a 9x13-inch baking dish with cooking spray and preheat the oven to 350oF.
2. In a large mixing bowl, add eggs and milk. Mix thoroughly.
3. With a paper towel, squeeze out the excess moisture from the spinach leaves and add to the bowl of eggs.
4. Into small pieces, break the artichoke hearts and separate the leaves. Add to the bowl of eggs.
5. Except for the ricotta cheese, add remaining ingredients in the bowl of eggs and mix thoroughly.
6. Pour egg mixture into the prepared dish.
7. Evenly add dollops of ricotta cheese on top of the eggs and then pop in the oven.
8. Bake until eggs are set and doesn't jiggle when shook, about 35 minutes.
9. Remove from the oven and evenly divide into suggested servings. Enjoy.

NUTRITION:
Calories: 302; Protein: 22.6g; Carbs: 10.8g; Fat: 18.7g

334. Brekky Egg-Potato Hash

Servings: 2 | Cooking Time: 25 minutes

1 zucchini, diced	1/2 cup chicken broth
½ pound cooked chicken	1 tablespoon olive oil
4 ounces shrimp	salt and ground black pepper to taste
1 large sweet potato, diced	2 eggs
1/4 teaspoon cayenne pepper	2 teaspoons garlic powder
1 cup fresh spinach (optional)	

1. In a skillet, add the olive oil.
2. Fry the shrimp, cooked chicken and sweet potato for 2 minutes.

3. Add the cayenne pepper, garlic powder and salt and toss for 4 minutes.
4. Add the zucchini and toss for another 3 minutes.
5. Whisk the eggs in a bowl and add to the skillet.
6. Season using salt and pepper. Cover with the lid.
7. Cook for 1 minute and add the chicken broth.
8. Cover and cook for another 8 minutes on high heat.
9. Add the spinach and toss for 2 more minutes.
10. Serve immediately.

NUTRITION:
Calories: 190; Protein: 11.7g; Carbs: 2.9g; Fat: 12.3g

335. Cooked Beef Mushroom Egg

Servings: 2 | Cooking Time: 15 minutes

¼ cup cooked beef, diced	6 eggs
4 mushrooms, diced	Salt and pepper to taste
12 ounces spinach	2 onions, chopped
A dash of onion powder	¼ green bell pepper, chopped
A dash of garlic powder	

1. In a skillet, toss the beef for 3 minutes or until crispy.
2. Take off the heat and add to a plate.
3. Add the onion, bell pepper, and mushroom in the skillet.
4. Add the rest of the ingredients.
5. Toss for about 4 minutes.
6. Return the beef to the skillet and toss for another minute.
7. Serve hot.

NUTRITION:
Calories: 213; Protein: 14.5g; Carbs: 3.4g; Fat: 15.7g

336. Curried Veggies and Poached Eggs

Servings: 4 | Cooking Time: 45 minutes

4 large eggs	½ tsp white vinegar
1/8 tsp crushed red pepper – optional	1 cup water
1 14-oz can chickpeas, drained	2 medium zucchinis, diced
½ lb sliced button mushrooms	1 tbsp yellow curry powder
2 cloves garlic, minced	1 large onion, chopped
2 tsps extra virgin olive oil	

1. On medium high fire, place a large saucepan and heat oil.
2. Sauté onions until tender around four to five minutes.
3. Add garlic and continue sautéing for another half minute.
4. Add curry powder, stir and cook until fragrant around one to two minutes.
5. Add mushrooms, mix, cover and cook for 5 to 8 minutes or until mushrooms are tender and have released their liquid.
6. Add red pepper if using, water, chickpeas and zucchini. Mix well to combine and bring to a boil.
7. Once boiling, reduce fire to a simmer, cover and cook until zucchini is tender around 15 to 20 minutes of simmering.
8. Meanwhile, in a small pot filled with 3-inches deep of water, bring to a boil on high fire.
9. Once boiling, reduce fire to a simmer and add vinegar.
10. Slowly add one egg, slipping it gently into the water. Allow to simmer until egg is cooked, around 3 to 5 minutes.
11. Remove egg with a slotted spoon and transfer to a plate, one plate one egg.
12. Repeat the process with remaining eggs.
13. Once the veggies are done cooking, divide evenly into 4 servings and place one serving per plate of egg.
14. Serve and enjoy.

NUTRITION:
Calories: 215; Protein: 13.8g; Carbs: 20.6g; Fat: 9.4g

337.   Dill and Tomato Frittata
Servings: 6 | Cooking Time: 35 minutes

pepper and salt to taste	1 tsp red pepper flakes
2 garlic cloves, minced	½ cup crumbled goat cheese – optional
2 tbsp fresh chives, chopped	2 tbsp fresh dill, chopped
4 tomatoes, diced	8 eggs, whisked
1 tsp coconut oil	

1. Grease a 9-inch round baking pan and preheat oven to 325F.
2. In a large bowl, mix well all ingredients and pour into prepped pan.
3. Pop into the oven and bake until middle is cooked through around 30-35 minutes.
4. Remove from oven and garnish with more chives and dill.

338.   Dill, Havarti & Asparagus Frittata
Servings: 4 | Cooking Time: 20 minutes

1 tsp dried dill weed or 2 tsp minced fresh dill	4-oz Havarti cheese cut into small cubes
6 eggs, beaten well	Pepper and salt to taste
1 stalk green onions sliced for garnish	3 tsp. olive oil
2/3 cup diced cherry tomatoes	6-8 oz fresh asparagus, ends trimmed and cut into 1 ½-inch lengths

1. On medium-high the fire, place a large cast-iron pan and add oil. Once oil is hot, stir-fry asparagus for 4 minutes.
2. Add dill weed and tomatoes. Cook for two minutes.
3. Meanwhile, season eggs with pepper and salt. Beat well.
4. Pour eggs over the tomatoes.
5. Evenly spread cheese on top.
6. Preheat broiler.
7. Lower the fire to low, cover pan, and let it cook for 10 minutes until the cheese on top has melted.
8. Turn off the fire and transfer pan in the oven and broil for 2 minutes or until tops are browned.
9. Remove from the oven, sprinkle sliced green onions, serve, and enjoy.

NUTRITION:
Calories: 244; Protein: 16.0g; Carbs: 3.7g; Fat: 18.3g

339.   Egg and Ham Breakfast Cup
Servings: 12 | Cooking Time: 12 minutes

INGREDIENTS

2 green onion bunch, chopped	12 eggs
6 thick pieces nitrate free ham	

1. Grease a 12-muffin tin and preheat oven to 400oF.
2. Add 2 hams per muffin compartment, press down to form a cup and add egg in middle. Repeat process to remaining muffin compartments.
3. Pop in the oven and bake until eggs are cooked to desired doneness, around 10 to 12 minutes.
4. To serve, garnish with chopped green onions.

NUTRITION:
Calories: 92; Protein: 7.3g; Carbs: 0.8g; Fat: 6.4g

340.   Egg Muffin Sandwich
Servings: 2 | Cooking Time: 10 minutes

1 large egg, free-range or organic	1/4 cup almond flour (25 g / 0.9 oz)
1/4 cup flax meal (38 g / 1.3 oz)	1/4 cup grated cheddar cheese (28 g / 1 oz)
1/4 tsp baking soda	2 tbsp heavy whipping cream or coconut milk
2 tbsp water	pinch salt
1 tbsp butter or 2 tbsp cream cheese for spreading	1 tbsp ghee
1 tsp Dijon mustard	2 large eggs, free-range or organic
2 slices cheddar cheese or other hard type cheese (56 g / 2 oz)	Optional: 1 cup greens (lettuce, kale, chard, spinach, watercress, etc.)
salt and pepper to taste	

1. Make the Muffin: In a small mixing bowl, mix well almond flour, flax meal, baking soda, and salt. Stir in water, cream, and eggs. Mix thoroughly.
2. Fold in cheese and evenly divide in two single-serve ramekins.
3. Pop in the microwave and cook for 75 seconds.
4. Make the filing: on medium the fire, place a small nonstick pan, heat ghee and cook the eggs to the desired doneness. Season with pepper and salt.
5. To make the muffin sandwiches, slice the muffins in half. Spread cream cheese on one side and mustard on the other side.
6. Add egg and greens. Top with the other half of sliced muffin.
7. Serve and enjoy.

NUTRITION:
Calories: 639; Protein: 26.5g; Carbs: 10.4g; Fat: 54.6g

341. Eggs Benedict and Artichoke Hearts
Servings: 2 | Cooking Time: 30 minutes

Salt and pepper to taste	¾ cup balsamic vinegar
4 artichoke hearts	¼ cup bacon, cooked
1 egg white	8 eggs
1 tablespoon lemon juice	¾ cup melted ghee or butter

1. Line a baking sheet with parchment paper or foil.
2. Preheat the oven to 3750F.
3. Deconstruct the artichokes and remove the hearts. Place the hearts in balsamic vinegar for 20 minutes. Set aside.
4. Prepare the hollandaise sauce by using four eggs and separate the yolk from the white. Reserve the egg white for the artichoke hearts. Add the yolks and lemon juice and cook in a double boiler while stirring constantly to create a silky texture of the sauce. Add the oil and season with salt and pepper. Set aside.
5. Remove the artichoke hearts from the balsamic vinegar marinade and place on the cookie sheet. Brush the artichokes with the egg white and cook in the oven for 20 minutes.
6. Poach the remaining four eggs. Turn up the heat and let the water boil. Crack the eggs one at a time and cook for a minute before removing the egg.
7. Assemble by layering the artichokes, bacon and poached eggs.
8. Pour over the hollandaise sauce.
9. Serve with toasted bread.

NUTRITION:
Calories: 640; Protein: 28.3g; Carbs: 36.0g; Fat: 42.5g

342.   Eggs over Kale Hash
Servings: 4 | Cooking Time: 20 minutes

4 large eggs	1 bunch chopped kale
Dash of ground nutmeg	2 sweet potatoes, cubed
1 14.5-ounce can of chicken broth	

1. In a large non-stick skillet, bring the chicken broth to a simmer. Add the sweet potatoes and season slightly with salt and pepper. Add a dash of nutmeg to improve the flavor.
2. Cook until the sweet potatoes become soft, around 10 minutes. Add kale and season with salt and pepper. Continue cooking for four minutes or until kale has wilted. Set aside.
3. Using the same skillet, heat 1 tablespoon of olive oil over medium high heat.
4. Cook the eggs sunny side up until the whites become opaque and the yolks have set. Top the kale hash with the eggs. Serve immediately.

NUTRITION:
Calories: 158; Protein: 9.8g; Carbs 18.5g; Fat: 5.6g

343. Eggs with Dill, Pepper, and Salmon

Servings: 6 | Cooking Time: 15 minutes

pepper and salt to taste	1 tsp red pepper flakes
2 garlic cloves, minced	½ cup crumbled goat cheese
2 tbsp fresh chives, chopped	2 tbsp fresh dill, chopped
4 tomatoes, diced	8 eggs, whisked
1 tsp coconut oil	

1. In a big bowl whisk the eggs. Mix in pepper, salt, red pepper flakes, garlic, dill and salmon.
2. On low fire, place a nonstick fry pan and lightly grease with oil.
3. Pour egg mixture and whisk around until cooked through to make scrambled eggs.
4. Serve and enjoy topped with goat cheese.

NUTRITION:
Calories: 141; Protein: 10.3g; Carbs: 6.7g; Fat: 8.5g

344. Fig and Walnut Skillet Frittata

Servings: 4 | Cooking Time: 15 minutes

1 cup figs, halved	4 eggs, beaten
1 teaspoon cinnamon	A pinch of salt
2 tablespoons almond flour	2 tablespoons coconut flour
1 cup walnut, chopped	2 tablespoons coconut oil
1 teaspoon cardamom	6 tablespoons raw honey

1. In a mixing bowl, beat the eggs.
2. Add the coconut flour, almond flour, cardamom, honey, salt and cinnamon.
3. Mix well. Heat the coconut oil in a skillet over medium heat.
4. Add the egg mixture gently.
5. Add the walnuts and figs on top.
6. Cover and cook on medium low heat for about 10 minutes.
7. Serve hot with more honey on top.

NUTRITION:
Calories: 221; Protein: 12.7g; Carbs: 5.9g; Fat: 16.3g

345. Frittata with Dill and Tomatoes

Servings: 4 | Cooking Time: 35 minutes

pepper and salt to taste	1 tsp red pepper flakes
2 garlic cloves, minced	½ cup crumbled goat cheese – optional
2 tbsp fresh chives, chopped	2 tbsp fresh dill, chopped
4 tomatoes, diced	8 eggs, whisked
1 tsp coconut oil	

1. Grease a 9-inch round baking pan and preheat oven to 325oF.
2. In a large bowl, mix well all ingredients and pour into prepped pan.
3. Pop into the oven and bake until middle is cooked through around 30-35 minutes.
4. Remove from oven and garnish with more chives and dill.

NUTRITION:
Calories: 309; Protein: 19.8g; Carbs: 8.0g; Fat: 22.0g

346. Italian Scrambled Eggs

Servings: 1 | Cooking Time: 7 minutes

1 teaspoon balsamic vinegar	2 large eggs
¼ teaspoon rosemary, minced	½ cup cherry tomatoes
1 ½ cup kale, chopped	½ teaspoon olive oil

1. Melt the olive oil in a skillet over medium high heat.
2. Sauté the kale and add rosemary and salt to taste. Add three tablespoons of water to prevent the kale from burning at the bottom of the pan. Cook for three to four minutes.
3. Add the tomatoes and stir.
4. Push the vegetables on one side of the skillet and add the eggs. Season with salt and pepper to taste.
5. Scramble the eggs then fold in the tomatoes and kales.

NUTRITION:
Calories: 230; Protein: 16.4g; Carbs: 15.0g; Fat: 12.4g

347. Kale and Red Pepper Frittata

Servings: 4 | Cooking Time: 23 minutes

Salt and pepper to taste	½ cup almond milk
8 large eggs	2 cups kale, rinsed and chopped
3 slices of crispy bacon, chopped	1/3 cup onion, chopped
½ cup red pepper, chopped	1 tablespoon coconut oil

1. Preheat the oven to 3500F.
2. In a medium bowl, combine the eggs and almond milk. Season with salt and pepper. Set aside.
3. In a skillet, heat the coconut oil over medium flame and sauté the onions and red pepper for three minutes or until the onion is translucent. Add in the kale and cook for 5 minutes more.
4. Add the eggs into the mixture along with the bacon and cook for four minutes or until the edges start to set.
5. Continue cooking the frittata in the oven for 15 minutes.

NUTRITION:
Calories: 242; Protein: 16.5g; Carbs: 7.0g; Fat: 16.45g

348. Lettuce Stuffed with Eggs 'n Crab Meat

Servings: 8 | Cooking Time: 10 minutes

24 butter lettuce leaves	1 tsp dry mustard
¼ cup finely chopped celery	1 cup lump crabmeat, around 5 ounces
3 tbsp plain Greek yogurt	2 tbsp extra virgin olive oil
¼ tsp ground pepper	8 large eggs
½ tsp salt, divided	1 tbsp fresh lemon juice, divided
2 cups thinly sliced radishes	

1. In a medium bowl, mix ¼ tsp salt, 2 tsps. juice and radishes. Cover and chill for half an hour.
2. On medium saucepan, place eggs and cover with water over an inch above the eggs. Bring the pan of water to a boil. Once boiling, reduce fire to a simmer and cook for ten minutes.
3. Turn off fire, discard hot water and place eggs in an ice water bath to cool completely.
4. Peel eggshells and slice eggs in half lengthwise and remove the yolks.
5. With a sieve on top of a bowl, place yolks and press through a sieve. Set aside a tablespoon of yolk.
6. On remaining bowl of yolks add pepper, ¼ tsp salt and 1 tsp juice. Mix well and as you are stirring, slowly add oil until well incorporated. Add yogurt, stir well to mix.
7. Add mustard, celery and crabmeat. Gently mix to combine. If needed, taste and adjust seasoning of the filling.
8. On a serving platter, arrange 3 lettuce in a fan for two egg slices. To make the egg whites sit flat, you can slice a bit of the bottom to make it flat. Evenly divide crab filling into egg white holes.
9. Then evenly divide into eight servings the radish salad and add on the side of the eggs, on top of the lettuce leaves. Serve and enjoy.

NUTRITION:
Calories: 121; Protein: 10.0g; Carbs: 1.6g; Fat: 8.3g

349. Mixed Greens and Ricotta Frittata

Servings: 8 | Cooking Time: 35 minutes

1 tbsp pine nuts	1 clove garlic, chopped
¼ cup fresh mint leaves	¾ cup fresh parsley leaves
1 cup fresh basil leaves	8-oz part-skim ricotta
1 tbsp red-wine vinegar	½ + 1/8 tsp freshly ground black pepper, divided
½ tsp salt, divided	10 large eggs
1 lb chopped mixed greens	Pinch of red pepper flakes
1 medium red onion, finely diced	1/3 cup + 2 tbsp olive oil, divided

1. Preheat oven to 350oF.
2. On medium high fire, place a nonstick skillet and heat 1 tbsp oil. Sauté onions until soft and translucent, around 4 minutes. Add half of greens and pepper flakes and sauté until tender and crisp, around 5 minutes. Remove cooked greens and place in colander. Add remaining uncooked greens in skillet and sauté until tender and crisp, when done add to colander. Allow cooked veggies to cool enough to handle, then squeeze dry and place in a bowl.

3. Whisk well ¼ tsp pepper, ¼ tsp salt, Parmesan and eggs in a large bowl.
4. In bowl of cooked vegetables, add 1/8 tsp pepper, ricotta and vinegar. Mix thoroughly. Then pour into bowl of eggs and mix well.
5. On medium fire, place same skillet used previously and heat 1 tbsp oil. Pour egg mixture and cook for 8 minutes or until sides are set. Turn off fire, place skillet inside oven and bake for 15 minutes or until middle of frittata is set.
6. Meanwhile, make the pesto by processing pine nuts, garlic, mint, parsley and basil in a food processor until coarsely chopped. Add 1/3 cup oil and continue processing. Season with remaining pepper and salt. Process once again until thoroughly mixed.
7. To serve, slice the frittata in 8 equal wedges and serve with a dollop of pesto.

NUTRITION:
Calories: 280; Protein: 14g; Carbs: 8g; Fat: 21.3g

350.   Mushroom Tomato Frittata
Servings: 8 | Cooking Time: 8 minutes

¼ cup mushroom, sliced	10 eggs
1 cup cherry tomatoes	Salt
Pepper	1 teaspoon olive oil

1. Whisk the eggs in a bowl.
2. Add the eggs in a skillet.
3. Add the mushroom, cherry tomatoes and season using salt and pepper.
4. Cover with lid and cook for about 5 to 8 minutes on low heat.

NUTRITION:
Calories: 190; Protein: 11.7g; Carbs: 2.9g; Fat: 12.3g

351. Mushroom, Spinach and Turmeric Frittata
Servings: 6 | Cooking Time: 35 minutes

½ tsp pepper	½ tsp salt
1 tsp turmeric	5-oz firm tofu
4 large eggs	6 large egg whites
¼ cup water	1 lb fresh spinach
6 cloves freshly chopped garlic	1 large onion, chopped
1 lb button mushrooms, sliced	

1. Grease a 10-inch nonstick and oven proof skillet and preheat oven to 350oF.
2. Place skillet on medium high fire and add mushrooms. Cook until golden brown.
3. Add onions, cook for 3 minutes or until onions are tender.
4. Add garlic, sauté for 30 seconds.
5. Add water and spinach, cook while covered until spinach is wilted, around 2 minutes.
6. Remove lid and continue cooking until water is fully evaporated.
7. In a blender, puree pepper, salt, turmeric, tofu, eggs and egg whites until smooth. Pour into skillet once liquid is fully evaporated.
8. Pop skillet into oven and bake until the center is set around 25-30 minutes.
9. Remove skillet from oven and let it stand for ten minutes before inverting and transferring to a serving plate.
10. Cut into 6 equal wedges, serve and enjoy.

NUTRITION:
Calories: 166; Protein: 15.9g; Carbs: 12.2g; Fat: 6.0g

352.   Paleo Almond Banana Pancakes
Servings: 3 | Cooking Time: 10 minutes

¼ cup almond flour	½ teaspoon ground cinnamon
3 eggs	1 banana, mashed
1 tablespoon almond butter	1 teaspoon vanilla extract
1 teaspoon olive oil	Sliced banana to serve

1. Whisk the eggs in a mixing bowl until they become fluffy.
2. In another bowl mash the banana using a fork and add to the egg mixture.
3. Add the vanilla, almond butter, cinnamon and almond flour.
4. Mix into a smooth batter.
5. Heat the olive oil in a skillet.
6. Add one spoonful of the batter and fry them from both sides.
7. Keep doing these steps until you are done with all the batter.
8. Add some sliced banana on top before serving.

NUTRITION:
Calories: 306; Protein: 14.4g; Carbs: 3.6g; Fat: 26.0g

353.   Parmesan and Poached Eggs on Asparagus
Servings: 4 | Cooking Time: 15 minutes

INGREDIENTS

4 tbsp coarsely grated fresh Parmesan cheese, divided	Freshly ground black pepper, to taste
2 tsps finely chopped fresh parsley	2 tbsp fresh lemon juice
1 tbsp unsalted butter	1 garlic clove, chopped
1 tbsp extra virgin olive oil	2 bunches asparagus spears, trimmed around 40
1 tsp salt, divided	1 tsp white vinegar
8 large eggs	

1. Break eggs and place in one paper cup per egg. On medium high fire, place a low sided pan filled 3/4 with water. Add ½ tsp salt and vinegar into water. Set aside.
2. On medium high fire bring another pot of water to boil. Once boiling, lower fire to a simmer and blanch asparagus until tender and crisp, around 3-4 minutes. With tongs transfer asparagus to a serving platter and set aside.
3. On medium fire, place a medium saucepan and heat olive oil. Once hot, for a minute sauté garlic and turn off fire. Add butter right away and swirl around pan to melt. Add remaining pepper, salt, parsley and lemon juice and mix thoroughly. Add asparagus and toss to combine well with garlic butter sauce. Transfer to serving platter along with sauce.
4. In boiling pan of water, poach the eggs by pouring eggs into the water slowly and cook for two minutes per egg. With a slotted spoon, remove egg, to remove excess water, tap slotted spoon several times on kitchen towel and place on top of asparagus.
5. To serve, top eggs with parmesan cheese and divide the asparagus into two and 2 eggs per plate. Serve and enjoy.

NUTRITION:
Calories: 256; Protein: 18g; Carbs: 8g; Fat: 16.9g

354.   Scrambled Eggs with Feta 'n Mushrooms
Servings: 1 | Cooking Time: 6 minutes

Pepper to taste	2 tbsp feta cheese
1 whole egg	2 egg whites
1 cup fresh spinach, chopped	½ cup fresh mushrooms, sliced
Cooking spray	

1. On medium high fire, place a nonstick fry pan and grease with cooking spray.
2. Once hot, add spinach and mushrooms.
3. Sauté until spinach is wilted, around 2-3 minutes.
4. Meanwhile, in a bowl whisk well egg, egg whites, and cheese. Season with pepper.
5. Pour egg mixture into pan and scramble until eggs are cooked through, around 3-4 minutes.
6. Serve and enjoy with a piece of toast or brown rice.

NUTRITION:
Calories: 211; Protein: 18.6g; Carbs: 7.4g; Fat: 11.9g

355.   Scrambled eggs with Smoked Salmon
Servings: 1 | Cooking Time: 8 minutes

1 tbsp coconut oil	Pepper and salt to taste
1/8 tsp red pepper flakes	1/8 tsp garlic powder
1 tbsp fresh dill, chopped finely	4 oz smoked salmon, torn apart
2 whole eggs + 1 egg yolk, whisked	

1. In a big bowl whisk the eggs. Mix in pepper, salt, red pepper flakes, garlic, dill and salmon.
2. On low fire, place a nonstick fry pan and lightly grease with oil.
3. Pour egg mixture and whisk around until cooked through to make scrambled eggs, around 8 minutes on medium fire.
4. Serve and enjoy.

NUTRITION:
Calories: 366; Protein: 32.0; Carbs: 1.0g; Fat: 26.0g

356. Spiced Breakfast Casserole

Servings: 6 | Cooking Time: 35 minutes

1 tablespoon nutrition al yeast	¼ cup water
6 large eggs	1 teaspoon coriander
1 teaspoon cumin	8 kale leaves, stems removed and torn into small pieces
2 sausages, cooked and chopped	1 large sweet potato, peeled and chopped

1. Preheat the oven to 375oF.
2. Grease an 8" x 8" baking pan with olive oil and set aside.
3. Place sweet potatoes in a microwavable bowl and add ¼ cup water. Cook the chopped sweet potatoes in the microwave for three to five minutes. Drain the excess water then set aside.
4. Fry in a skillet heated over medium flame the sausage and cook until brown. Mix in the kale and cook until wilted.
5. Add the coriander, cumin and cooked sweet potatoes.
6. In another bowl, mix together the eggs, water and nutritional yeast. Add the vegetable and meat mixture into the bowl and mix completely.
7. Place the mixture in the baking dish and make sure that the mixture is evenly distributed within the pan.
8. Bake for 20 minutes or until the eggs are done.
9. Slice into squares.

NUTRITION:
Calories: 137; Protein: 10.1g; Carbs: 10.0g; Fat: 6.6g

357. Spinach, Mushroom and Sausage Frittata

Servings: 4 | Cooking Time: 30 minutes

Salt and pepper to taste	10 eggs
½ small onion, chopped	1 mushroom, sliced
1 cup fresh spinach, chopped	½ pound sausage, ground
2 tablespoon coconut oil	

1. Preheat the oven to 3500F.
2. Heat a skillet over medium high flame and add the coconut oil.
3. Sauté the onions until softened. Add in the sausage and cook for two minutes
4. Add in the spinach and mushroom. Stir constantly until the spinach has wilted.
5. Turn off the stove and distribute the vegetable mixture evenly.
6. Pour in the beaten eggs and transfer to the oven.
7. Cook for twenty minutes or until the eggs are completely cooked through.

NUTRITION:
Calories: 383; Protein: 24.9g; Carbs: 8.6g; Fat: 27.6g

358. Tomato-Bacon Quiche

Servings: 6 | Cooking Time: 47 minutes

Topping INGREDIENTS	2 small medium sized tomatoes, sliced
Quiche INGREDIENTS	¼ tsp black pepper
¼ tsp salt	¼ tsp ground mustard
½ cup fresh spinach, chopped	2/4 cups cauliflower, ground into rice
5 slices nitrate free bacon, cooked and chopped	3 tbsp unsweetened plain almond milk
½ cup organic white eggs	5 eggs, beaten
Zucchini Hash Crust:	1/8 tsp sea salt
1 tbsp butter	1 tsp flax meal

1 ½ tbsp coconut flour	1 egg, beaten
2 small to medium sized organic zucchini, grated	

1. Grease a pie dish and preheat oven to 400oF.
2. Grate zucchini, drain and squeeze dry.
3. In a bowl, add dry zucchini and remaining crust ingredients and mix well.
4. Place in bottom of pie plate and press down as if making a pie crust. Pop in the oven and bake for 9 minutes.
5. Meanwhile in a large mixing bowl, whisk well black pepper, salt, mustard, almond milk, egg whites, and egg.
6. Add bacon, spinach, and cauliflower rice. Mix well. Pour into baked zucchini crust, top with tomato slices.
7. Pop back in the oven and bake for 28 minutes. If at 20 minutes baking time top is browning too much, cover with parchment paper for remainder of cooking time.
8. Once done cooking, remove from oven, let it stand for at least ten minutes.
9. Slice into equal triangles, serve and enjoy.

NUTRITION:
Calories: 154; Protein: 11.6g; Carbs: 3.4g; Fat: 10.3g

359. Your Standard Quiche

Servings: 6 | Cooking Time: 45 minutes

4 oz sliced Portobello mushrooms	pepper and salt to taste
½ tbsp dried basil	½ tbsp dried parsley
6 eggs, whisked	¾ lb pork breakfast sausage

1. Grease a 9-inch round pie plate or baking pan and preheat oven to 350oF.
2. On medium fire, place a nonstick fry pan and cook sausage. Stir fry until cooked as you break them into pieces. Discard excess oil once cooked.
3. In a big bowl, whisk pepper, salt, basil, parsley and eggs. Pour into prepped baking plate.
4. Pop into the oven and bake until middle is firm around 30-35 minutes.
5. Once done, remove from oven; let it stand for 10 minutes before slicing and serving.

NUTRITION:
Calories: 283; Protein: 15.0g; Carbs: 3.2g; Fat: 23.3g

360. Zucchini Tomato Frittata

Servings: 8 | Cooking Time: 30 minutes

3 lbs tomatoes, thinly sliced crosswise	¾ cup cheddar cheese, shredded
¼ cup milk	8 large eggs
1 tbsp fresh thyme leaves	3 zucchinis, cut into ¼-inch thick rounds
1 onion, finely chopped	1 tbsp olive oil
Salt and pepper to taste	

1. Preheat the oven to 425 degrees Fahrenheit.
2. Prepare a non-stick skillet and heat it over medium heat.
3. Sauté the zucchini, onion and thyme. Cook and stir often for 8 to 10 minutes. Let the liquid in the pan evaporate and season with salt and pepper to taste. Remove the skillet from heat.
4. In a bowl, whisk the milk, cheese, eggs, salt and pepper together. Pour the egg mixture over the zucchini in the skillet. Lift the zucchini to allow the eggs to coat the pan. Arrange the tomato slices on top.
5. Return to the skillet and heat to medium low fire and cook until the sides are set or golden brown, around 7 minutes.
6. Place the skillet inside the oven and cook for 10 to 15 minutes or until the center of the frittata is cooked through. To check if the egg is cooked through, insert a wooden skewer in the middle and it should come out clean.
7. Remove from the oven and loosen the frittata from the skillet. Serve warm.

NUTRITION:
Calories: 175; Protein: 12.0g; Carbs: 13.6g; Fat: 8.1g

VEGETARIAN RECIPES

361. Creamy Carrot Chowder
Servings: 8 | Cooking Time: 40 minutes

8 fresh mint sprigs
1 tsp fresh ginger, peeled and grated
1 lb. baby carrots, peeled and cut into 2-inch lengths
2 tsp sesame oil

½ cup 2% Greek Style Plain yogurt
2 cups chicken broth
1/3 cup sliced shallots

1. On medium fire, place a medium heavy bottom pot and heat oil.
2. Sauté shallots until tender around 2 minutes.
3. Add carrots and sauté for another 4 minutes.
4. Pour broth, cover and bring to a boil. Once soup is boiling, slow fire to a simmer and cook carrots until tender around 22 minutes.
5. Add ginger and continue cooking while covered for another eight minutes.
6. Turn off fire and let it cool for 10 minutes.
7. Pour mixture into blender and puree. If needed, puree carrots in batches then return to pot.
8. Heat pureed carrots until heated through around 2 minutes.
9. Turn off fire and evenly pour into 8 serving bowls.
10. Serve and enjoy. Or you can store in the freezer in 8 different lidded containers for a quick soup in the middle of the week.

NUTRITION:
Calories: 47; Carbs: 6.5g; Protein: 2.2g; Fat: 1.6g

362. Creamy Corn Soup
Servings: 4 | Cooking Time: 20 minutes

4 slices crisp cooked bacon, crumbled
1/4 cup water
4 cups chicken broth
2 egg whites
1 tbsp sherry

2 tbsp cornstarch
2 tsp soy sauce
1 (14.75 oz) can cream-style corn
1/4 tsp salt
1/2 lb. skinless, boneless chicken breast meat, finely chopped

1. Combine chicken with the sherry, egg whites, salt in a bowl. Stir in the cream style corn. Mix well.
2. Boil the soy sauce and chicken broth in a wok. Then stir in the chicken mixture, while continue boiling. Then simmer for about 3 minutes, stir frequently to avoid burning.
3. Mix corn starch and water until well combined. Mix to the simmering broth, while constantly stirring until it slightly thickens. Cook for about 2 minutes more.
4. Serve topped with the crumbled bacon.

NUTRITION:
Calories: 305; Carbs: 28.0g; Protein: 21.1g; Fat: 13.0g

363. Creamy Kale and Mushrooms
Servings: 3 | Cooking Time: 15 minutes

3 tablespoons coconut oil
1 onion, chopped
5 white button mushrooms, chopped
Salt and pepper to taste

3 cloves of garlic, minced
1 bunch kale, stems removed and leaves chopped
1 cup coconut milk

1. Heat oil in a pot.
2. Sauté the garlic and onion until fragrant for 2 minutes.
3. Stir in mushrooms. Season with pepper and salt. Cook for 8 minutes.
4. Stir in kale and coconut milk. Simmer for 5 minutes.
5. Adjust seasoning to taste.

NUTRITION:
Calories: 365; Carbs: 17.9g; Protein: 6g; Fat: 33.5g

364. Crunchy Kale Chips
Servings: 8 | Cooking Time: 2 hours

2 tbsp filtered water
1 tbsp raw honey
1 lemon, juiced
1 cup fresh cashews, soaked 2 hours

½ tsp sea salt
2 tbsp nutrition al yeast
1 cup sweet potato, grated
2 bunches green curly kale, washed, ribs and stems removed, leaves torn into bite sized pieces

1. Prepare a baking sheet by covering with an unbleached parchment paper. Preheat oven to 150oF.
2. In a large mixing bowl, place kale.
3. In a food processor, process remaining ingredients until smooth. Pour over kale.
4. With your hands, coat kale with marinade.
5. Evenly spread kale onto parchment paper and pop in the oven. Dehydrate for 2 hours and turn leaves after the first hour of baking.
6. Remove from oven; let it cool completely before serving.

NUTRITION:
Calories: 209; Carbs: 13.0g; Protein: 7.0g; Fat: 15.9g

365. Delicious and Healthy Roasted Eggplant
Servings: 6 | Cooking Time: 30 minutes

Pinch of sugar
¼ tsp cayenne pepper or to taste
2 tbsp fresh basil, chopped
½ cup red onion, finely chopped
¼ cup extra virgin olive oil
1 medium eggplant, around 1 lb.

¼ tsp salt
1 tbsp parsley, flat leaf and chopped finely
1 small chili pepper, seeded and minced, optional
½ cup Greek feta cheese, crumbled
2 tbsp lemon juice

1. Preheat broiler and position rack 6 inches away from heat source.
2. Pierce the eggplant with a knife or fork. Then with a foil, line a baking pan and place the eggplant and broil. Make sure to turn eggplant every five minutes or until the skin is charred and eggplant is soft which takes around 14 to 18 minutes of broiling. Once done, remove from heat and let cool.
3. In a medium bowl, add lemon. Then cut eggplant in half, lengthwise, and scrape the flesh and place in the bowl with lemon. Add oil and mix until well combined. Then add salt, cayenne, parsley, basil, chili pepper, bell pepper, onion and feta. Toss until well combined and add sugar to taste if wanted.

NUTRITION:
Calories: 97; Carbs: 7.4g; Protein: 2.9g; Fat: 6.7g

366. Delicious Stuffed Squash
Servings: 4 servings | Cooking Time: 30minutes

¼ cup sour cream
3 tbsp taco sauce
½ small green bell pepper, seeded and chopped
1 tsp cumin
¼ tsp cayenne
1 can 15-oz black beans, drained and rinsed
1 tbsp olive oil

½ cup shredded cheddar
1 small tomato, chopped
½ medium onion, chopped
1 tsp onion powder
1 ½ tsp chili powder
1 clove garlic, minced
2 medium zucchinis

2 medium yellow squash	Salt and pepper

1. Boil until tender in a large pot of water zucchini and yellow squash, then drain. Lengthwise, slice the squash and trim the ends. Take out the center flesh and chop.
2. On medium high fire, place skillet with oil and sauté garlic until fragrant. Add onion and tomato and sauté for 8 minutes. Add chopped squash, bell pepper, cumin, onion powder, cayenne, chilli powder and black beans and continue cooking until veggies are tender.
3. Season with pepper and salt to taste. Remove from fire.
4. Spread 1 tsp of taco sauce on each squash shell, fill with half of the cooked filling, top with cheese and garnish with sour cream. Repeat procedure on other half of squash shell. Serve and enjoy.

NUTRITION:
Calories: 318; Carbs: 28.0g; Protein: 21.0g; Fat: 16.0g

367. Easy and Healthy Baked Vegetables

Servings: 6 | Cooking Time: 1 hour and 15 minutes

2 lbs. Brussels sprouts, trimmed	3 lbs. Butternut Squash, peeled, seeded and cut into same size as sprouts
1 lb Pork breakfast sausage	1 tbsp fat from fried sausage

1. Grease a 9x13 inch baking pan and preheat oven to 350oF.
2. On medium high fire, place a large nonstick saucepan and cook sausage. Break up sausages and cook until browned.
3. In a greased pan mix browned sausage, squash, sprouts, sea salt and fat. Toss to mix well. Pop into the oven and cook for an hour.
4. Remove from oven and serve warm.

NUTRITION:
Calories: 364; Carbs: 41.2g; Protein: 19.0g; Fat: 16.5g

368. Eggplant Bolognese With Zucchini Noodles

Servings: 4 | Cooking Time: 20 minutes

6 leaves of fresh basil, chopped	1 28-ounce can plum tomatoes
½ cup red wine	1 tablespoon tomato paste
4 sprigs of thyme, chopped	2 bay leaves
3 cloves garlic, minced	1 large yellow onion, chopped
Salt and pepper to taste	2 tablespoon extra-virgin olive oil
½ pound ground beef	1 ½ pounds eggplant, diced
2 cups zucchini noodles	

1. Heat the skillet over medium high heat and add oil. Sauté the onion and beef and sprinkle with salt and pepper. Sauté for 10 minutes until the meat is brown. Add in the eggplants, bay leaves, garlic and thyme. Cook for another 15 minutes.
2. Once the eggplant is tender, add the tomato paste and wine. Add the tomatoes and crush using a spoon. Bring to a boil and reduce the heat to low. Simmer for 10 minutes.
3. In a skillet, add oil and sauté the zucchini noodles for five minutes. Turn off the heat.
4. Pour the tomato sauce over the zucchini noodles and garnish with fresh basil.

NUTRITION:
Calories: 320; Carbs: 24.8g; Protein: 19.2g; Fat: 17.0g

369. Feta and Roasted Eggplant Dip

Servings: 12 | Cooking Time: 20 minutes

¼ tsp salt	¼ tsp cayenne pepper
1 tbsp finely chopped flat leaf parsley	2 tbsp chopped fresh basil
1 small Chile pepper	1 small red bell pepper, finely chopped
½ cup finely chopped red onion	½ cup crumbled Greek nonfat feta

	cheese
¼ cup extra-virgin olive oil	2 tbsp lemon juice
1 medium eggplant, around 1 lb.	

1. Preheat broiler, position rack on topmost part of oven, and line a baking pan with foil.
2. With a fork or knife, poke eggplant, place on prepared baking pan, and broil for 5 minutes per side until skin is charred all around.
3. Once eggplant skin is charred, remove from broiler and allow to cool to handle.
4. Once eggplant is cool enough to handle, slice in half lengthwise, scoop out flesh, and place in a medium bowl.
5. Pour in lemon juice and toss eggplant to coat with lemon juice and prevent it from discoloring.
6. Add oil; continue mixing until oil is absorbed by eggplant.
7. Stir in salt, cayenne pepper, parsley, basil, Chile pepper, bell pepper, onion, and feta.
8. Toss to mix well and serve.

NUTRITION: Calories: 58; Carbs: 3.7g; Protein: 1.2g; Fat: 4.6g

370. Garlic 'n Sour Cream Zucchini Bake

Servings: 3 | Cooking Time: 20 minutes

1/4 cup grated Parmesan cheese	paprika to taste
1 tablespoon minced garlic	1 large zucchini, cut lengthwise then in half
1 cup sour cream	1 (8 ounce) package cream cheese, softened

1. Lightly grease a casserole dish with cooking spray.
2. Place zucchini slices in a single layer in dish.
3. In a bowl whisk well, remaining ingredients except for paprika. Spread on top of zucchini slices. Sprinkle paprika.
4. Cover dish with foil.
5. For 10 minutes, cook in preheated 390oF oven.
6. Remove foil and cook for 10 minutes.
7. Serve and enjoy.

NUTRITION:
Calories: 385; Carbs: 13.5g; Protein: 11.9g; Fat: 32.4g

371. Garlicky Rosemary Potatoes

Servings: 4 | Cooking Time: 2 minutes

1-pound potatoes, peeled and sliced thinly	2 garlic cloves
½ teaspoon salt	1 tablespoon olive oil
2 sprigs of rosemary	

1. Place a trivet or steamer basket in the Instant Pot and pour in a cup of water.
2. In a baking dish that can fit inside the Instant Pot, combine all ingredients and toss to coat everything.
3. Cover the baking dish with aluminum foil and place on the steamer basket.
4. Close the lid and press the Steam button.
5. Adjust the cooking time to 30 minutes
6. Do quick pressure release.
7. Once cooled, evenly divide into serving size, keep in your preferred container, and refrigerate until ready to eat.

NUTRITION:
Calories: 119; Carbs: 20.31g; Protein: 2.39g; Fat: 3.48g

372. Ginger and Spice Carrot Soup

Servings: 6 | Cooking Time: 40 minutes

¼ cup Greek yogurt	2 tsp fresh lime juice
5 cups low-salt chicken broth	1 ½ tsp finely grated lime peel
4 cups of carrots, peeled, thinly sliced into rounds	2 cups chopped onions

1 tbsp minced and peeled fresh ginger

½ tsp curry powder

3 tbsp expeller-pressed sunflower oil

½ tsp yellow mustard seeds

1 tsp coriander seeds

1. In a food processor, grind mustard seeds and coriander into a powder.
2. On medium high fire, place a large pot and heat oil.
3. Add curry powder and powdered seeds and sauté for a minute.
4. Add ginger, cook for a minute.
5. Add lime peel, carrots and onions. Sauté for 3 minutes or until onions are softened.
6. Season with pepper and salt.
7. Add broth and bring to a boil. Reduce fire to a simmer and simmer uncovered for 30 minutes or until carrots are tender.
8. Cool broth slightly, and puree in batches. Return pureed carrots into pot.
9. Add lime juice, add more pepper and salt to taste.
10. Transfer to a serving bowl, drizzle with yogurt and serve.

NUTRITION:
Calories: 129; Carbs: 13.6g; Protein: 2.8g; Fat: 7.7g

373. Ginger-Egg Drop Soup with Zoodle
Servings: 4 | Cooking Time: 15 minutes

½ teaspoons red pepper flakes

2 cups thinly sliced scallions, divided

2 cups, plus 1 tablespoon water, divided

2 tablespoons extra virgin olive oil

2 tablespoons minced ginger

3 tablespoons corn starch

4 large eggs, beaten

4 medium to large zucchini, spiralized into noodles

5 cups shiitake mushrooms, sliced

5 tablespoons low-sodium tamari sauce or soy sauce

8 cups vegetable broth, divided

Salt & pepper to taste

1. On medium-high the fire, place a large pot and add oil.
2. Once oil is hot, stir in ginger and sauté for two minutes.
3. Stir in a tablespoon of water and shiitake mushrooms. Cook for 5 minutes or until mushrooms start to give off liquid.
4. Stir in 1 ½ cups scallions, tamari sauce, red pepper flakes, remaining water, and 7 cups of the vegetable broth. Mix well and bring to a boil.
5. Meanwhile, in a small bowl whisk well cornstarch and remaining cup of vegetable broth and set aside.
6. Once pot is boiling, slowly pour in eggs while stirring pot continuously. Mix well.
7. Add the cornstarch slurry in pot and mix well. Continue mixing every now and then until thickened, about 5 minutes.
8. Taste and adjust seasoning with pepper and salt.
9. Stir in zoodles and cook until heated through, about 2 minutes.
10. Serve with a sprinkle of remaining scallions and enjoy.

NUTRITION:
Calories: 238; Protein: 10.6g; Carbs: 34.3g; Sugar: 12.8g; Fat: 8.6g

374. Ginger Vegetable Stir Fry
Servings: 4 | Cooking Time: 5 minutes

1 tablespoon oil

3 cloves of garlic, minced

1 onion, chopped

1 thumb-size ginger, sliced

1 tablespoon water

1 large carrots, peeled and julienned

1 large green bell pepper, seeded and julienned

1 large yellow bell pepper, seeded and julienned

1 large red bell pepper, seeded and julienned

1 zucchini, julienned

Salt and pepper to taste

1. Heat oil in a skillet over medium flame and sauté the garlic, onion, and ginger until fragrant.
2. Stir in the rest of the ingredients and adjust the flame to high.
3. Keep on stirring for at least 5 minutes until vegetables are half-cooked.
4. Place in individual containers.
5. Put a label and store in the fridge.

6. Allow to thaw at room temperature before heating in the microwave oven.

NUTRITION:
Calories: 102; Carbs: 13.6g; Protein:0 g; Fat: 2g; Fiber: 7.6g

375. Gobi Masala Soup
Servings: 4 | Cooking Time: 35 minutes

1 tsp salt

1 tsp ground turmeric

1 tsp ground coriander

2 tsp cumin seeds

3 tsp dark mustard seeds

1 cup water

3 cups beef broth

1 head cauliflower, chopped

3 carrots, chopped

1 large onion, chopped

2 tbsp coconut oil

Chopped cilantro for topping

Crushed red pepper to taste

Black pepper to taste

1 tbsp lemon juice

1. On medium high fire, place a large heavy bottomed pot and heat coconut oil.
2. Once hot, sauté garlic cloves for a minute. Add carrots and continue sautéing for 4 minutes more.
3. Add turmeric, coriander, cumin, mustard seeds, and cauliflower. Sauté for 5 minutes.
4. Add water and beef broth and simmer for 10 to 15 minutes.
5. Turn off fire and transfer to blender. Puree until smoot and creamy.
6. Return to pot, continue simmering for another ten minutes.
7. Season with crushed red pepper, lemon juice, pepper, and salt.
8. To serve, garnish with cilantro, and enjoy.

NUTRITION:
Calories: 148; Carbs: 16.1g; Protein: 3.7g; Fat: 8.8g

376. Greek Styled Veggie-Rice
Servings: 6 | Cooking Time: 20 minutes

pepper and salt to taste

¼ cup extra virgin olive oil

3 tbsp chopped fresh mint

½ cup grape tomatoes, halved

½ red bell pepper, diced small

1 head cauliflower, cut into large florets

¼ cup fresh lemon juice

½ yellow onion, minced

1. In a bowl mix lemon juice and onion and leave for 30 minutes. Then drain onion and reserve the juice and onion bits.
2. In a blender, shred cauliflower until the size of a grain of rice.
3. On medium fire, place a medium nonstick skillet and for 8-10 minutes cook cauliflower while covered.
4. Add grape tomatoes and bell pepper and cook for 3 minutes while stirring occasionally.
5. Add mint and onion bits. Cook for another three minutes.
6. Meanwhile, in a small bowl whisk pepper, salt, 3 tbsp reserved lemon juice and olive oil until well blended.
7. Remove cooked cauliflower, transfer to a serving bowl, pour lemon juice mixture and toss to mix.
8. Before serving, if needed season with pepper and salt to taste.

NUTRITION:
Calories: 120; Carbs: 8.0g; Protein: 2.3g; Fat: 9.5g

377. Green Vegan Soup
Servings: 6 | Cooking Time: 20 minutes

1 medium head cauliflower, cut into bite-sized florets

1 medium white onion, peeled and diced

2 cloves garlic, peeled and diced

1 bay leaf crumbled

5-oz watercress

fresh spinach or frozen spinach

1-liter vegetable stock or bone broth

1 cup cream or coconut milk + 6 tbsp for garnish

1/4 cup ghee or coconut oil

1 tsp salt or to taste

freshly ground black pepper

Optional: fresh herbs such as parsley or chives for garnish

1. On medium-high the fire, place a Dutch oven greased with ghee. Once hot, sauté garlic for a minute. Add onions and sauté until soft and translucent, about 5 minutes.
2. Add cauliflower florets and crumbled bay leaf. Mix well and cook for 5 minutes.
3. Stir in watercress and spinach. Sauté for 3 minutes.
4. Add vegetable stock and bring to a boil.
5. When cauliflower is crisp-tender, stir in coconut milk.
6. Season with pepper and salt.
7. With a hand blender, puree soup until smooth and creamy.
8. Serve and enjoy.

NUTRITION:
Calories: 392; Protein: 4.9g; Carbs: 9.7g; Sugar: 6.8g; Fat: 37.6g

378. Grilled Eggplant Caprese
Servings: 4 | Cooking Time: 10 minutes

- 1 eggplant aubergine, small/medium
- 1 tomato large
- 2 basil leaves or a little more as needed
- 4-oz mozzarella
- good quality olive oil
- Pepper and salt to taste

1. Cut the ends of the eggplant and then cut it lengthwise into ¼-inch thick slices. Discard the smaller pieces that's mostly skin and short.
2. Slice the tomatoes and mozzarella into thin slices just like the eggplant.
3. On medium-high the fire, place a griddle and let it heat up.
4. Brush eggplant slices with olive oil and place on grill. Grill for 3 minutes. Turnover and grill for a minute. Add a slice of cheese on one side and tomato on the other side. Continue cooking for another 2 minutes.
5. Sprinkle with basil leaves. Season with pepper and salt.
6. Fold eggplant in half and skewer with a cocktail stick.
7. Serve and enjoy.

NUTRITION:
Calories: 59; Protein: 3.0g; Carbs: 4.0g; Sugar: 2.0g; Fat: 3.0g

379. Grilled Zucchini Bread and Cheese Sandwich
Servings: 2 | Cooking Time: 40 minutes

1 large egg	1/2 cup freshly grated Parmesan
1/4 cup almond flour	2 cup grated zucchini
2 cup shredded Cheddar	2 green onions thinly sliced
Freshly ground black pepper	kosher salt
Vegetable oil, for cooking	

1. With a paper towel, squeeze dry the zucchinis and place in a bowl. Add almond flour, green onions, Parmesan, and egg. Season with pepper and salt. Whisk well to combine.
2. Place a large nonstick pan on medium the fire and add oil to cover pan. Once hot, add ¼ cup of zucchini mixture and shape into a square like a bread. Add another batch as many as you can put in the pan. If needed, cook in batches. Cook for four minutes per side and place on a paper towel lined plate.
3. Once done cooking zucchinis, wipe off oil from the pan. Place one zucchini piece on the pan, spread ½ of shredded cheese, and then top with another piece of zucchini. Grill for two minutes per side. Repeat process to make 2 sandwiches.
4. Serve and enjoy.

NUTRITION:
Calories: 667; Protein: 41.5g; Carbs: 14.4g; Fat: 49.9g

380. Hoemade Egg Drop Soup
Servings: 4 | Cooking Time: 15 minutes

1 tbsp cornstarch	1 tbsp dried minced onion
1 tsp dried parsley	2 eggs

4 cubes chicken bouillon	4 cups water
1 cup chopped carrots	½ cup thinly shredded cabbage

1. Combine water, bouillon, parsley, cabbage, carrots, and onion flakes in a saucepan, and then bring to a boil.
2. Beat the eggs lightly and stir into the soup.
3. Dissolve cornstarch with a little water. Stir until smooth and stir into the soup. Let it boil until the soup thickens.

NUTRITION:
Calories: 98; Carbs: 6.9g; Protein: 5.1g; Fat: 5.3g

381. Hot and Sour Soup
Servings: 4 | Cooking Time: 25 minutes

½ tsp sesame oil	1 cup fresh bean sprouts
1 egg, lightly beaten	1 tsp black pepper
1 tsp ground ginger	3 tbsp white vinegar
3 tbsp soy sauce	¼ lb. sliced mushrooms
½ lb. tofu, cubed	2 tbsp corn starch
3 ½ cups chicken broth	

1. Mix corn starch and ¼ cup chicken broth and put aside.
2. Over high heat place a pot then combine and boil: pepper, ginger, vinegar, soy sauce, mushrooms, tofu and chicken broth.
3. Once boiling, add the corn starch mixture. Stir constantly and reduce fire. Once concoction is thickened, drop the slightly beaten egg while stirring vigorously.
4. Add bean sprouts and for one to two minutes allow simmering.
5. Remove from fire and transfer to serving bowls and enjoy while hot.

NUTRITION:
Calories: 141; Carbs: 12.9g; Protein: 10.0g; Fat: 6.6g

382. Indian Bell Peppers and Potato Stir Fry
Servings: 2 | Cooking Time: 15 minutes

1 tablespoon oil	½ teaspoon cumin seeds
4 cloves of garlic, minced	4 potatoes, scrubbed and halved
Salt and pepper to taste	5 tablespoons water
2 bell peppers, seeded and julienned	Chopped cilantro for garnish

1. Heat oil in a skillet over medium flame and toast the cumin seeds until fragrant.
2. Add the garlic until fragrant.
3. Stir in the potatoes, salt, pepper, water, and bell peppers.
4. Close the lid and allow to simmer for at least 10 minutes.
5. Garnish with cilantro before cooking time ends.
6. Place in individual containers.
7. Put a label and store in the fridge.
8. Allow to thaw at room temperature before heating in the microwave oven.

NUTRITION:
Calories: 83; Carbs: 7.3g; Protein: 2.8g; Fat: 6.4g; Fiber:1.7

383. Indian Style Okra
Servings: 4 | Cooking Time: 12 minutes

1 lb. small to medium okra pods, trimmed	¼ tsp curry powder
½ tsp kosher salt	1 tsp finely chopped serrano chili
1 tsp ground coriander	1 tbsp canola oil
¾ tsp brown mustard seeds	

1. On medium high fire, place a large and heavy skillet and cook mustard seeds until fragrant, around 30 seconds.
2. Add canola oil. Add okra, curry powder, salt, chili, and coriander. Sauté for a minute while stirring every once in a while.
3. Cover and cook low fire for at least 8 minutes. Stir occasionally.
4. Uncover, increase fire to medium high and cook until okra is lightly browned, around 2 minutes more.
5. Serve and enjoy.

NUTRITION:
Calories: 78; Carbs: 6.4g; Protein: 2.1g; Fat: 5.7g

384.   Instant Pot Artichoke Hearts

Servings: 6 | Cooking Time: 30 minutes

4 artichokes, rinsed and trimmed

2 cups bone broth
1 stalk, celery
Salt and pepper to taste

Juice from 2 small lemons, freshly squeezed
1 tablespoon tarragon leaves
½ cup extra virgin olive oil

1. Place all ingredients in a pressure cooker.
2. Give a good stir.
3. Close the lid and seal the valve.
4. Pressure cook for 4 minutes.
5. Allow pressure cooker to release steam naturally.
6. Then serve and enjoy.

NUTRITION:
Calories: 133; Carbs: 14.3g; Protein: 4.4g; Fat: 11.7g

385.   Instant Pot Fried Veggies

Servings: 3 | Cooking Time: 6 minutes

1 tablespoon olive oil
4 cloves of garlic, minced
1 zucchini, julienned
½ cup chopped tomatoes
Salt and pepper to taste

1 onion, chopped
2 carrots, peeled and julienned
1 large potato, peeled and julienned
1 teaspoon rosemary sprig

1. Press the Sauté button and heat the oil.
2. Sauté the onion and garlic until fragrant.
3. Stir in the rest of the ingredients.

4. Close the lid and make sure that the vents are sealed.
5. Press the Manual button and adjust the cooking time to 1 minute.
6. Do a quick pressure release.
7. Once the lid is open, press the Sauté button and continue stirring until the liquid has reduced.
8. Once cooled, evenly divide into serving size, keep in your preferred container, and refrigerate until ready to eat.

NUTRITION:
Calories: 97; Carbs: 10.4g; Protein: 0.5g; Fat: 4.2g

386.   Instant Pot Sautéed Kale

Servings: 6 | Cooking Time: minutes

3 tablespoons coconut oil
1 onion, chopped

4cups kale, chopped
Salt and pepper to taste

2 cloves of garlic, minced
2 teaspoons crushed red pepper flakes
¼ cup water

1. Press the "Sauté" button on the Instant Pot.
2. Heat the oil and sauté the garlic and onions until fragrant.
3. Stir in the rest of the ingredients.
4. Close the lid and make sure that the steam release valve is set to "Sealing."
5. Press the "Manual" button and adjust the cooking time to 4 minutes.
6. Do a quick pressure release.

NUTRITION:
Calories: 82; Carbs: 5.1g; Protein: 1.1g; Fat: 7.9g

387.   Fig Relish Panini

Servings: 4 | Cooking Time: 40 minutes

Grated parmesan cheese, for garnish	Olive oil
Fig relish (recipe follows)	Arugula
Basil leaves	Toma cheese, grated or sliced
Sweet butter	4 ciabatta slices
Fig Relish INGREDIENTS	1 tsp dry mustard
Pinch of salt	1 tsp mustard seed
½ cup apple cider vinegar	½ cup sugar
½ lb. Mission figs, stemmed and peeled	

1. Create fig relish by mincing the figs. Then put in all ingredients, except for the dry mustard, in a small pot and simmer for 30 minutes until it becomes jam like. Season with dry mustard according to taste and let cool before refrigerating.
2. Spread sweet butter on two slices of ciabatta rolls and layer on the following: cheese, basil leaves, arugula and fig relish then cover with the remaining bread slice.
3. Grill in a Panini press until cheese is melted and bread is crisped and ridged.

NUTRITION:
Calories: 264; Carbs: 55.1g; Protein: 6.0g; Fat: 4.2g

388.   Fruity and Cheesy Quesadilla

Servings: 1 | Cooking Time: 15 minutes

¼ cup hand grated jack cheese	½ cup finely chopped fresh mango
1 large whole-grain tortilla	1 tbsp chopped fresh cilantro

1. In a medium bowl, mix cilantro and mango.
2. Place mango mixture inside tortilla and top with cheese.
3. Pop in a preheated 350oF oven and bake until cheese is melted completely around 10 to 15 minutes.

NUTRITION:
Calories: 169; Fat: 9g; Protein: 7g; Carbohydrates: 15g

389.   Garlic & Tomato Gluten Free Focaccia

Servings: 8 | Cooking Time: 20 minutes

1 egg	½ tsp lemon juice
1 tbsp honey	4 tbsp olive oil
A pinch of sugar	1 ¼ cup warm water
1 tbsp active dry yeast	2 tsp rosemary, chopped
2 tsp thyme, chopped	2 tsp basil, chopped
2 cloves garlic, minced	1 ¼ tsp sea salt
2 tsp xanthan gum	½ cup millet flour
1 cup potato starch, not flour	1 cup sorghum flour
Gluten free cornmeal for dusting	

1. For 5 minutes, turn on the oven and then turn it off, while keeping oven door closed.
2. In a small bowl, mix warm water and pinch of sugar. Add yeast and swirl gently. Leave for 7 minutes.
3. In a large mixing bowl, whisk well herbs, garlic, salt, xanthan gum, starch, and flours.
4. Once yeast is done proofing, pour into bowl of flours. Whisk in egg, lemon juice, honey, and olive oil.
5. Mix thoroughly and place in a well-greased square pan, dusted with cornmeal.
6. Top with fresh garlic, more herbs, and sliced tomatoes.
7. Place in the warmed oven and let it rise for half an hour.

8. Turn on oven to 375oF and after preheating time it for 20 minutes. Focaccia is done once tops are lightly browned.
9. Remove from oven and pan immediately and let it cool.
10. Best served when warm.

NUTRITION:
Calories: 251; Carbs: 38.4g; Protein: 5.4g; Fat: 9.0g

390.   Garlic-Rosemary Dinner Rolls

Servings: 8 | Cooking Time: 20 minutes

2 garlic cloves, minced	1 tsp dried crushed rosemary
½ tsp apple cider vinegar	2 tbsp olive oil
2 eggs	1 ¼ tsp salt
1 ¾ tsp xanthan gum	½ cup tapioca starch
¾ cup brown rice flour	1 cup sorghum flour
2 tsp dry active yeast	1 tbsp honey
¾ cup hot water	

1. Mix well water and honey in a small bowl and add yeast. Leave it for exactly 7 minutes.
2. In a large bowl, mix the following with a paddle mixer: garlic, rosemary, salt, xanthan gum, sorghum flour, tapioca starch, and brown rice flour.
3. In a medium bowl, whisk well vinegar, olive oil, and eggs.
4. Into bowl of dry ingredients pour in vinegar and yeast mixture and mix well.
5. Grease a 12-muffin tin with cooking spray. Transfer dough evenly into 12 muffin tins and leave it 20 minutes to rise.
6. Then preheat oven to 375oF and bake dinner rolls until tops are golden brown, around 17 to 19 minutes.
7. Remove dinner rolls from oven and muffin tins immediately and let it cool.
8. Best served when warm.

NUTRITION:
Calories: 200; Carbs: 34.3g; Protein: 4.2g; Fat: 5.4g

391. Grilled Burgers with Mushrooms

Servings: 4 | Cooking Time: 10 minutes

2 Bibb lettuce, halved	4 slices red onion
4 slices tomato	4 whole wheat buns, toasted
2 tbsp olive oil	¼ tsp cayenne pepper, optional
1 garlic clove, minced	1 tbsp sugar
½ cup water	1/3 cup balsamic vinegar
4 large Portobello mushroom caps, around 5-inches in diameter	

1. Remove stems from mushrooms and clean with a damp cloth. Transfer into a baking dish with gill-side up.
2. In a bowl, mix thoroughly olive oil, cayenne pepper, garlic, sugar, water and vinegar. Pour over mushrooms and marinate mushrooms in the ref for at least an hour.
3. Once the one hour is nearly up, preheat grill to medium high fire and grease grill grate.
4. Grill mushrooms for five minutes per side or until tender. Baste mushrooms with marinade so it doesn't dry up.
5. To assemble, place ½ of bread bun on a plate, top with a slice of onion, mushroom, tomato and one lettuce leaf. Cover with the other top half of the bun. Repeat process with remaining ingredients, serve and enjoy.

NUTRITION:
Calories: 244.1; Carbs: 32g; Protein: 8.1g; Fat: 9.3g

393.   Grilled Sandwich with Goat Cheese
Servings: 4 | Cooking Time: 8 minutes

½ cup soft goat cheese	4 Kaiser rolls 2-oz
¼ tsp freshly ground black pepper	¼ tsp salt
1/3 cup chopped basil	Cooking spray
4 big Portobello mushroom caps	1 yellow bell pepper, cut in half and seeded
1 red bell pepper, cut in half and seeded	1 garlic clove, minced
1 tbsp olive oil	¼ cup balsamic vinegar

1. In a large bowl, mix garlic, olive oil and balsamic vinegar. Add mushroom and bell peppers. Gently mix to coat. Remove veggies from vinegar and discard vinegar mixture.
2. Coat with cooking spray a grill rack and the grill preheated to medium high fire.
3. Place mushrooms and bell peppers on the grill and grill for 4 minutes per side. Remove from grill and let cool a bit.
4. Into thin strips, cut the bell peppers.
5. In a small bowl, combine black pepper, salt, basil and sliced bell peppers.
6. Horizontally, cut the Kaiser rolls and evenly spread cheese on the cut side. Arrange 1 Portobello per roll, top with 1/3 bell pepper mixture and cover with the other half of the roll.
7. Grill the rolls as you press down on them to create a Panini like line on the bread. Grill until bread is toasted.

NUTRITION:
Calories: 317; Carbs: 41.7g; Protein: 14.0g; Fat: 10.5g

394.   Halibut Sandwiches Mediterranean Style
Servings: 4 | Cooking Time: 23 minutes

2 packed cups arugula or 2 oz.	Grated zest of 1 large lemon
1 tbsp capers, drained and mashed	2 tbsp fresh flat leaf parsley, chopped
¼ cup fresh basil, chopped	¼ cup sun dried tomatoes, chopped
¼ cup reduced fat mayonnaise	1 garlic clove, halved
1 pc of 14 oz of ciabatta loaf bread with ends trimmed and split in half, horizontally	2 tbsp plus 1 tsp olive oil, divided
Kosher salt and freshly ground pepper	2 pcs or 6 oz halibut fillets, skinned
Cooking spray	

1. Heat oven to 450oF.
2. With cooking spray, coat a baking dish. Season halibut with a pinch of pepper and salt plus rub with a tsp of oil and place on baking dish. Then put in oven and bake until cooked or for ten to fifteen minutes. Remove from oven and let cool.
3. Get a slice of bread and coat with olive oil the sliced portions. Put in oven and cook until golden, around six to eight minutes. Remove from heat and rub garlic on the bread.
4. Combine the following in a medium bowl: lemon zest, capers, parsley, basil, sun dried tomatoes and mayonnaise. Then add the halibut, mashing with fork until flaked. Spread the mixture on one side of bread, add arugula and cover with the other bread half and serve.

NUTRITION:
Calories: 125; Carbs: 8.0g; Protein: 3.9g; Fat: 9.2g

395.   Herbed Panini Fillet O'Fish
Servings: 4 | Cooking Time: 25 minutes

4 slices thick sourdough bread	4 slices mozzarella cheese
1 portabella mushroom, sliced	1 small onion, sliced
6 tbsp oil	4 garlic and herb fish fillets

1. Prepare your fillets by adding salt, pepper and herbs (rosemary, thyme, parsley whatever you like). Then dredged in flour before deep frying in very hot oil. Once nicely browned, remove from oil and set aside.

2. On medium high fire, sauté for five minutes the onions and mushroom in a skillet with 2 tbsp oil.
3. Prepare sourdough breads by layering the following over it: cheese, fish fillet, onion mixture and cheese again before covering with another bread slice.
4. Grill in your Panini press until cheese is melted and bread is crisped and ridged.

NUTRITION:
Calories: 422; Carbs: 13.2g; Protein: 51.2g; Fat: 17.2g

396.   Italian Flat Bread Gluten Free
Servings: 8 | Cooking Time: 30 minutes

1 tbsp apple cider	2 tbsp water
½ cup yogurt	2 tbsp butter
2 tbsp sugar	2 eggs
1 tsp xanthan gum	½ tsp salt
1 tsp baking soda	1 ½ tsp baking powder
½ cup potato starch, not potato flour	½ cup tapioca flour
¼ cup brown rice flour	1/3 cup sorghum flour

1. With parchment paper, line an 8 x 8-inch baking pan and grease parchment paper. Preheat oven to 375oF.
2. Mix xanthan gum, salt, baking soda, baking powder, all flours, and starch in a large bowl.
3. Whisk well sugar and eggs in a medium bowl until creamed. Add vinegar, water, yogurt, and butter. Whisk thoroughly.
4. Pour in egg mixture into bowl of flours and mix well.
5. Transfer sticky dough into prepared pan and bake in the oven for 25 to 30 minutes.
6. If tops of bread start to brown a lot, cover top with foil and continue baking until done.
7. Remove from oven and pan right away and let it cool.
8. Best served when warm.

NUTRITION:
Calories: 166; Carbs: 27.8g; Protein: 3.4g; Fat: 4.8g

397.   Lemon Aioli and Swordfish Panini
Servings: 4 | Cooking Time: 25 minutes

Swordfish Panini INGREDIENTS	
1 loaf focaccia bread	2 oz fresh arugula greens
1 tbsp herbes de Provence	2 cloves garlic minced
4 pcs of 6oz swordfish fillet	Pepper and salt
Lemon Aioli INGREDIENTS	1 ½ tbsp olive oil
¼ tsp salt	¼ tsp freshly ground black pepper
2 tbsp fresh lemon juice	1 clove garlic, minced
2/3 cup mayonnaise	1 lemon, zested

1. In a small bowl, mix well all lemon Aioli ingredients and put aside.
2. Over medium high fire, heat olive oil in skillet. Season with pepper, salt, minced garlic and herbs de Provence the swordfish. Then pan fry fish until golden brown on both sides, around 5 minutes per side.
3. Slice bread into four slices. Smear on the lemon aioli mixture on two bread slices, layer with arugula leaves and fried fish then cover with the remaining bread slices before grilling in a Panini press.
4. Grill until bread is crisped and ridged.

NUTRITION:
Calories: 433; Carbs: 15.0g; Protein: 36.2g; Fat: 25.1g

398.   Lemon, Buttered Shrimp Panini
Servings: 4 | Cooking Time: 10 minutes

3 tbsp butter	1 baguette
1 tsp hot sauce	1 tbsp parsley
2 tbsp lemon juice	4 garlic cloves, minced
1 lb. shrimp peeled	

1. Make a hollowed portion on your baguette.
2. Sauté the following on a skillet with melted butter: parsley, hot sauce, lemon juice and garlic. After a minute or two mix in the shrimps and sautéing for five minutes.
3. Scoop shrimps into baguette and grill in a Panini press until baguette is crisped and ridged.

NUTRITION:
Calories: 262; Carbs: 14.1g; Protein: 26.1g; Fat: 10.8g

399. Mediterranean Baba Ghanoush
Servings: 4 | Cooking Time: 25 minutes

1 bulb garlic	1 red bell pepper, halved and seeded
1 tbsp chopped fresh basil	1 tbsp olive oil
1 tsp black pepper	2 eggplants, sliced lengthwise
2 rounds of flatbread or pita	Juice of 1 lemon

1. Grease grill grate with cooking spray and preheat grill to medium high.
2. Slice tops of garlic bulb and wrap in foil. Place in the cooler portion of the grill and roast for at least 20 minutes.
3. Place bell pepper and eggplant slices on the hottest part of grill.
4. Grill for at least two to three minutes each side.
5. Once bulbs are done, peel off skins of roasted garlic and place peeled garlic into food processor.
6. Add olive oil, pepper, basil, lemon juice, grilled red bell pepper and grilled eggplant.
7. Puree until smooth and transfer into a bowl.
8. Grill bread at least 30 seconds per side to warm.
9. Serve bread with the pureed dip and enjoy.

NUTRITION:
Calories: 213.6; Carbs: 36.3g; Protein: 6.3g; Fat: 4.8g

400. Multi Grain & Gluten Free Dinner Rolls
Servings: 8 | Cooking Time: 20 minutes

½ tsp apple cider vinegar	3 tbsp olive oil
2 eggs	1 tsp baking powder
1 tsp salt	2 tsp xanthan gum
½ cup tapioca starch	¼ cup brown teff flour
¼ cup flax meal	¼ cup amaranth flour
¼ cup sorghum flour	¾ cup brown rice flour

1. Mix well water and honey in a small bowl and add yeast. Leave it for exactly 10 minutes.
2. In a large bowl, mix the following with a paddle mixer: baking powder, salt, xanthan gum, flax meal, sorghum flour, teff flour, tapioca starch, amaranth flour, and brown rice flour.
3. In a medium bowl, whisk well vinegar, olive oil, and eggs.
4. Into bowl of dry ingredients pour in vinegar and yeast mixture and mix well.
5. Grease a 12-muffin tin with cooking spray. Transfer dough evenly into 12 muffin tins and leave it for an hour to rise.
6. Then preheat oven to 375oF and bake dinner rolls until tops are golden brown, around 20 minutes.
7. Remove dinner rolls from oven and muffin tins immediately and let it cool.
8. Best served when warm.

NUTRITION:
Calories: 207; Carbs: 28.4g; Protein: 4.6g; Fat: 8.3g

401. Mushroom and Eggplant Vegan Panini
Servings: 4 | Cooking Time: 18 minutes

4 thin slices Asiago Cheese	4 thin slices Swiss cheese
¼ cup fat free ranch dressing	8 slices focaccia bread
2 tsp grated parmesan cheese	1 tsp onion powder
1 tsp garlic powder	4 slices ½-inch thick eggplant, peeled
1 cup fat-free balsamic vinaigrette	4 portobello mushroom caps

2 red bell peppers

1. Broil peppers in oven for five minutes or until its skin has blistered and blackened. Remove peppers and place in bowl while quickly covering with plastic wrap, let cool for twenty minutes before peeling off the skin and refrigerating overnight.
2. In a re-sealable bag, place mushrooms and vinaigrette and marinate in the ref for a night.
3. Next day, grill mushrooms while discarding marinade. While seasoning eggplant with onion and garlic powder then grill along with mushrooms until tender, around four to five minutes.
4. Remove mushrooms and eggplant from griller and top with parmesan.
5. On four slices of focaccia, smear ranch dressing evenly then layer: cheese, mushroom, roasted peppers and eggplant slices and cover with the remaining focaccia slices.
6. Grill in a Panini press until cheese has melted and bread is crisped and ridged.

NUTRITION:
Calories: 574; Carbs: 77.1g; Protein: 29.6g; Fat: 19.9g

402. Open Face Egg and Bacon Sandwich
Servings: 1 | Cooking Time: 20 minutes

¼ oz reduced fat cheddar, shredded	½ small jalapeno, thinly sliced
½ whole grain English muffin, split	1 large organic egg
1 thick slice of tomato	1-piece turkey bacon
2 thin slices red onion	4-5 sprigs fresh cilantro
Cooking spray	Pepper to taste

1. On medium fire, place a skillet, cook bacon until crisp tender and set aside.
2. In same skillet, drain oils, and place ½ of English muffin and heat for at least a minute per side. Transfer muffin to a serving plate.
3. Coat the same skillet with cooking spray and fry egg to desired doneness. Once cooked, place egg on top of muffin.
4. Add cilantro, tomato, onion, jalapeno and bacon on top of egg. Serve and enjoy.

NUTRITION:
Calories: 245; Carbs: 24.7g; Protein: 11.8g; Fat: 11g

403. Paleo Chocolate Banana Bread
Servings: 10 | Cooking Time: 50 minutes

¼ cup dark chocolate, chopped	½ cup almond butter
½ cup coconut flour, sifted	½ teaspoon cinnamon powder
1 teaspoon baking soda	1 teaspoon vanilla extract
4 bananas, mashed	4 eggs
4 tablespoon coconut oil, melted	A pinch of salt

1. Preheat the oven to 350oF.
2. Grease an 8" x 8" square pan and set aside.
3. In a large bowl, mix together the eggs, banana, vanilla extract, almond butter and coconut oil. Mix well until well combined.
4. Add the cinnamon powder, coconut flour, baking powder, baking soda and salt to the wet ingredients. Fold until well combined. Add in the chopped chocolates then fold the batter again.
5. Pour the batter into the greased pan. Spread evenly.
6. Bake in the oven for about 50 minutes or until a toothpick inserted in the center comes out clean.
7. Remove from the hot oven and cool in a wire rack for an hour.

NUTRITION:
Calories: 150.3; Carbs: 13.9g; Protein: 3.2g; Fat: 9.1g

405. Panini and Eggplant Caponata

Servings: 4 | Cooking Time: 10 minutes

¼ cup packed fresh basil leaves
4 oz thinly sliced mozzarella
1 ciabatta roll 6-7-inch length, horizontally split
¼ of a 7oz can of eggplant caponata
1 tbsp olive oil

1. Spread oil evenly on the sliced part of the ciabatta and layer on the following: cheese, caponata, basil leaves and cheese again before covering with another slice of ciabatta.
2. Then grill sandwich in a Panini press until cheese melts and bread gets crisped and ridged.

NUTRITION:
Calories: 295; Carbs: 44.4g; Protein: 16.4g; Fat: 7.3g

406. Panini with Chicken-Fontina

Servings: 2 | Cooking Time: 45 minutes

¼ Cup Arugula
3 oz fontina cheese thinly sliced
1 ciabatta roll
1 tbsp + 1 tsp olive oil
2 oz sliced cooked chicken
1 tbsp Dijon mustard
¼ cup water
1 large onion, diced

DIRECTIONS
1. On medium low fire, place a skillet and heat 1 tbsp oil. Sauté onion and cook for 5 minutes. Pour in water while stirring and cooking continuously for 30 minutes until onion is golden brown and tender.
2. Slice bread roll lengthwise and spread the following on one bread half, on the cut side: mustard, caramelized onion, chicken, arugula and cheese. Cover with the remaining bread half.
3. Place the sandwich in a Panini maker and grill for 5 to 8 minutes or until cheese is melted and bread is ridged and crisped.

NUTRITION:
Calories: 216; Carbs: 18.7g; Protein: 22.3g; Fat: 24.5g

407. Pesto, Avocado and Tomato Panini

Servings: 4 | Cooking Time: 10 minutes

Panini INGREDIENTS
8 oz fresh buffalo mozzarella cheese

2 avocados, peeled, pitted, quartered and cut into thin strips
Pesto INGREDIENTS
½ lemon
1/3 cup parmesan cheese
1 ½ bunches fresh basil leaves
2 tbsp extra virgin olive oil
2 vine-ripened tomatoes cut into ¼ inch thick slices
1 ciabatta loaf

Pepper and salt
1/3 cup extra virgin olive oil
1/3 cup pine nuts, toasted
2 garlic cloves, peeled

1. To make the pesto, puree garlic in a food processor and transfer to a mortar and pestle and add in basil and smash into a coarse paste like consistency. Mix in the pine nuts and continue crushing. Once paste like, add the parmesan cheese and mix. Pour in olive oil and blend thoroughly while adding lemon juice. Season with pepper and salt. Put aside.
2. Prepare Panini by slicing ciabatta loaf in three horizontal pieces. To prepare Panini, over bottom loaf slice layer the following: avocado, tomato, pepper, salt and mozzarella cheese. Then top with the middle ciabatta slice and repeat layering process again and cover with the topmost ciabatta bread slice.
3. Grill in a Panini press until cheese is melted and bred is crisped and ridged.

NUTRITION:
Calories: 577; Carbs: 15.5g; Protein: 24.2g; Fat: 49.3g

408. Quinoa Pizza Muffins

Servings: 4 | Cooking Time: 30 minutes

1 cup uncooked quinoa
2 large eggs

½ medium onion, diced
1 cup shredded mozzarella cheese
1 tbsp dried oregano
1/8 tsp salt
½ cup roasted red pepper, chopped*
1 cup diced bell pepper
1 tbsp dried basil
2 tsp garlic powder
1 tsp crushed red peppers
Pizza Sauce, about 1-2 cups

1. Preheat oven to 350oF.
2. Cook quinoa according to directions.
3. Combine all ingredients (except sauce) into bowl. Mix all ingredients well.
4. Scoop quinoa pizza mixture into muffin tin evenly. Makes 12 muffins.
5. Bake for 30 minutes until muffins turn golden in color and the edges are getting crispy.
6. Top with 1 or 2 tbsp pizza sauce and enjoy!

NUTRITION:
Calories: 303; Carbs: 41.3g; Protein: 21.0g; Fat: 6.1g

409. Rosemary-Walnut Loaf Bread

Servings: 8 | Cooking Time: 45 minutes

½ cup chopped walnuts
1 1/3 cups lukewarm carbonated water
½ cup extra virgin olive oil
3 eggs
1 tsp salt
¼ cup buttermilk powder
1 cup tapioca starch
1 ¼ cups all-purpose Bob's Red Mill gluten-free flour mix
4 tbsp fresh, chopped rosemary
1 tbsp honey

1 tsp apple cider vinegar
5 tsp instant dry yeast granules
1 tbsp xanthan gum
1 cup white rice flour
1 cup arrowroot starch

1. In a large mixing bowl, whisk well eggs. Add 1 cup warm water, honey, olive oil, and vinegar.
2. While beating continuously, add the rest of the ingredients except for rosemary and walnuts.
3. Continue beating. If dough is too stiff, add a bit of warm water. Dough should be shaggy and thick.
4. Then add rosemary and walnuts continue kneading until evenly distributed.
5. Cover bowl of dough with a clean towel, place in a warm spot, and let it rise for 30 minutes.
6. Fifteen minutes into rising time, preheat oven to 400oF.
7. Generously grease with olive oil a 2-quart Dutch oven and preheat inside oven without the lid.
8. Once dough is done rising, remove pot from oven, and place dough inside. With a wet spatula, spread top of dough evenly in pot.
9. Brush tops of bread with 2 tbsp of olive oil, cover Dutch oven and bake for 35 to 45 minutes.
10. Once bread is done, remove from oven. And gently remove bread from pot.
11. Allow bread to cool at least ten minutes before slicing.
12. Serve and enjoy.

NUTRITION:
Calories: 424; Carbs: 56.8g; Protein: 7.0g; Fat: 19.0g

410. Sandwich with Hummus

Servings: 4 | Cooking Time: 0 minutes

4 cups alfalfa sprouts

4 red onion sliced ¼-inch thick
2 cups shredded Bibb lettuce
1 can 15.5-oz chickpeas, drained
¼ tsp salt
1 tbsp tahini
2 tbsp water
1 cup cucumber sliced 1/8 inch thick
8 tomatoes sliced ¼-inch thick
12 slices 1-oz whole wheat bread
2 garlic cloves, peeled
½ tsp ground cumin
1 tbsp lemon juice
3 tbsp plain fat free yogurt

1. In a food processor, blend chickpeas, garlic, salt, cumin, tahini, lemon juice, water and yogurt until smooth to create hummus.
2. On 1 slice of bread, spread 2 tbsp hummus, top with 1 onion slice, 2 tomato slices, ½ cup lettuce, another bread slice, 1 cup sprouts, ¼ cup

cucumber and cover with another bread slice. Repeat procedure for the rest of the ingredients.

NUTRITION:
Calories: 407; Carbs: 67.7g; Protein: 18.8 g; Fat: 6.8g

411. Sandwich with Spinach and Tuna Salad

Servings: 4 | Cooking Time: 0 minutes

1 cup fresh baby spinach	8 slices 100% whole wheat sandwich bread
¼ tsp freshly ground black pepper	½ tsp salt free seasoning blend
Juice of one lemon	2 tbsp olive oil
½ tsp dill weed	2 ribs celery, diced

1. In a medium bowl, mix well dill weed, celery, onion, cucumber and tuna.
2. Add lemon juice and olive oil and mix thoroughly.
3. Season with pepper and salt-free seasoning blend.
4. To assemble sandwich, you can toast bread slices, on top of one bread slice layer ½ cup tuna salad, top with ¼ cup spinach and cover with another slice of bread.
5. Repeat procedure to remaining ingredients, serve and enjoy.

NUTRITION:
Calories: 272.5; Carbs: 35.9g; Protein: 10.4g; Fat: 9.7g

412. Spiced Roast Beef Panini

Servings: 2 | Cooking Time: 15 minutes

Creamy horseradish sauce	Butter
1 roasted red peppers	1 crusty bread, halved lengthwise
2 slices Havarti cheese	4 Slices deli roast beef

1. On one bread slice, butter one side, spread over the horseradish sauce, then add evenly the cheese and roast beef and topped with roasted peppers.
2. Cover the filling with the other bread half and start grilling in a Panini press for around three to five minutes while pressing down for a ridged effect.
3. Serve and enjoy.

NUTRITION:
Calories: 311; Carbs: 33.8g; Protein: 17.3g; Fat: 11.7g

413. Sun-Dried Tomatoes Panini

Servings: 4 | Cooking Time: 15 minutes

½ cup shredded mozzarella cheese	8 slices country style Italian bread
1/8 tsp freshly ground black pepper	Cooking spray
3/8 tsp salt, divided	1 6oz package fresh baby spinach
8 garlic cloves, thinly sliced	1/8 tsp crushed red pepper
¼ cup chopped drained oil packed sun-dried tomato	4 4oz chicken cutlets
1 tsp chopped rosemary	2 tbsp extra virgin olive oil, divided

1. In a re-sealable bag mix chicken, rosemary and 2 tsp olive oil. Allow to marinate for 30 minutes in the ref.
2. On medium high fire, place a skillet and heat 4 tsp oil. Sauté for a minute garlic, red pepper and sun-dried tomato. Add 1/8 tsp salt and spinach and cook for a minute and put aside.
3. On a grill pan coated with cooking spray, grill chicken for three minutes per side. Season with black pepper and salt.
4. To assemble the sandwich, evenly layer the following on one bread slice: cheese, spinach mixture, and chicken cutlet. Cover with another bread slice.
5. Place sandwich in a Panini press and grill for around five minutes or until cheese is melted and bread is crisped and ridged.

NUTRITION:
Calories: 369; Carbs: 25.7g; Protein: 42.7g; Fat: 10.1g

414. Sunflower Gluten Free Bread

Servings: 8 | Cooking Time: 30 minutes

1 tsp apple cider vinegar	3 tbsp olive oil
3 egg whites	Extra seeds for sprinkling on top of loaf
1 ¼ tsp sea salt	2 ¾ tsp xanthan gum
2 tbsp hemp seeds	2 tbsp poppy seeds
¼ cup flax meal	¼ cup buckwheat flour
½ cup brown rice flour	1 cup tapioca starch
1 ½ cups sorghum flour	2 ½ tsp dry active yeast
1 tbsp honey	1 ¼ cup hot water

1. Mix honey and water in a small bowl. Add yeast and stir a bit and leave on for 7 minutes.
2. In a large mixing bowl, mix well salt, xanthan gum, hemp, poppy, flax meal, buckwheat flour, brown rice four, tapioca starch, and sorghum flour and beat with a paddle mixer.
3. In a medium bowl, beat well vinegar, oil, and eggs.
4. In bowl of dry ingredients, pour in bowl of egg mixture and yeast mixture and mix well until you have a smooth dough.
5. In a greased 10-inch cast iron skillet, transfer dough. Lightly wet hands with warm water and smoothen surface of dough until the surface is even. (A 9-inch cake pan will also do nicely if you don't have a cast iron skillet).
6. Sprinkle extra seeds on top of dough and leave dough in a warm corner for 45 to 60 minutes to rise.
7. Then pop risen dough in a 375oF preheated oven until tops are golden brown, around 30 minutes.
8. Once done cooking, immediately remove dough from pan and let it cool a bit before slicing and serving.

NUTRITION:
Calories: 291; Carbs: 49.1g; Protein: 6.0g; Fat: 8.5g

415. Tasty Crabby Panini

Servings: 4 | Cooking Time: 10 minutes

1 tbsp Olive oil	French bread split and sliced diagonally
1 lb. blue crab meat or shrimp or spiny lobster or stone crab	½ cup celery
¼ cup green onion chopped	1 tsp Worcestershire sauce
1 tsp lemon juice	1 tbsp Dijon mustard
½ cup light mayonnaise	

1. In a medium bowl mix the following thoroughly: celery, onion, Worcestershire, lemon juice, mustard and mayonnaise. Season with pepper and salt. Then gently add in the almonds and crabs.
2. Spread olive oil on sliced sides of bread and smear with crab mixture before covering with another bread slice.
3. Grill sandwich in a Panini press until bread is crisped and ridged.

NUTRITION:
Calories: 248; Carbs: 12.0g; Protein: 24.5g; Fat: 10.9g

416. Tuna Melt Panini

Servings: 4 | Cooking Time: 10 minutes

2 tbsp softened unsalted butter	16 pcs of 1/8-inch kosher dill pickle
8 pcs of ¼ inch thick cheddar or Swiss cheese	Mayonnaise and Dijon mustard
4 ciabatta rolls, split	Pepper and salt
½ tsp crushed red pepper	1 tbsp minced basil
1 tbsp balsamic vinegar	¼ cup extra virgin olive oil
¼ cup finely diced red onion	2 cans of 6oz albacore tuna

1. Combine thoroughly the following in a bowl: salt pepper, crushed red pepper, basil, vinegar, olive oil, onion and tuna.
2. Smear with mayonnaise and mustard the cut sides of the bread rolls then layer on: cheese, tuna salad and pickles. Cover with the remaining slice of roll.

3. Grill in a Panini press ensuring that cheese is melted and bread is crisped and ridged.

NUTRITION:
Calories: 539; Carbs: 27.7g; Protein: 21.6g; Fat: 38.5g

417. Tuscan Bread Dipper

Servings: 8 | Cooking Time: 0 minutes

¼ cup balsamic vinegar	¼ cup extra virgin olive oil
¼ teaspoon salt	½ tbsp fresh basil, minced
½ teaspoon pepper	1 ½ teaspoon Italian seasoning
2 cloves garlic minced	8 pieces Food for Life Brown Rice English Muffins

1. In a small bowl mix well all ingredients except for bread. Allow herbs to steep in olive oil-balsamic vinegar mixture for at least 30 minutes.
2. To serve, toast bread, cut each muffin in half and serve with balsamic vinegar dip.

NUTRITION:
Calories: 168.5; Carbs: 27.7g; Protein: 5.2g; Fat: 4.1g

418. Keto Breakfast Pizza

Servings: 6 | Preparation time: 30 mins

2 tablespoons coconut flour	2 cups cauliflower, grated
½ teaspoon salt	1 tablespoon psyllium husk powder
4 eggs	**Toppings:**
Avocado	Smoked Salmon
Herbs	Olive oil
Spinach	

1. Preheat the oven to 360 degrees and grease a pizza tray.
2. Mix together all ingredients in a bowl, except toppings, and keep aside.
3. Pour the pizza dough onto the pan and mold it into an even pizza crust using hands.
4. Top the pizza with toppings and transfer in the oven.
5. Bake for about 15 minutes until golden brown and remove from the oven to serve.

NUTRITION:
Calories: 454 Carbs: 16g Fats: 31g Proteins: 22g Sodium: 1325mg Sugar: 4.4g

419. Coconut Flour Pizza

Servings: 4 | Preparation time: 35 mins

2 tablespoons psyllium husk powder	¾ cup coconut flour
1 teaspoon garlic powder	½ teaspoon salt
½ teaspoon baking soda	1 cup boiling water
1 teaspoon apple cider vinegar	3 eggs
Toppings	3 tablespoons tomato sauce
1½ oz. Mozzarella cheese	1 tablespoon basil, freshly chopped

1. Preheat the oven to 350 degrees F and grease a baking sheet.
2. Mix coconut flour, salt, psyllium husk powder, and garlic powder until fully combined.
3. Add eggs, apple cider vinegar, and baking soda and knead with boiling water.
4. Place the dough out on a baking sheet and top with the toppings.
5. Transfer in the oven and bake for about 20 minutes.
6. Dish out and serve warm.

NUTRITION:
Calories: 173 Carbs: 16.8g Fats: 7.4g Proteins: 10.4g Sodium: 622mg Sugar: 0.9g

420. Mini Pizza Crusts

Servings: 4 | Preparation time: 20 mins

1 cup coconut flour, sifted	8 large eggs, 5 whole eggs and 3 egg whites
½ teaspoon baking powder	Italian spices, to taste
Salt and black pepper, to taste	For the pizza sauce
2 garlic cloves, crushed	1 teaspoon dried basil
½ cup tomato sauce	¼ teaspoon sea salt

1. Preheat the oven to 350 degrees F and grease a baking tray.
2. Whisk together eggs and egg whites in a large bowl and stir in the coconut flour, baking powder, Italian spices, salt, and black pepper.
3. Make small dough balls from this mixture and press on the baking tray.
4. Transfer in the oven and bake for about 20 minutes.
5. Allow pizza bases to cool and keep aside.
6. Combine all ingredients for the pizza sauce together and sit at room temperature for half an hour.
7. Spread this pizza sauce over the pizza crusts and serve.

NUTRITION:
Calories: 170 Carbs: 5.7g Fats: 10.5g Proteins: 13.6g Sodium: 461mg Sugar: 2.3g

421. Keto Pepperoni Pizza

Servings: 4 | Preparation time: 40 mins

Crust	6 oz. mozzarella cheese, shredded
4 eggs	Topping
1 teaspoon dried oregano	1½ oz. pepperoni
3 tablespoons tomato paste	5 oz. mozzarella cheese, shredded
Olives	

1. Preheat the oven to 400 degrees F and grease a baking sheet.
2. Whisk together eggs and cheese in a bowl and spread on a baking sheet.
3. Transfer in the oven and bake for about 15 minutes until golden.
4. Remove from the oven and allow it to cool.
5. Increase the oven temperature to 450 degrees F.
6. Spread the tomato paste on the crust and top with oregano, pepperoni, cheese, and olives on top.
7. Bake for another 10 minutes and serve hot.

NUTRITION:
Calories: 356 Carbs: 6.1g Fats: 23.8g Proteins: 30.6g Sodium: 790mg Sugar: 1.8g

422. Thin Crust Low Carb Pizza

Servings: 6 | Preparation time: 25 mins

2 tablespoons tomato sauce	1/8 teaspoon black pepper
1/8 teaspoon chili flakes	1 piece low-carb pita bread
2 ounces low-moisture mozzarella cheese	1/8 teaspoon garlic powder
Toppings:	Bacon, roasted red peppers, spinach, olives, pesto, artichokes, salami, pepperoni, roast beef, prosciutto, avocado, ham, chili paste, Sriracha

1. Preheat the oven to 450 degrees F and grease a baking dish.
2. Mix together tomato sauce, black pepper, chili flakes, and garlic powder in a bowl and keep aside.
3. Place the low-carb pita bread in the oven and bake for about 2 minutes.
4. Remove from oven and spread the tomato sauce on it.
5. Add mozzarella cheese and top with your favorite toppings.
6. Bake again for 3 minutes and dish out.

NUTRITION:
Calories: 254 Carbs: 12.9g Fats: 16g Proteins: 19.3g Sodium: 255mg Sugar: 2.8g

423. BBQ Chicken Pizza

Servings: 4 | Preparation time: 30 mins

Dairy Free Pizza Crust	6 tablespoons Parmesan cheese
6 large eggs	3 tablespoons psyllium husk powder
Salt and black pepper, to taste	1½ teaspoons Italian seasoning
Toppings	6 oz. rotisserie chicken, shredded
4 oz. cheddar cheese	1 tablespoon mayonnaise
4 tablespoons tomato sauce	4 tablespoons BBQ sauce

1. Preheat the oven to 400 degrees F and grease a baking dish.
2. Place all Pizza Crust ingredients in an immersion blender and blend until smooth.
3. Spread dough mixture onto the baking dish and transfer in the oven.
4. Bake for about 10 minutes and top with favorite toppings.
5. Bake for about 3 minutes and dish out.

NUTRITION:
Calories: 356 Carbs: 2.9g Fats: 24.5g Proteins: 24.5g Sodium: 396mg Sugar: 0.6g

424. Buffalo Chicken Crust Pizza

Servings: 6 | Preparation time: 25 mins

1 cup whole milk mozzarella, shredded	1 teaspoon dried oregano
2 tablespoons butter	1 pound chicken thighs, boneless and skinless
1 large egg	¼ teaspoon black pepper
¼ teaspoon salt	1 stalk celery
3 tablespoons Franks Red Hot Original	1 stalk green onion
1 tablespoon sour cream	1 ounce bleu cheese, crumbled

1. Preheat the oven to 400 degrees F and grease a baking dish.
2. Process chicken thighs in a food processor until smooth.
3. Transfer to a large bowl and add egg, ½ cup of shredded mozzarella, oregano, black pepper, and salt to form a dough.
4. Spread the chicken dough in the baking dish and transfer in the oven.
5. Bake for about 25 minutes and keep aside.
6. Meanwhile, heat butter and add celery, and cook for about 4 minutes.
7. Mix Franks Red Hot Original with the sour cream in a small bowl.
8. Spread the sauce mixture over the crust, layer with the cooked celery and remaining ½ cup of mozzarella and the bleu cheese.
9. Bake for another 10 minutes, until the cheese is melted

NUTRITION:
Calories: 172 Carbs: 1g Fats: 12.9g Proteins: 13.8g Sodium: 172mg Sugar: 0.2g

425. Fresh Bell Pepper Basil Pizza

Servings: 3 | Preparation time: 25 mins

Pizza Base	½ cup almond flour
2 tablespoons cream cheese	1 teaspoon Italian seasoning
½ teaspoon black pepper	6 ounces mozzarella cheese
2 tablespoons psyllium husk	2 tablespoons fresh Parmesan cheese
1 large egg	½ teaspoon salt
Toppings	4 ounces cheddar cheese, shredded
¼ cup Marinara sauce	2/3 medium bell pepper
1 medium vine tomato	3 tablespoons basil, fresh chopped

1. Preheat the oven to 400 degrees F and grease a baking dish.
2. Microwave mozzarella cheese for about 30 seconds and top with the remaining pizza crust.
3. Add the remaining pizza ingredients to the cheese and mix together.
4. Flatten the dough and transfer in the oven.
5. Bake for about 10 minutes and remove pizza from the oven.
6. Top the pizza with the toppings and bake for another 10 minutes.
7. Remove pizza from the oven and allow to cool.

NUTRITION:

Calories: 411 Carbs: 6.4g Fats: 31.3g Proteins: 22.2g Sodium: 152mg Sugar: 2.8g

426. Keto Thai Chicken Flatbread Pizza

Servings: 12 | Preparation time: 25 mins

Peanut Sauce	2 tablespoons rice wine vinegar
4 tablespoons reduced sugar ketchup	4 tablespoons soy sauce
4 tablespoons coconut oil	½ lime, juiced
1 teaspoon fish sauce	Pizza Base
¾ cup almond flour	3 tablespoons cream cheese
½ teaspoon garlic powder	8 oz. mozzarella cheese
1 tablespoon psyllium husk powder	1 large egg
½ teaspoon onion powder	½ teaspoon ginger
½ teaspoon black pepper	½ teaspoon salt
Toppings	3 oz. mung bean sprouts
2 medium green onions	2 tablespoons peanuts
2 chicken thighs	6 oz. mozzarella cheese
1½ oz. carrots, shredded	

1. Preheat oven to 400 degrees F and grease a baking tray.
2. Mix together all peanut sauce ingredients and set aside.
3. Microwave cream cheese and mozzarella cheese for the pizza base for 1 minute.
4. Add eggs, then mix together with all dry ingredients.
5. Arrange dough onto a baking tray and bake for about 15 minutes.
6. Flip pizza and top with sauce, chopped chicken, shredded carrots, and mozzarella.
7. Bake again for 10 minutes, or until cheese has melted.
8. Top with bean sprouts, spring onion, peanuts, and cilantro.

NUTRITION:
Calories: 268 Carbs: 3.2g Fats: 21g Proteins: 15g Sodium: 94mg Sugar: 0.2g

427. Apple and Ham Flatbread Pizza

Servings: 8 | Preparation time: 15 mins

For the crust:	¾ cup almond flour
½ teaspoon sea salt	2 cups mozzarella cheese, shredded
2 tablespoons cream cheese	1/8 teaspoon dried thyme
For the topping:	½ small red onion, cut into thin slices
4 ounces low carbohydrate ham, cut into chunks	Salt and black pepper, to taste
1 cup Mexican blend cheese, grated	¼ medium apple, sliced
1/8 teaspoon dried thyme	

1. Preheat the oven to 425 degrees F and grease a 12-inch pizza pan.
2. Boil water and steam cream cheese, mozzarella cheese, almond flour, thyme, and salt.
3. When the cheese melts enough, knead for a few minutes to thoroughly mix dough.
4. Make a ball out of the dough and arrange in the pizza pan.
5. Poke holes all over the dough with a fork and transfer in the oven.
6. Bake for about 8 minutes until golden brown and reset the oven setting to 350 degrees F.
7. Sprinkle ¼ cup of the Mexican blend cheese over the flatbread and top with onions, apples, and ham.
8. Cover with the remaining ¾ cup of the Mexican blend cheese and sprinkle with the thyme, salt, and black pepper.
9. Bake for about 7 minutes until cheese is melted and crust is golden brown.
10. Remove the flatbread from the oven and allow to cool before cutting.
11. Slice into desired pieces and serve.

NUTRITION:
Calories: 179 Carbs: 5.3g Fats: 13.6g Proteins: 10.4g Sodium: 539mg Sugar: 2.1g   Air Fryer Breakfast Recipes

428. Ham, Spinach & Egg in a Cup
Servings: 8 | Preparation time: 35 mins

2 tablespoons olive oil	2 tablespoons unsalted butter, melted
2 pounds fresh baby spinach	8 eggs
8 teaspoons milk	14-ounce ham, sliced
Salt and black pepper, to taste	

1. Preheat the Airfryer to 360 degrees F and grease 8 ramekins with butter.
2. Heat oil in a skillet on medium heat and add spinach.
3. Cook for about 3 minutes and drain the liquid completely from the spinach.
4. Divide the spinach into prepared ramekins and layer with ham slices.
5. Crack 1 egg over ham slices into each ramekin and drizzle evenly with milk.
6. Sprinkle with salt and black pepper and bake for about 20 minutes.

NUTRITION:
Calories: 228 Carbs: 6.6g Fats: 15.6g Proteins: 17.2g Sodium: 821mg Sugar: 1.1g

429. Eggs with Sausage & Bacon
Servings: 2 | Preparation time: 25 mins

4 chicken sausages	4 bacon slices
2 eggs	Salt and freshly ground black pepper, to taste

1. Preheat the Airfryer to 330 degrees F and place sausages and bacon slices in an Airfryer basket.
2. Cook for about 10 minutes and lightly grease 2 ramekins.
3. Crack 1 egg in each prepared ramekin and season with salt and black pepper.
4. Cook for about 10 minutes and divide sausages and bacon slices in serving plates.

NUTRITION:
Calories: 245 Carbs: 5.7g Fats: 15.8g Proteins: 17.8g Sodium: 480mg Sugar: 0.7g

430. Tropical Almond Pancakes
Servings: 8 | Preparation time: 15 mins

2 cups creamy milk	3½ cups almond flour
1 teaspoon baking soda	½ teaspoon salt
1 teaspoon allspice	2 tablespoons vanilla
1 teaspoon cinnamon	1 teaspoon baking powder
½ cup club soda	

1. Preheat the Air fryer at 290 degrees F and grease the cooking basket of the air fryer.
2. Whisk together salt, almond flour, baking soda, allspice and cinnamon in a large bowl.
3. Mix together the vanilla, baking powder and club soda and add to the flour mixture.
4. Stir the mixture thoroughly and pour the mixture into the cooking basket.
5. Cook for about 10 minutes and dish out in a serving platter.

NUTRITION:
Calories: 324 Carbs: 12.8g Fats: 24.5g Proteins: 11.4g Sodium: 342mg Sugar: 1.6g

431. Bacon & Hot Dogs Omelet
Servings: 4 | Preparation time: 15 mins

4 hot dogs, chopped	8 eggs
2 bacon slices, chopped	4 small onions, chopped

1. Preheat the Airfryer to 325 degrees F.
2. Crack the eggs in an Airfryer baking pan and beat well.

3. Stir in the remaining ingredients and cook for about 10 minutes until completely done.

NUTRITION:
Calories: 298 Carbs: 9g Fats: 21.8g Proteins: 16.9g Sodium: 628mg Sugar: 5.1g

432. Toasted Bagels
Servings: 6 | Preparation time: 10 mins

6 teaspoons butter	3 bagels, halved

1. Preheat the Airfryer to 375 degrees F and arrange the bagels into an Airfryer basket.
2. Cook for about 3 minutes and remove the bagels from Airfryer.
3. Spread butter evenly over bagels and cook for about 3 more minutes.

NUTRITION:
Calories: 169 Carbs: 26.5g Fats: 4.7g Proteins: 5.3g Sodium: 262mg Sugar: 2.7g

433. Eggless Spinach & Bacon Quiche
Servings: 8 | Preparation time: 20 mins

1 cup fresh spinach, chopped	4 slices of bacon, cooked and chopped
½ cup mozzarella cheese, shredded	4 tablespoons milk
4 dashes Tabasco sauce	1 cup Parmesan cheese, shredded
Salt and freshly ground black pepper, to taste	

1. Preheat the Airfryer to 325 degrees F and grease a baking dish.
2. Put all the ingredients in a bowl and mix well.
3. Transfer the mixture into prepared baking dish and cook for about 8 minutes.
4. Dish out and serve.

NUTRITION:
Calories: 72 Carbs: 0.9g Fats: 5.2g Proteins: 5.5g Sodium: 271mg Sugar: 0.4g

434. Ham Casserole
Servings: 4 | Preparation time: 25 mins

4-ounce ham, sliced thinly	4 teaspoons unsalted butter, softened
8 large eggs, divided	4 tablespoons heavy cream
¼ teaspoon smoked paprika	4 teaspoons fresh chives, minced
Salt and freshly ground black pepper, to taste	6 tablespoons Parmesan cheese, grated finely

1. Preheat the Airfryer to 325 degrees F and spread butter in the pie pan.
2. Place ham slices in the bottom of the pie pan.
3. Whisk together 2 eggs, cream, salt and black pepper until smooth.
4. Place the egg mixture evenly over the ham slices and crack the remaining eggs on top.
5. Season with paprika, salt and black pepper.
6. Top evenly with chives and cheese and place the pie pan in an Airfryer.
7. Cook for about 12 minutes and serve with toasted bread slices.

NUTRITION:
Calories: 410 Carbs: 3.9g Fats: 30.8g Proteins: 31.2g Sodium: 933mg Sugar: 0.8g

435. Sausage & Bacon with Beans
Servings: 12 | Preparation time: 30 mins

12 medium sausages	12 bacon slices
8 eggs	2 cans baked beans
12 bread slices, toasted	

1. Preheat the Airfryer at 325 degrees F and place sausages and bacon in a fryer basket.
2. Cook for about 10 minutes and place the baked beans in a ramekin.
3. Place eggs in another ramekin and the Airfryer to 395 degrees F.
4. Cook for about 10 more minutes and divide the sausage mixture, beans and eggs in serving plates
5. Serve with bread slices.

NUTRITION:
Calories: 276 Carbs: 14.1g Fats: 17g Proteins: 16.3g Sodium: 817mg Sugar: 0.6g

436. French Toasts
Servings: 4 | Preparation time: 15 mins

½ cup evaporated milk	4 eggs
6 tablespoons sugar	¼ teaspoon vanilla extract
8 bread slices	4 teaspoons olive oil

1. Preheat the Airfryer to 395 degrees F and grease a pan.
2. Put all the ingredients in a large shallow dish except the bread slices.
3. Beat till well combined and dip each bread slice in egg mixture from both sides.
4. Arrange the bread slices in the prepared pan and cook for about 3 minutes per side.

NUTRITION:
Calories: 261 Carbs: 30.6g Fats: 12g Proteins: 9.1g Sodium: 218mg Sugar: 22.3g

437. Veggie Hash
Servings: 8 | Preparation time: 55 mins

2 medium onions, chopped	2 teaspoons dried thyme, crushed
4 teaspoons butter	1 green bell pepper, seeded and chopped
3 pounds russet potatoes, peeled and cubed	Salt and freshly ground black pepper, to taste
10 eggs	

1. Preheat the Airfryer to 395 degrees F and grease the Airfryer pan with butter.
2. Add bell peppers and onions and cook for about 5 minutes.
3. Add the herbs, potatoes, salt and black pepper and cook for about 30 minutes.
4. Heat a greased skillet on medium heat and add beaten eggs.
5. Cook for about 1 minute on each side and remove from the skillet.
6. Cut it into small pieces and add egg pieces into Airfryer pan.
7. Cook for about 5 more minutes and dish out.

NUTRITION:
Calories: 229 Carbs: 31g Fats: 7.6g Proteins: 10.3g Sodium: 102mg Sugar: 4.3g

438. Parmesan Garlic Rolls
Servings: 4 | Preparation time: 15 mins

1 cup Parmesan cheese, grated	4 dinner rolls
4 tablespoons unsalted butter, melted	1 tablespoon garlic bread seasoning mix

1. Preheat the Airfryer at 360 degrees F and cut the dinner rolls into cross style.
2. Stuff the slits evenly with the cheese and coat the tops of each roll with butter.
3. Sprinkle with the seasoning mix and cook for about 5 minutes until cheese is fully melted.

NUTRITION:
Calories: 391 Carbs: 45g Fats: 18.6g Proteins: 11.7g Sodium: 608mg Sugar: 4.8g

439. Pickled Toasts
Servings: 4 | Preparation time: 25 mins

4 tablespoons unsalted butter, softened	8 bread slices, toasted
4 tablespoons Branston pickle	½ cup Parmesan cheese, grated

1. Preheat the Airfryer to 385 degrees F and place the bread slice in a fryer basket.
2. Cook for about 5 minutes and spread butter evenly over bread slices.
3. Layer with Branston pickle and top evenly with cheese.
4. Cook for about 5 minutes until cheese is fully melted.

NUTRITION:
Calories: 186 Carbs: 16.3g Fats: 12.9g Proteins: 2.6g Sodium: 397mg Sugar: 6.8g

440. Potato Rosti
Servings: 4 | Preparation time: 15 mins

½ pound russet potatoes, peeled and grated roughly	Salt and freshly ground black pepper, to taste
3.5 ounces smoked salmon, cut into slices	k1 teaspoon olive oil
1 tablespoon chives, chopped finely	2 tablespoons sour cream

1. Preheat the Airfryer to 360 degrees F and grease a pizza pan with the olive oil.
2. Add chives, potatoes, salt and black pepper in a large bowl and mix until well combined.
3. Place the potato mixture into the prepared pizza pan and transfer the pizza pan in an Airfryer basket.
4. Cook for about 15 minutes and cut the potato rosti into wedges.
5. Top with the smoked salmon slices and sour cream and serve.

NUTRITION:
Calories: 91 Carbs: 9.2g Fats: 3.6g Proteins: 5.7g Sodium: 503mg Sugar: 0.7g

441. Pumpkin Pancakes
Servings: 8 | Preparation time: 20 mins

2 squares puff pastry	6 tablespoons pumpkin filling
2 small eggs, beaten	¼ teaspoon cinnamon

1. Preheat the Airfryer to 360 degrees F and roll out a square of puff pastry.
2. Layer it with pumpkin pie filling, leaving about ¼-inch space around the edges.
3. Cut it up into equal sized square pieces and cover the gaps with beaten egg.
4. Arrange the squares into a baking dish and cook for about 12 minutes.
5. Sprinkle some cinnamon and serve.

NUTRITION:
Calories: 51 Carbs: 5g Fats: 2.5g Proteins: 2.4g Sodium: 48mg Sugar: 0.5g

442. Simple Cheese Sandwiches
Servings: 4 | Preparation time: 10 mins

8 American cheese slices	8 bread slices
8 teaspoons butter	

1. Preheat the Air fryer to 365 degrees F and arrange cheese slices between bread slices.
2. Spread butter over outer sides of sandwich and repeat with the remaining butter, slices and cheese.
3. Arrange the sandwiches in an Air fryer basket and cook for about 8 minutes, flipping once in the middle way.

NUTRITION:
Calories: 254 Carbs: 12.4g Fats: 18.8g Proteins: 9.2g Sodium: 708mg Sugar: 3.9g

SNACKS

443. Light & Creamy Garlic Hummus

Preparation Time: 10 minutes | **Cooking Time:** 40 minutes | **Servings:** 12

1 1/2 cups dry chickpeas, rinsed
1 tbsp garlic, minced
6 cups of water
Salt

2 1/2 tbsp fresh lemon juice
1/2 cup tahini
Pepper

1. Add water and chickpeas into the instant pot.
2. Seal pot with a lid and select manual and set timer for 40 minutes.
3. Once done, allow to release pressure naturally. Remove lid.
4. Drain chickpeas well and reserved 1/2 cup chickpeas liquid.
5. Transfer chickpeas, reserved liquid, lemon juice, garlic, tahini, pepper, and salt into the food processor and process until smooth.
6. Serve and enjoy.

NUTRITION:
Calories 152 Fat 6.9 g Carbohydrates 17.6 g Sugar 2.8 g Protein 6.6 g Cholesterol 0 mg

444. Perfect Queso

Preparation Time: 10 minutes | **Cooking Time:** 15 minutes | **Servings:** 16

1 lb ground beef
10 oz can tomatoes, diced
1 tsp chili powder
Pepper

32 oz Velveeta cheese, cut into cubes
1 1/2 tbsp taco seasoning
1 onion, diced
Salt

1. Set instant pot on sauté mode.
2. Add meat, onion, taco seasoning, chili powder, pepper, and salt into the pot and cook until meat is no longer pink.
3. Add tomatoes and stir well. Top with cheese and do not stir.
4. Seal pot with lid and cook on high for 4 minutes.
5. Once done, release pressure using quick release. Remove lid.
6. Stir everything well and serve.

NUTRITION:
Calories 257 Fat 15.9 g Carbohydrates 10.2 g Sugar 4.9 g Protein 21 g Cholesterol 71 mg

445. Creamy Potato Spread

Preparation Time: 10 minutes | **Cooking Time:** 15 minutes | **Servings:** 6

1 lb sweet potatoes, peeled and chopped
1/2 tsp paprika
1 cup tomato puree
Salt

3/4 tbsp fresh chives, chopped
1 tbsp garlic, minced
Pepper

1. Add all ingredients except chives into the inner pot of instant pot and stir well.
2. Seal pot with lid and cook on high for 15 minutes.
3. Once done, allow to release pressure naturally for 10 minutes then release remaining using quick release. Remove lid.
4. Transfer instant pot sweet potato mixture into the food processor and process until smooth.
5. Garnish with chives and serve.

NUTRITION:
Calories 108 Fat 0.3 g Carbohydrates 25.4 g Sugar 2.4 g Protein 2 g Cholesterol 0 mg

446. Cucumber Tomato Okra Salsa

Preparation Time: 10 minutes | **Cooking Time:** 15 minutes | **Servings:** 4

1 lb tomatoes, chopped
1/4 cup fresh lemon juice
1 tbsp fresh oregano, chopped
1 tbsp olive oil
1 tbsp garlic, chopped
Pepper

1/4 tsp red pepper flakes
1 cucumber, chopped
1 tbsp fresh basil, chopped
1 onion, chopped
1 1/2 cups okra, chopped
Salt

1. Add oil into the inner pot of instant pot and set the pot on sauté mode.
2. Add onion, garlic, pepper, and salt and sauté for 3 minutes.
3. Add remaining ingredients except for cucumber and stir well.
4. Seal pot with lid and cook on high for 12 minutes.
5. Once done, allow to release pressure naturally for 10 minutes then release remaining using quick release. Remove lid.
6. Once the salsa mixture is cool then add cucumber and mix well.
7. Serve and enjoy.

NUTRITION:
Calories 99 Fat 4.2 g Carbohydrates 14.3 g Sugar 6.4 g Protein 2.9 g Cholesterol 0 mg

447. Parmesan Potatoes

Preparation Time: 10 minutes | **Cooking Time:** 6 minutes | **Servings:** 4

2 lb potatoes, rinsed and cut into chunks
2 tbsp olive oil
1/2 tsp Italian seasoning
1 cup vegetable broth

2 tbsp parmesan cheese, grated
1/2 tsp parsley
1 tsp garlic, minced
1/2 tsp salt

1. Add all ingredients except cheese into the instant pot and stir well.
2. Seal pot with lid and cook on high for 6 minutes.
3. Once done, release pressure using quick release. Remove lid.
4. Add parmesan cheese and stir until cheese is melted.
5. Serve and enjoy.

NUTRITION:
Calories 237 Fat 8.3 g Carbohydrates 36.3 g Sugar 2.8 g Protein 5.9 g Cholesterol 2 mg

448. Creamy Artichoke Dip

Preparation Time: 10 minutes | **Cooking Time:** 5 minutes | **Servings:** 8

28 oz can artichoke hearts, drain and quartered
1 cup sour cream
3.5 oz can green chilies
Pepper

1 1/2 cups parmesan cheese, shredded
1 cup mayonnaise
1 cup of water
Salt

1. Add artichokes, water, and green chilies into the instant pot.
2. Seal pot with the lid and select manual and set timer for 1 minute.
3. Once done, release pressure using quick release. Remove lid. Drain excess water.
4. Set instant pot on sauté mode. Add remaining ingredients and stir well and cook until cheese is melted.
5. Serve and enjoy.

NUTRITION:
Calories 262 Fat 7.6 g Carbohydrates 14.4 g Sugar 2.8 g Protein 8.4 g Cholesterol 32 mg

449. Homemade Salsa

Preparation Time: 10 minutes | Cooking Time: 5 minutes | Servings: 8

12 oz grape tomatoes, halved	1/4 cup fresh cilantro, chopped
1 fresh lime juice	28 oz tomatoes, crushed
1 tbsp garlic, minced	1 green bell pepper, chopped
1 red bell pepper, chopped	2 onions, chopped
6 whole tomatoes	Salt

1. Add whole tomatoes into the instant pot and gently smash the tomatoes.
2. Add remaining ingredients except cilantro, lime juice, and salt and stir well.
3. Seal pot with lid and cook on high for 5 minutes.
4. Once done, allow to release pressure naturally for 10 minutes then release remaining using quick release. Remove lid.
5. Add cilantro, lime juice, and salt and stir well.
6. Serve and enjoy.

NUTRITION:
Calories 146 Fat 1.2 g Carbohydrates 33.2 g Sugar 4 g Protein 6.9 g Cholesterol 0 mg

450. Delicious Eggplant Caponata

Preparation Time: 10 minutes | Cooking Time: 5 minutes | Servings: 8

1 eggplant, cut into 1/2-inch chunks	1 lb tomatoes, diced
1/2 cup tomato puree	1/4 cup dates, chopped
2 tbsp vinegar	1/2 cup fresh parsley, chopped
2 celery stalks, chopped	1 small onion, chopped
2 zucchini, cut into 1/2-inch chunks	Pepper
Salt	

1. Add all ingredients into the inner pot of instant pot and stir well.
2. Seal pot with lid and cook on high for 5 minutes.
3. Once done, release pressure using quick release. Remove lid.
4. Stir well and serve.

NUTRITION:
Calories 60 Fat 0.4 g Carbohydrates 14 g Sugar 8.8 g Protein 2.3 g Cholesterol 0.4 mg

451. Flavorful Roasted Baby Potatoes

Preparation Time: 10 minutes | Cooking Time: 10 minutes | Servings: 4

2 lbs baby potatoes, clean and cut in half	1/2 cup vegetable stock
1 tsp paprika	3/4 tsp garlic powder
1 tsp onion powder	2 tsp Italian seasoning
1 tbsp olive oil	Pepper
Salt	

1. Add oil into the inner pot of instant pot and set the pot on sauté mode.
2. Add potatoes and sauté for 5 minutes. Add remaining ingredients and stir well.
3. Seal pot with lid and cook on high for 5 minutes.
4. Once done, release pressure using quick release. Remove lid.
5. Stir well and serve.

NUTRITION:
Calories 175 Fat 4.5 g Carbohydrates 29.8 g Sugar 0.7 g Protein 6.1 g Cholesterol 2 mg

452. Perfect Italian Potatoes

Preparation Time: 10 minutes | Cooking Time: 7 minutes | Servings: 6

2 lbs baby potatoes, clean and cut in	3/4 cup vegetable broth

half
6 oz Italian dry dressing mix

1. Add all ingredients into the inner pot of instant pot and stir well.
2. Seal pot with lid and cook on high for 7 minutes.
3. Once done, allow to release pressure naturally for 3 minutes then release remaining using quick release. Remove lid.
4. Stir well and serve.

NUTRITION:
Calories 149 Fat 0.3 g Carbohydrates 41.6 g Sugar 11.4 g Protein 4.5 g Cholesterol 0 mg

453. Garlic Pinto Bean Dip

Preparation Time: 10 minutes | Cooking Time: 43 minutes | Servings: 6

1 cup dry pinto beans, rinsed	1/2 tsp cumin
1/2 cup salsa	2 garlic cloves
2 chipotle peppers in adobo sauce	5 cups vegetable stock
Pepper	Salt

1. Add beans, stock, garlic, and chipotle peppers into the instant pot.
2. Seal pot with lid and cook on high for 43 minutes.
3. Once done, release pressure using quick release. Remove lid.
4. Drain beans well and reserve 1/2 cup of stock.
5. Transfer beans, reserve stock, and remaining ingredients into the food processor and process until smooth.
6. Serve and enjoy.

NUTRITION:
Calories 129 Fat 0.9 g Carbohydrates 23 g Sugar 1.9 g Protein 8 g Cholesterol 2 mg

454. Creamy Eggplant Dip

Preparation Time: 10 minutes | Cooking Time: 20 minutes | Servings: 4

1 eggplant	1/2 tsp paprika
1 tbsp olive oil	1 tbsp fresh lime juice
2 tbsp tahini	1 garlic clove
1 cup of water	Pepper
Salt	

1. Add water and eggplant into the instant pot.
2. Seal pot with the lid and select manual and set timer for 20 minutes.
3. Once done, release pressure using quick release. Remove lid.
4. Drain eggplant and let it cool.
5. Once the eggplant is cool then remove eggplant skin and transfer eggplant flesh into the food processor.
6. Add remaining ingredients into the food processor and process until smooth.
7. Serve and enjoy.

NUTRITION:
Calories 108 Fat 7.8 g Carbohydrates 9.7 g Sugar 3.7 g Protein 2.5 g Cholesterol 0 mg

455. Jalapeno Chickpea Hummus

Preparation Time: 10 minutes | Cooking Time: 25 minutes | Servings: 4

1 cup dry chickpeas, soaked overnight and drained	1 tsp ground cumin
1/4 cup jalapenos, diced	1/2 cup fresh cilantro
1 tbsp tahini	1/2 cup olive oil
Pepper	Salt

1. Add chickpeas into the instant pot and cover with vegetable stock.
2. Seal pot with lid and cook on high for 25 minutes.
3. Once done, allow to release pressure naturally. Remove lid.
4. Drain chickpeas well and transfer into the food processor along with remaining ingredients and process until smooth.

5. Serve and enjoy.

NUTRITION:
Calories 425 Fat 30.4 g Carbohydrates 31.8 g Sugar 5.6 g Protein 10.5 g Cholesterol 0 mg

456. Tasty Black Bean Dip

Preparation Time: 10 minutes | Cooking Time: 18 minutes | Servings: 6

2 cups dry black beans, soaked overnight and drained	1 1/2 cups cheese, shredded
1 tsp dried oregano	1 1/2 tsp chili powder
2 cups tomatoes, chopped	2 tbsp olive oil
1 1/2 tbsp garlic, minced	1 medium onion, sliced
4 cups vegetable stock	Pepper
Salt	

1. Add all ingredients except cheese into the instant pot.
2. Seal pot with lid and cook on high for 18 minutes.
3. Once done, allow to release pressure naturally. Remove lid. Drain excess water.
4. Add cheese and stir until cheese is melted.
5. Blend bean mixture using an immersion blender until smooth.
6. Serve and enjoy.

NUTRITION:
Calories 402 Fat 15.3 g Carbohydrates 46.6 g Sugar 4.4 g Protein 22.2 g Cholesterol 30 mg

457. Healthy Kidney Bean Dip

Preparation Time: 10 minutes | Cooking Time: 10 minutes | Servings: 6

1 cup dry white kidney beans, soaked overnight and drained	1 tbsp fresh lemon juice
2 tbsp water	1/2 cup coconut yogurt
1 roasted garlic clove	1 tbsp olive oil
1/4 tsp cayenne	1 tsp dried parsley
Pepper	Salt

1. Add soaked beans and 1 3/4 cups of water into the instant pot.
2. Seal pot with lid and cook on high for 10 minutes.
3. Once done, allow to release pressure naturally. Remove lid.
4. Drain beans well and transfer them into the food processor.
5. Add remaining ingredients into the food processor and process until smooth.
6. Serve and enjoy.

NUTRITION:
Calories 136 Fat 3.2 g Carbohydrates 20 g Sugar 2.1 g Protein 7.7 g Cholesterol 0 mg

458. Creamy Pepper Spread

Preparation Time: 10 minutes | Cooking Time: 15 minutes | Servings: 4

1 lb red bell peppers, chopped and remove seeds	1 1/2 tbsp fresh basil
1 tbsp olive oil	1 tbsp fresh lime juice
1 tsp garlic, minced	Pepper
Salt	

1. Add all ingredients into the inner pot of instant pot and stir well.
2. Seal pot with lid and cook on high for 15 minutes.
3. Once done, allow to release pressure naturally for 10 minutes then release remaining using quick release. Remove lid.
4. Transfer bell pepper mixture into the food processor and process until smooth.
5. Serve and enjoy.

NUTRITION:

Calories 41 Fat 3.6 g Carbohydrates 3.5 g Sugar 1.7 g Protein 0.4 g Cholesterol 0 mg

459. Healthy Spinach Dip

Preparation Time: 10 minutes | Cooking Time: 8 minutes | Servings: 4

14 oz spinach	2 tbsp fresh lime juice
1 tbsp garlic, minced	2 tbsp olive oil
2 tbsp coconut cream	Pepper
Salt	

1. Add all ingredients except coconut cream into the instant pot and stir well.
2. Seal pot with lid and cook on low pressure for 8 minutes.
3. Once done, allow to release pressure naturally for 5 minutes then release remaining using quick release. Remove lid.
4. Add coconut cream and stir well and blend spinach mixture using a blender until smooth.
5. Serve and enjoy.

NUTRITION:
Calories 109 Fat 9.2 g Carbohydrates 6.6 g Sugar 1.1 g Protein 3.2 g Cholesterol 0 mg

460. Kidney Bean Spread

Preparation Time: 10 minutes | Cooking Time: 18 minutes | Servings: 4

1 lb dry kidney beans, soaked overnight and drained	1 tsp garlic, minced
2 tbsp olive oil	1 tbsp fresh lemon juice
1 tbsp paprika	4 cups vegetable stock
1/2 cup onion, chopped	Pepper
Salt	

1. Add beans and stock into the instant pot.
2. Seal pot with lid and cook on high for 18 minutes.
3. Once done, allow to release pressure naturally. Remove lid.
4. Drain beans well and reserve 1/2 cup stock.
5. Transfer beans, reserve stock, and remaining ingredients into the food processor and process until smooth.
6. Serve and enjoy.

NUTRITION:
Calories 461 Fat 8.6 g Carbohydrates 73 g Sugar 4 g Protein 26.4 g Cholesterol 0 mg

461. Tomato Cucumber Salsa

Preparation Time: 10 minutes | Cooking Time: 5 minutes | Servings: 4

1 cucumber, chopped	1 1/2 lbs grape tomatoes, chopped
1 tbsp fresh chives, chopped	1 tbsp fresh parsley, chopped
1 tbsp fresh basil, chopped	2 onion, chopped
1/4 cup vinegar	2 tbsp olive oil
1/4 cup vegetable stock	2 chili peppers, chopped
Pepper	Salt

1. Add tomatoes, stock, and chili peppers into the instant pot and stir well.
2. Seal pot with lid and cook on low pressure for 5 minutes.
3. Once done, allow to release pressure naturally for 5 minutes then release remaining using quick release. Remove lid.
4. Transfer tomato mixture into the mixing bowl.
5. Add remaining ingredients into the bowl and mix well.
6. Serve and enjoy.

NUTRITION:
Calories 129 Fat 7.5 g Carbohydrates 15 g Sugar 8.3 g Protein 2.7 g Cholesterol 0 mg

462. Spicy Berry Dip

Preparation Time: 10 minutes | Cooking Time: 15 minutes | Servings: 4

10 oz cranberries	1/4 cup fresh orange juice
3/4 tsp paprika	1/2 tsp chili powder
1 tsp lemon zest	1 tbsp lemon juice

1. Add all ingredients into the inner pot of instant pot and stir well.
2. Seal pot with lid and cook on high for 15 minutes.
3. Once done, allow to release pressure naturally for 5 minutes then release remaining using quick release. Remove lid.
4. Blend cranberry mixture using a blender until getting the desired consistency.
5. Serve and enjoy.

NUTRITION:
Calories 49 Fat 0.2 g Carbohydrates 8.6 g Sugar 4.1 g Protein 0.3 g Cholesterol 0 mg

463. Rosemary Cauliflower Dip

Preparation Time: 10 minutes | Cooking Time: 15 minutes | Servings: 4

1 lb cauliflower florets	1 tbsp fresh parsley, chopped
1/2 cup heavy cream	1/2 cup vegetable stock
1 tbsp garlic, minced	1 tbsp rosemary, chopped
1 tbsp olive oil	1 onion, chopped
Pepper	Salt

1. Add oil into the inner pot of instant pot and set the pot on sauté mode.
2. Add onion and sauté for 5 minutes.
3. Add remaining ingredients except for parsley and heavy cream and stir well.
4. Seal pot with lid and cook on high for 10 minutes.
5. Once done, allow to release pressure naturally for 10 minutes then release remaining using quick release. Remove lid.
6. Add cream and stir well. Blend cauliflower mixture using immersion blender until smooth.
7. Garnish with parsley and serve.

NUTRITION:
Calories 128 Fat 9.4 g Carbohydrates 10.4 g Sugar 4 g Protein 3.1 g Cholesterol 21 mg

464. Tomato Olive Salsa

Preparation Time: 10 minutes | Cooking Time: 5 minutes | Servings: 4

2 cups olives, pitted and chopped	1/4 cup fresh parsley, chopped
1/4 cup fresh basil, chopped	2 tbsp green onion, chopped
1 cup grape tomatoes, halved	1 tbsp olive oil
1 tbsp vinegar	Pepper
Salt	

1. Add all ingredients into the inner pot of instant pot and stir well.
2. Seal pot with lid and cook on high for 5 minutes.
3. Once done, allow to release pressure naturally for 5 minutes then release remaining using quick release. Remove lid.
4. Stir well and serve.

NUTRITION:
Calories 119 Fat 10.8 g Carbohydrates 6.5 g Sugar 1.3 g Protein 1.2 g Cholesterol 0 mg

465. Easy Tomato Dip

Preparation Time: 10 minutes | Cooking Time: 13 minutes | Servings: 4

2 cups tomato puree	1/2 tsp ground cumin
1 tsp garlic, minced	1/4 cup vinegar
1 onion, chopped	1 tbsp olive oil
Pepper	Salt

1. Add oil into the inner pot of instant pot and set the pot on sauté mode.
2. Add onion and sauté for 3 minutes.
3. Add remaining ingredients and stir well.
4. Seal pot with lid and cook on high for 10 minutes.
5. Once done, allow to release pressure naturally for 10 minutes then release remaining using quick release. Remove lid.
6. Blend tomato mixture using an immersion blender until smooth.
7. Serve and enjoy.

NUTRITION:
Calories 94 Fat 3.9 g Carbohydrates 14.3 g Sugar 7.3 g Protein 2.5 g Cholesterol 0 mg

466. Balsamic Bell Pepper Salsa

Preparation Time: 10 minutes | Cooking Time: 6 minutes | Servings: 2

2 red bell peppers, chopped and seeds removed	1 cup grape tomatoes, halved
1/2 tbsp cayenne	1 tbsp balsamic vinegar
2 cup vegetable broth	1/2 cup sour cream
1/2 tsp garlic powder	1/2 onion, chopped
Salt	

1. Add all ingredients except cream into the instant pot and stir well.
2. Seal pot with lid and cook on high for 6 minutes.
3. Once done, release pressure using quick release. Remove lid.
4. Add sour cream and stir well.
5. Blend the salsa mixture using an immersion blender until smooth.
6. Serve and enjoy.

NUTRITION:
Calories 235 Fat 14.2 g Carbohydrates 19.8 g Sugar 10.7 g Protein 9.2 g Cholesterol 25 mg

467. Spicy Chicken Dip

Preparation Time: 10 minutes | Cooking Time: 15 minutes | Servings: 10

1 lb chicken breast, skinless and boneless	1/2 cup sour cream
8 oz cheddar cheese, shredded	1/2 cup chicken stock
2 jalapeno pepper, sliced	8 oz cream cheese
Pepper	Salt

1. Add chicken, stock, jalapenos, and cream cheese into the instant pot.
2. Seal pot with lid and cook on high for 12 minutes.
3. Once done, release pressure using quick release. Remove lid.
4. Shred chicken using a fork.
5. Set pot on sauté mode. Add remaining ingredients and stir well and cook until cheese is melted.

NUTRITION:
Calories 248 Fat 19 g Carbohydrates 1.6 g Sugar 0.3 g Protein 17.4 g Cholesterol 83 mg

468. Slow Cooked Cheesy Artichoke Dip

Preparation Time: 10 minutes | Cooking Time: 60 minutes | Servings: 6

10 oz can artichoke hearts, drained and chopped	4 cups spinach, chopped
8 oz cream cheese	3 tbsp sour cream
1/4 cup mayonnaise	3/4 cup mozzarella cheese, shredded
1/4 cup parmesan cheese, grated	3 garlic cloves, minced
1/2 tsp dried parsley	Pepper
Salt	

1. Add all ingredients into the inner pot of instant pot and stir well.
2. Seal the pot with the lid and select slow cook mode and set the timer for 60 minutes. Stir once while cooking.
3. Serve and enjoy.

NUTRITION:

Calories 226 Fat 19.3 g Carbohydrates 7.5 g Sugar 1.2 g Protein 6.8 g Cholesterol 51 mg

469. Olive Eggplant Spread

Preparation: 10 minutes Cooking Time: 8 minutes Servings: 12

1 3/4 lbs eggplant, chopped	1/2 tbsp dried oregano
1/4 cup olives, pitted and chopped	1 tbsp tahini
1/4 cup fresh lime juice	1/2 cup water
2 garlic cloves	1/4 cup olive oil
Salt	

1. Add oil into the inner pot of instant pot and set the pot on sauté mode.
2. Add eggplant and cook for 3-5 minutes. Turn off sauté mode.
3. Add water and salt and stir well.

4. Seal pot with lid and cook on high for 3 minutes.
5. Once done, release pressure using quick release. Remove lid.
6. Drain eggplant well and transfer into the food processor.
7. Add remaining ingredients into the food processor and process until smooth.
8. Serve and enjoy.

NUTRITION:

Calories 65 Fat 5.3 g Carbohydrates 4.7 g Sugar 2 g Protein 0.9 g Cholesterol 0 mg

470. Pepper Tomato Eggplant Spread

Preparation Time: 10 minutes | Cooking Time: 10 minutes | Servings: 3

2 cups eggplant, chopped	1/4 cup vegetable broth
2 tbsp tomato paste	1/4 cup sun-dried tomatoes, minced
1 cup bell pepper, chopped	1 tsp garlic, minced
1 cup onion, chopped	3 tbsp olive oil
Salt	

1. Add oil into the inner pot of instant pot and set the pot on sauté mode.
2. Add onion and sauté for 3 minutes.
3. Add eggplant, bell pepper, and garlic and sauté for 2 minutes.
4. Add remaining ingredients and stir well.
5. Seal pot with lid and cook on high for 5 minutes.
6. Once done, release pressure using quick release. Remove lid.
7. Lightly mash the eggplant mixture using a potato masher.
8. Stir well and serve.

NUTRITION:

Calories 178 Fat 14.4 g Carbohydrates 12.8 g Sugar 7 g Protein 2.4 g Cholesterol 0 mg

471. Vanilla Apple Compote

Preparation Time: 10 minutes | Cooking Time: 15 minutes | Servings: 6

3 cups apples, cored and cubed
3/4 cup coconut sugar
2 tbsp fresh lime juice
1 tsp vanilla
1 cup of water

1. Add all ingredients into the inner pot of instant pot and stir well.
2. Seal pot with lid and cook on high for 15 minutes.
3. Once done, allow to release pressure naturally for 10 minutes then release remaining using quick release. Remove lid.
4. Stir and serve.

NUTRITION:
Calories 76 Fat 0.2 g Carbohydrates 19.1 g Sugar 11.9 g Protein 0.5 g Cholesterol 0 mg

472. Apple Dates Mix

Preparation Time: 10 minutes | Cooking Time: 15 minutes | Servings: 4

4 apples, cored and cut into chunks
1 tsp cinnamon
1 1/2 cups apple juice
1 tsp vanilla
1/2 cup dates, pitted

1. Add all ingredients into the inner pot of instant pot and stir well.
2. Seal pot with lid and cook on high for 15 minutes.
3. Once done, allow to release pressure naturally for 10 minutes then release remaining using quick release. Remove lid.
4. Stir and serve.

NUTRITION:
Calories 226 Fat 0.6 g Carbohydrates 58.6 g Sugar 46.4 g Protein 1.3 g Cholesterol 0 mg

473. Choco Rice Pudding

Preparation Time: 10 minutes | Cooking Time: 20 minutes | Servings: 4

1 1/4 cup rice
1 tsp vanilla
1 tsp liquid stevia
1/4 cup dark chocolate, chopped
1/3 cup coconut butter
2 1/2 cups almond milk

1. Add all ingredients into the inner pot of instant pot and stir well.
2. Seal pot with lid and cook on high for 20 minutes.
3. Once done, allow to release pressure naturally. Remove lid.
4. Stir well and serve.

NUTRITION:
Calories 632 Fat 39.9 g Carbohydrates 63.5 g Sugar 12.5 g Protein 8.6 g Cholesterol 2 mg

474. Grapes Stew

Preparation: 10 minutes   Cooking: 15 minutes   Servings: 4

1 cup grapes, halved
1 tbsp fresh lemon juice
2 cups rhubarb, chopped
1 tsp vanilla
1 tbsp honey
2 cups of water

1. Add all ingredients into the inner pot of instant pot and stir well.
2. Seal pot with lid and cook on high for 15 minutes.
3. Once done, allow to release pressure naturally for 10 minutes then release remaining using quick release. Remove lid.
4. Stir and serve.

NUTRITION:
Calories 48 Fat 0.2 g Carbohydrates 11.3 g Sugar 8.9 g Protein 0.7 g Cholesterol 0 mg

475. Chocolate Rice

Preparation Time: 10 minutes | Cooking Time: 20 minutes | Servings: 4

1 cup of rice
2 tbsp maple syrup
1 tbsp cocoa powder
2 cups almond milk

1. Add all ingredients into the inner pot of instant pot and stir well.
2. Seal pot with lid and cook on high for 20 minutes.
3. Once done, allow to release pressure naturally for 10 minutes then release remaining using quick release. Remove lid.
4. Stir and serve.

NUTRITION:
Calories 474 Fat 29.1 g Carbohydrates 51.1 g Sugar 10 g Protein 6.3 g Cholesterol 0 mg

476. Raisins Cinnamon Peaches

Preparation Time: 10 minutes | Cooking Time: 15 minutes | Servings: 4

4 peaches, cored and cut into chunks
1 tsp cinnamon
1 cup of water
1 tsp vanilla
1/2 cup raisins

1. Add all ingredients into the inner pot of instant pot and stir well.
2. Seal pot with lid and cook on high for 15 minutes.
3. Once done, allow to release pressure naturally for 10 minutes then release remaining using quick release. Remove lid.
4. Stir and serve.

NUTRITION:
Calories 118 Fat 0.5 g Carbohydrates 29 g Sugar 24.9 g Protein 2 g Cholesterol 0 mg

477. Lemon Pear Compote

Preparation Time: 10 minutes | Cooking Time: 15 minutes | Servings: 6

3 cups pears, cored and cut into chunks
1 tsp liquid stevia
2 tbsp lemon juice
1 tsp vanilla
1 tbsp lemon zest, grated

1. Add all ingredients into the inner pot of instant pot and stir well.
2. Seal pot with lid and cook on high for 15 minutes.
3. Once done, allow to release pressure naturally for 10 minutes then release remaining using quick release. Remove lid.
4. Stir and serve.

NUTRITION:
Calories 50 Fat 0.2 g Carbohydrates 12.7 g Sugar 8.1 g Protein 0.4 g Cholesterol 0 mg

478. Strawberry Stew

Preparation Time: 10 minutes | Cooking Time: 15 minutes | Servings: 4

12 oz fresh strawberries, sliced	1 tsp vanilla
1 1/2 cups water	1 tsp liquid stevia
2 tbsp lime juice	

1. Add all ingredients into the inner pot of instant pot and stir well.
2. Seal pot with lid and cook on high for 15 minutes.
3. Once done, allow to release pressure naturally for 10 minutes then release remaining using quick release. Remove lid.
4. Stir and serve.

NUTRITION:
Calories 36 Fat 0.3 g Carbohydrates 8.5 g Sugar 4.7 g Protein 0.7 g Cholesterol 0 mg

479. Walnut Apple Pear Mix

Preparation Time: 10 minutes | Cooking Time: 10 minutes | Servings: 4

2 apples, cored and cut into wedges	1/2 tsp vanilla
1 cup apple juice	2 tbsp walnuts, chopped
2 apples, cored and cut into wedges	

1. Add all ingredients into the inner pot of instant pot and stir well.
2. Seal pot with lid and cook on high for 10 minutes.
3. Once done, allow to release pressure naturally for 10 minutes then release remaining using quick release. Remove lid.
4. Serve and enjoy.

NUTRITION:
Calories 132 Fat 2.6 g Carbohydrates 28.3 g Sugar 21.9 g Protein 1.3 g Cholesterol 0 mg

480. Cinnamon Pear Jam

Preparation Time: 10 minutes | Cooking Time: 4 minutes | Servings: 12

8 pears, cored and cut into quarters	1 tsp cinnamon
1/4 cup apple juice	2 apples, peeled, cored and diced

1. Add all ingredients into the inner pot of instant pot and stir well.
2. Seal pot with lid and cook on high for 4 minutes.
3. Once done, allow to release pressure naturally. Remove lid.
4. Blend pear apple mixture using an immersion blender until smooth.
5. Serve and enjoy.

NUTRITION:
Calories 103 Fat 0.3 g Carbohydrates 27.1 g Sugar 18 g Protein 0.6 g Cholesterol 0 mg

481. Delicious Apple Pear Cobbler

Preparation Time: 10 minutes | Cooking Time: 12 minutes | Servings: 4

3 apples, cored and cut into chunks	1 cup steel-cut oats
2 pears, cored and cut into chunks	1/4 cup maple syrup
1 1/2 cups water	1 tsp cinnamon

1. Spray instant pot from inside with cooking spray.
2. Add all ingredients into the inner pot of instant pot and stir well.
3. Seal pot with lid and cook on high for 12 minutes.
4. Once done, release pressure using quick release. Remove lid.
5. Sere and enjoy.

NUTRITION:
Calories 278 Fat 1.8 g Carbohydrates 66.5 g Sugar 39.5 g Protein 3.5 g Cholesterol 0 mg

482. Coconut Rice Pudding

Preparation Time: 10 minutes | Cooking Time: 3 minutes | Servings: 4

1/2 cup rice	1/4 cup shredded coconut
3 tbsp swerve	1 1/2 cups water
14 oz can coconut milk	Pinch of salt

1. Spray instant pot from inside with cooking spray.
2. Add all ingredients into the inner pot of instant pot and stir well.
3. Seal pot with lid and cook on high for 3 minutes.
4. Once done, allow to release pressure naturally for 10 minutes then release remaining using quick release. Remove lid.
5. Serve and enjoy.

NUTRITION:
Calories 298 Fat 23 g Carbohydrates 33.3 gSugar 11.6 g Protein 3.8 g Cholesterol 0 mg

483. Pear Sauce

Preparation Time: 10 minutes | Cooking Time: 15 minutes | Servings: 6

10 pears, sliced	1 cup apple juice
1 1/2 tsp cinnamon	1/4 tsp nutmeg

1. Add all ingredients into the instant pot and stir well.
2. Seal pot with lid and cook on high for 15 minutes.
3. Once done, allow to release pressure naturally for 10 minutes then release remaining using quick release. Remove lid.
4. Blend the pear mixture using an immersion blender until smooth.
5. Serve and enjoy.

NUTRITION:
Calories 222 Fat 0.6 g Carbohydrates 58.2 g Sugar 38 g Protein 1.3 g Cholesterol 0 mg

484. Sweet Peach Jam

Preparation Time: 10 minutes | Cooking Time: 16 minutes | Servings: 20

1 1/2 lb fresh peaches, pitted and chopped	1/2 tbsp vanilla
1/4 cup maple syrup	

1. Add all ingredients into the instant pot and stir well.
2. Seal pot with lid and cook on high for 1 minute.
3. Once done, allow to release pressure naturally. Remove lid.
4. Set pot on sauté mode and cook for 15 minutes or until jam thickened.
5. Pour into the container and store it in the fridge.

NUTRITION:
Calories 16 Fat 0 g Carbohydrates 3.7 g Sugar 3.4 g Protein 0.1 g Cholesterol 0 mg

485. Warm Peach Compote

Preparation Time: 10 minutes | Cooking Time: 1 minute | Servings: 4

4 peaches, peeled and chopped	1 tbsp water
1/2 tbsp cornstarch	1 tsp vanilla

1. Add water, vanilla, and peaches into the instant pot.
2. Seal pot with lid and cook on high for 1 minute.
3. Once done, allow to release pressure naturally. Remove lid.
4. In a small bowl, whisk together 1 tablespoon of water and cornstarch and pour into the pot and stir well.
5. Serve and enjoy.

NUTRITION:
Calories 66 Fat 0.4 g Carbohydrates 15 g Sugar 14.1 g Protein 1.4 g Cholesterol 0 mg

486. Spiced Pear Sauce

Preparation Time: 10 minutes | Cooking Time: 6 hours | Servings: 12

8 pears, cored and diced
1/4 tsp ground nutmeg
1 cup of water
1/2 tsp ground cinnamon
1/4 tsp ground cardamom

1. Add all ingredients into the instant pot and stir well.
2. Seal the pot with a lid and select slow cook mode and cook on low for 6 hours.
3. Mash the sauce using potato masher.
4. Pour into the container and store it in the fridge.

NUTRITION:
Calories 81 Fat 0.2 g Carbohydrates 21.4 g Sugar 13.6 g Protein 0.5 g Cholesterol 0 mg

487. Honey Fruit Compote

Preparation Time: 10 minutes | Cooking Time: 3 minutes | Servings: 4

1/3 cup honey
1 1/2 cups raspberries
1 1/2 cups blueberries

1. Add all ingredients into the instant pot and stir well.
2. Seal pot with lid and cook on high for 3 minutes.
3. Once done, allow to release pressure naturally. Remove lid.
4. Serve and enjoy.

NUTRITION:
Calories 141 Fat 0.5 g Carbohydrates 36.7 g Sugar 30.6 g Protein 1 g Cholesterol 0 mg

488. Creamy Brown Rice Pudding

Preparation Time: 10 minutes | Cooking Time: 20 minutes | Servings: 8

1 cup of rice
1 cup of water
1/2 cup pecans, chopped
1 tbsp coconut butter
Pinch of salt
1 cup of brown rice
1 cup half and half
2 tsp vanilla
1/2 cup heavy cream

1. Add coconut butter into the instant pot and set the pot on sauté mode.
2. Add pecans into the pot and stir until toasted.
3. Add remaining ingredients except for heavy cream and vanilla. Stir well.
4. Seal pot with lid and cook on high for 20 minutes.
5. Once done, allow to release pressure naturally for 10 minutes then release remaining using quick release. Remove lid.
6. Add vanilla and heavy cream. Stir well and serve.

NUTRITION:
Calories 276 Fat 10.9 g Carbohydrates 39.2 g Sugar 0.5 g Protein 5 g Cholesterol 21 mg

489. Lemon Cranberry Sauce

Preparation Time: 10 minutes | Cooking Time: 14 minutes | Servings: 8

10 oz fresh cranberries
1/4 cup water
1 tsp vanilla extract
3/4 cup Swerve
1 tsp lemon zest

1. Add cranberries and water into the instant pot.
2. Seal pot with lid and cook on high for 1 minute.
3. Once done, allow to release pressure naturally for 10 minutes then release remaining using quick release. Remove lid.
4. Set pot on sauté mode.
5. Add remaining ingredients and cook for 2-3 minutes.
6. Pour in container and store in fridge.

NUTRITION:

Calories 21 Carbohydrates 25.8 g Sugar 23.9 g Protein 0 g

490. Blackberry Jam

Preparation Time: 10 minutes | Cooking Time: 6 hours | Servings: 6

3 cups fresh blackberries
4 tbsp Swerve
1/4 cup coconut butter
1/4 cup chia seeds
1/4 cup fresh lemon juice

1. Add all ingredients into the instant pot and stir well.
2. Seal the pot with a lid and select slow cook mode and cook on low for 6 hours.
3. Pour in container and store in fridge.

NUTRITION:
Calories 101 Fat 6.8 g Carbohydrates 20 g Sugar 14.4 g Protein 2 g Cholesterol 0 mg

491. Chunky Apple Sauce

Preparation: 10 minutes   Cooking: 12 minutes   Servings: 16

4 apples, peeled, cored and diced
4 pears, diced
1/4 cup maple syrup
1 tsp vanilla
2 tbsp cinnamon
3/4 cup water

1. Add all ingredients into the instant pot and stir well.
2. Seal pot with lid and cook on high for 12 minutes.
3. Once done, allow to release pressure naturally for 10 minutes then release remaining using quick release. Remove lid.
4. Serve and enjoy.

NUTRITION:
Calories 75 Fat 0.2 g Carbohydrates 19.7 g Sugar 13.9 g Protein 0.4 g Cholesterol 0 mg

492. Maple Syrup Cranberry Sauce

Preparation: 10 minutes   Cooking: 5 minutes   Servings: 8

12 oz fresh cranberries, rinsed
1/2 cup maple syrup
1 tsp orange zest, grated
1 apple, peeled, cored, and chopped
1/2 cup apple cider
1 orange juice

1. Add all ingredients into the instant pot and stir well.
2. Seal pot with lid and cook on high for 5 minutes.
3. Once done, allow to release pressure naturally for 10 minutes then release remaining using quick release. Remove lid.
4. Pour in container and store in fridge.

NUTRITION:
Calories 101 Fat 0.1 g Carbohydrates 23.9 g Sugar 18.8 g Protein 0.2 g Cholesterol 0 mg

493. Raisin Pecan Baked Apples

Preparation: 10 minutes   Cooking: 4 minutes   Servings: 6

6 apples, cored and cut into wedges
1/4 cup pecans, chopped
1/4 tsp nutmeg
1/3 cup honey
1 cup red wine
1/4 cup raisins
1 tsp cinnamon

1. Add all ingredients into the instant pot and stir well.
2. Seal pot with lid and cook on high for 4 minutes.
3. Once done, allow to release pressure naturally for 10 minutes then release remaining using quick release. Remove lid.
4. Stir well and serve.

NUTRITION:
Calories 229 Fat 0.9 g Carbohydrates 52.6 g Sugar 42.6 g Protein 1 g Cholesterol 0 mg

494. Healthy Zucchini Pudding

Preparation: 10 minutes   Cooking: 10 minutes   Servings: 4

2 cups zucchini, shredded	1/4 tsp cardamom powder
5 oz half and half	5 oz almond milk
1/4 cup Swerve	

1. Add all ingredients except cardamom into the instant pot and stir well.
2. Seal pot with lid and cook on high for 10 minutes.
3. Once done, allow to release pressure naturally for 10 minutes then release remaining using quick release. Remove lid.
4. Stir in cardamom and serve.

NUTRITION:

Calories 137 Fat 12.6 g Carbohydrates 20.5 g Sugar 17.2 g Protein 2.6 g Cholesterol 13 mg

495. Cinnamon Apple Rice Pudding

Preparation: 10 minutes Cooking: 15 minutes Servings: 8

1 cup of rice	1 tsp vanilla
1/4 apple, peeled and chopped	1/2 cup water
1 1/2 cup almond milk	1 tsp cinnamon
1 cinnamon stick	

1. Add all ingredients into the instant pot and stir well.
2. Seal pot with lid and cook on high for 15 minutes.
3. Once done, release pressure using quick release. Remove lid.
4. Stir and serve.

NUTRITION:

Calories 206 Fat 11.5 g Carbohydrates 23.7 g Sugar 2.7 g Protein 3 g Cholesterol 0 mg

496. Coconut Risotto Pudding

Preparation: 10 minutes Cooking: 20 minutes Servings: 6

3/4 cup rice	1/2 cup shredded coconut
1 tsp lemon juice	1/2 tsp vanilla
oz can coconut milk	1/4 cup maple syrup
1 1/2 cups water	

1. Add all ingredients into the instant pot and stir well.
2. Seal pot with lid and cook on high for 20 minutes.
3. Once done, allow to release pressure naturally for 10 minutes then release remaining using quick release. Remove lid.
4. Blend pudding mixture using an immersion blender until smooth.
5. Serve and enjoy.

NUTRITION:

Calories 205 Fat 8.6 g Carbohydrates 29.1 g Sugar 9 g Protein 2.6 g Cholesterol 0 mg

497. Mediterranean Baked Apples

Servings: 4, Cooking Time: 25 minutes

1.5 pounds apples, peeled and sliced	Juice from ½ lemon
A dash of cinnamon	

1. Preheat the oven to 2500F.
2. Line a baking sheet with parchment paper then set aside.
3. In a medium bowl, apples with lemon juice and cinnamon.
4. Place the apples on the parchment paper-lined baking sheet.
5. Bake for 25 minutes until crisp.

NUTRITION:

Calories: 90; Carbs: 23.9g; Protein: 0.5g; Fat: 0.3g

498. Mediterranean Diet Cookie Recipe

Servings: 12, Cooking Time: 40 minutes

1 tsp vanilla extract	½ tsp salt
4 large egg whites	1 ¼ cups sugar
2 cups toasted and skinned hazelnuts	

1. Preheat oven to 325oF and position oven rack in the center. Then line with baking paper your baking pan.
2. In a food processor, finely grind the hazelnuts and then transfer into a medium sized bowl.
3. In a large mixing bowl, on high speed beat salt and egg whites until stiff and there is formation of peaks. Then gently fold in the ground nut and vanilla until thoroughly mixed.
4. Drop a spoonful of the mixture onto prepared pan and bake the cookies for twenty minutes or until lightly browned per batch. Bake 6 cookies per cookie sheet.
5. Let it cool on pan for five minutes before removing.

NUTRITION:

Calorie per Servings: 173; Carbs: 23.0g; Protein: 3.1g; Fats: 7.6g

499. Mediterranean Style Fruit Medley

Servings: 7, Cooking Time: 5 minutes

4 fuyu persimmons, sliced into wedges	1 ½ cups grapes, halved
8 mint leaves, chopped	1 tablespoon lemon juice
1 tablespoon honey	½ cups almond, toasted and chopped

1. Combine all Ingredients in a bowl.
2. Toss then chill before serving.

NUTRITION:

Calories per serving: 159; Carbs: 32g; Protein: 3g; Fat: 4g

500. Mediterranean Watermelon Salad

Servings: 6, Cooking Time: 2 minutes

6 cups mixed salad greens, torn	3 cups watermelon, seeded and cubed
½ cup onion, sliced	1 tablespoon extra-virgin olive oil
1/3 cup feta cheese, crumbled	Cracked black pepper

1. In a large bowl, mix all ingredients.
2. Toss to combine everything.
3. Allow to chill before serving.

NUTRITION:

Calories: 91; Carbs: 15.2g; Protein: 1.9g; Fat: 2.8g

501. Melon Cucumber Smoothie

Servings: 2, Cooking Time: 5 minutes

½ cucumber	2 slices of melon
2 tablespoons lemon juice	1 pear, peeled and sliced
3 fresh mint leaves	½ cup almond milk

1. Place all Ingredients in a blender.
2. Blend until smooth.
3. Pour in a glass container and allow to chill in the fridge for at least 30 minutes.

NUTRITION:

Calories: 253; Carbs: 59.3g; Protein: 5.7g; Fat: 2.1g

502.   Peanut Banana Yogurt Bowl
Servings: 4, Cooking Time: 15 minutes

4 cups Greek yogurt
¼ cup creamy natural peanut butter
1 teaspoon nutmeg

2 medium bananas, sliced
¼ cup flax seed meal

1. Divide the yogurt between four bowls and top with banana, peanut butter, and flax seed meal.
2. Garnish with nutmeg.
3. Chill before serving.

NUTRITION:
Calories: 370; Carbs: 47.7g; Protein: 22.7g; Fat: 10.6g

503.   Pomegranate and Lychee Sorbet
Servings: 6, Cooking Time: 5 minutes

¾ cup dragon fruit cubes
Juice from 1 lemon
2 tablespoons pomegranate seeds

8 lychees, peeled and pitted
3 tablespoons stevia sugar

1. In a blender, combine, the dragon fruit, lychees, lemon, and stevia sugar.
2. Pulse until smooth.
3. Pour the mixture in a container with lid and place inside the fridge.
4. Allow sorbet to harden for at least 8 hours.
5. Sprinkle with pomegranate seeds before serving.

NUTRITION:
Calories per serving: 214; Carbs: 30.4g; Protein: 1.9g; Fat: 1.2g

504.   Pomegranate Granita with Lychee
Servings: 7, Cooking Time: 5 minutes

500 millimeters pomegranate juice, organic and sugar-free
½ cup lychee syrup
4 mint leaves

1 cup water

2 tablespoons lemon juice
1 cup fresh lychees, pitted and sliced

1. Place all Ingredients in a large pitcher.
2. Place inside the fridge to cool before serving.

NUTRITION:
Calories: 96; Carbs: 23.8g; Protein: 0.4g; Fat: 0.4g

505.   Roasted Berry and Honey Yogurt Pops
Servings: 8, Cooking Time: 15 minutes

12 ounces mixed berries
2 tablespoons honey
½ small lemon, juice

A dash of sea salt
2 cups whole Greek yogurt

1. Preheat the oven to 3500F.
2. Line a baking sheet with parchment paper then set aside.
3. In a medium bowl, toss the berries with sea salt and honey.
4. Pour the berries on the prepared baking sheet.
5. Roast for 30 minutes while stirring halfway.
6. While the fruit is roasting, blend the Greek yogurt and lemon juice. Add honey to taste if desired.
7. Once the berries are done, cool for at least ten minutes.
8. Fold the berries into the yogurt mixture.
9. Pour into popsicle molds and allow to freeze for at least 8 hours.
10. Serve chilled.

NUTRITION:
Calories: 177; Carbs: 24.8g; Protein: 3.2g; Fat: 7.9g

506.   Scrumptious Cake with Cinnamon
Servings: 8, Cooking Time: 40 minutes

1 lemon
1 tsp cinnamon
½ lb. ground almonds

4 eggs
¼ lb. sugar

1. Preheat oven to 350oF. Then grease a cake pan and set aside.
2. On high speed, beat for three minutes the sugar and eggs or until the volume is doubled.
3. Then with a spatula, gently fold in the lemon zest, cinnamon and almond flour until well mixed.
4. Then pour batter on prepared pan and bake for forty minutes or until golden brown.
5. Let cool before serving.

NUTRITION:
Calorie per Servings: 253; Carbs: 21.1g; Protein: 8.8g; Fats: 16.3g

507.   Smoothie Bowl with Dragon Fruit
Servings: 4, Cooking Time: 5 minutes

¼ of dragon fruit, peeled and sliced
2 cups baby greens (mixed)

1 cup frozen berries
½ cup coconut meat

1. Place all Ingredients in a blender and pulse until smooth.
2. Place on a bowl and allow to cool in the fridge for at least 20 minutes.
3. Garnish with whatever fruits or nuts available in your fridge.

NUTRITION:
Calories: 190; Carbs: 19g; Protein: 5g; Fat: 13g

508.   Soothing Red Smoothie
Servings: 2, Cooking Time: 3 minutes

4 plums, pitted
¼ cup blueberry
1 tablespoon linseed oil

¼ cup raspberry
1 tablespoon lemon juice

1. Place all Ingredients in a blender.
2. Blend until smooth.
3. Pour in a glass container and allow to chill in the fridge for at least 30 minutes.

NUTRITION:
Calories: 201; Carbs: 36.4g; Protein: 0.8g; Fat: 7.1g

509.   Strawberry and Avocado Medley
Servings: 4, Cooking Time: 5 minutes

2 cups strawberry, halved
2 tablespoons slivered almonds

1 avocado, pitted and sliced

1. Place all Ingredients in a mixing bowl.
2. Toss to combine.
3. Allow to chill in the fridge before serving.

NUTRITION:
Calories: 107; Carbs: 9.9g; Protein: 1.6g; Fat: 7.8g

510. Strawberry Banana Greek Yogurt Parfaits
Servings: 4, Cooking Time: 5 minutes

1 cup plain Greek yogurt, chilled
½ cup chopped strawberries

1 cup pepitas
½ banana, sliced

1. In a parfait glass, add the yogurt at the bottom of the glass.
2. Add a layer of pepitas, strawberries, and bananas.
3. Continue to layer the Ingredients until the entire glass is filled.

NUTRITION:
Calories per serving: 387; Carbs: 69.6g; Protein: 18.1g; Fat: 1g

511. Summertime Fruit Salad

Servings: 6, Cooking Time: 5 minutes

1-pound strawberries, hulled and sliced thinly
6 ounces blueberries
2 tablespoons lemon juice
2 teaspoons balsamic vinegar

3 medium peaches, sliced thinly
1 tablespoon fresh mint, chopped
1 tablespoon honey

1. In a salad bowl, combine all ingredients.
2. Gently toss to coat all ingredients.
3. Chill for at least 30 minutes before serving.

NUTRITION:
Calories: 146; Carbs: 22.8g; Protein: 8.1g; Fat: 3.4g

512. Sweet Tropical Medley Smoothie

Servings: 4, Preparation Time: 10 minutes Cooking time: 5 minutes

1 banana, peeled
1 cup fresh pineapple

1 sliced mango
½ cup coconut water

1. Place all Ingredients in a blender.
2. Blend until smooth.
3. Pour in a glass container and allow to chill in the fridge for at least 30 minutes.

NUTRITION:
Calories per serving: 73; Carbs: 18.6g; Protein: 0.8g; Fat: 0.5g.

CONCLUSION

The Mediterranean diet is the regime you've been waiting for that won't break your bank, isolate you from your friends and family, or cause you to bounce back to a size seventeen after only a few months. By now, you should have a keen understanding of what eating like a Mediterranean's means - and if you weren't entirely won over by the promise of carbs for life, we hope the weight loss and health benefits alone have swayed you in the direction of changing your life. When you commit to a Mediterranean diet, you commit to lots of healthy fats and oils, lots of time with your friends and family, and lots more years of health to come in the future. Don't give up, and don't forget that your body is yours, and yours only – so treat it kindly! Thanks for sticking with us as we walked you through all the ins and outs of the Mediterranean diet, and we wish you the best of luck on your journey towards a healthier, thinner, and more coastal-minded you

THE SUPER EASY
MEDITERRANEAN
DIET COOKBOOK
FOR BEGINNERS

250

QUICK AND SCRUMPTIOUS RECIPES WITH 5 OR
LESS INGREDIENTS
2-WEEK MEAL PLAN INCLUDED

By

Wilda Buckley

INTRODUCTION

The Mediterranean diet is straightforward, easy to follow, and delicious; your transition to this diet will be a lot easier and smoother if you do a little bit of preparation beforehand.

You must have the right ingredients on hand, know about some of the foods you'll be eating, and have an idea of the meals you'd like to prepare. You'll also want to gradually (or immediately, if you're eager) rid the house of the foods that you'll no longer be eating.

While there are no supplements or specially packaged foods to buy, there are several key ingredients that you'll need to stock up on, and you'll also want to locate sources for the freshest and most healthful fruits, vegetables, and fish.

Preparing for the Mediterranean diet is largely about preparing yourself for a new way of eating, adjusting your attitude toward food into one of joyful expectation and appreciation of good meals and good company. It's like a mindset as anything else, so you'll want to make your environment one in which the Mediterranean way of eating can be naturally followed and easily enjoyed.

Preparing for the Mediterranean diet can be as simple as getting out the good dishes so that you can fully enjoy your meals or visiting a few local markets to check out the freshness and prices of their offerings.

You can take a month to prepare your pantry and yourself, or you can take just a few days, but a little time spent in advance can make all the difference in those first few weeks of your healthful new lifestyle.

You don't need to go out and buy special appliances, hard-to-find or expensive ingredients, special supplements, or even new workout gear on the Mediterranean diet. Still, a few things will make your transition to the diet easier and more fun.

Before starting the diet, it would be helpful to spend a week or two cutting back on the least healthy foods you are currently eating. You might start with fast food if you frequent the drive-through or eliminate cream-based sauces and soups. You can then start cutting back on processed foods like chips, boxed dinners, and frozen meals.

Some other things to start trimming might be sodas, coffee with a lot of milk and sugar, butter, and red meats such as beef, pork, and lamb. You don't have to eliminate these things during this period, but you'd be surprised at how quickly your body adjusts if you gradually wean yourself from them. It can make it much easier to adapt to the diet once you do begin in earnest.

The Mediterranean diet isn't just a way to eat; it's a way to love eating. Don't just engage in the diet, consider trying out their culture as well; where seasonal and fresh ingredients are cherished, dishes are generously shared and simply prepared, and lastly, time is very well-spent by lingering over a conversation, food, and wine.

Having the lifestyle in the Mediterranean way can not only improve your health and help you lose weight, but it can also encourage you to slow down, at least two or three times a day, and take a break from a hectic schedule and a busy life.

Have fun discovering the Mediterranean diet; consider spending weekends at your local farmers' market and have an adventure trying out various ingredients. Have more quality time with your family and friends by simply sharing your delicious meals.

The Mediterranean diet isn't just about having a healthy life; it's about having great pleasure and happiness!

APPETIZER AND SNACK RECIPES

513. Light & Creamy Garlic Hummus

Preparation 10 minutes Cooking: 40 minutes Servings: 12

1 1/2 cups dry chickpeas, rinsed
1 tbsp. garlic, minced
6 cups of water

2 1/2 tbsp. fresh lemon juice
1/2 cup tahini

1. Add water and chickpeas into the instant pot.
2. Seal pot with a lid and select manual and set timer for 40 minutes.
3. Once done, allow to release pressure naturally. Remove lid.
4. Drain chickpeas well and reserved 1/2 cup chickpeas liquid.
5. Transfer chickpeas, reserved liquid, lemon juice, garlic, tahini, pepper, and salt into the food processor and process until smooth.
6. Serve and enjoy.

Nutrition:
152 Calories 6.9g Fat 17g Carbohydrates

514. Perfect Queso

Preparation: 10 minutes Cooking: 15 minutes Servings: 16

1 lb. ground beef
10 oz. can tomato, diced
1 tsp chili powder

32 oz. Velveeta cheese, cut into cubes
1 1/2 tbsp. taco seasoning

1. Set instant pot on sauté mode.
2. Add meat, 1 onion, taco seasoning, chili powder, pepper, and salt into the pot and cook until meat is no longer pink.
3. Add tomatoes and stir well. Top with cheese and do not stir.
4. Seal pot with lid and cook on high for 4 minutes.
5. Once done, release pressure using quick release. Remove lid.
6. Stir everything well and serve.

Nutrition:
257 Calories 15.9g Fat 10.2g Carbohydrates

515. Creamy Potato Spread

Preparation Time: 10 minutes Cooking Time: 15 minutes Servings: 6

1 lb. sweet potatoes, peeled and chopped
1/2 tsp paprika
1 cup tomato puree

3/4 tbsp. fresh chives, chopped
1 tbsp. garlic, minced

1. Add all ingredients except chives into the inner pot of instant pot and stir well.
2. Seal pot with lid and cook on high for 15 minutes.
3. When done, release pressure naturally for 10 minutes then releases remaining using quick release. Remove lid.
4. Transfer instant pot sweet potato mixture into the food processor and process until smooth.
5. Garnish with chives and serve.

Nutrition:
108 Calories 0.3g Fat 25.4g Carbohydrates

516. Creamy Artichoke Dip

Preparation: 10 minutes Cooking: 5 minutes Servings: 8

28 oz. can artichoke hearts, drain and quartered
1 cup sour cream, mayonnaise
1 cup of water

1 1/2 cups parmesan cheese, shredded
3.5 oz. can green chilies

1. Add artichokes, water, and green chilies into the instant pot.
2. Seal pot with the lid and select manual and set timer for 1 minute.
3. Once done, release pressure using quick release. Remove lid. Drain excess water.
4. Set instant pot on sauté mode. Cook the remaining ingredients and stir well until cheese is melted.
5. Serve and enjoy.

Nutrition:
262 Calories 7.6g Fat 14.4g Carbohydrates

517. Flavorful Roasted Baby Potatoes

Preparation Time: 10 minutes Cooking Time: 10 minutes Servings: 4

2 lbs. baby potatoes, clean and cut in half
3/4 tsp garlic powder
2 tsp Italian seasoning

1/2 cup vegetable stock
1 tsp onion powder, paprika

1. Pour oil into the inner pot of instant pot and set the pot on sauté mode.
2. Add potatoes and sauté for 5 minutes. Add remaining ingredients and stir well.
3. Seal pot with lid and cook on high for 5 minutes.
4. Once done, release pressure using quick release. Remove lid.
5. Stir well and serve.

Nutrition:
175 Calories 4.5g Fat 29.3g Carbohydrates

518. Perfect Italian Potatoes

Preparation Time: 10 minutes Cooking Time: 7 minutes Servings: 6

2 lbs. baby potatoes, clean and cut in half
6 oz. Italian dry dressing mix

3/4 cup vegetable broth

1. Incorporate all ingredients into the inner pot of instant pot and stir well.
2. Seal pot with lid and cook on high for 7 minutes.
3. Once done, allow to release pressure naturally for 3 minutes then release remaining using quick release. Remove lid.
4. Stir well and serve.

Nutrition:
149 Calories 0.3g Fat 41.6g Carbohydrates

519. Garlic Pinto Bean Dip

Preparation Time: 10 minutes Cooking Time: 43 minutes Servings: 6

1 cup dry pinto beans, rinsed
1/2 cup salsa
5 cups vegetable stock

1/2 tsp cumin
2 chipotle peppers in adobo sauce

1. Add beans, stock, 2 garlic cloves, and chipotle peppers into the instant pot.
2. Seal pot with lid and cook on high for 43 minutes.
3. Once done, release pressure using quick release. Remove lid.
4. Drain beans well and reserve 1/2 cup of stock.
5. Transfer beans, reserve stock, and remaining ingredients into the food processor and process until smooth.
6. Serve and enjoy.

Nutrition:
129 Calories 0.9g Fat 23g Carbohydrates

520. Creamy Eggplant Dip

Preparation Time: 10 minutes Cooking Time: 20 minutes Servings: 4

1 eggplant	1/2 tsp paprika
1 tbsp. fresh lime juice	2 tbsp. tahini
1 garlic clove	

1. Add 1 cup of water and eggplant into the instant pot.
2. Seal pot with the lid and select manual and set timer for 20 minutes.
3. Once done, release pressure using quick release. Remove lid.
4. Drain eggplant and let it cool.
5. Once the eggplant is cool then remove eggplant skin and transfer eggplant flesh into the food processor.
6. Pulse the remaining ingredients with food processor and process until smooth.

Nutrition:
108 Calories 7.8g Fat 9.7g Carbohydrates

521. Jalapeno Chickpea Hummus

Preparation Time: 10 minutes Cooking Time: 25 minutes Servings: 4

1 cup dry chickpeas, soaked overnight and drained	1 tsp ground cumin
1/4 cup jalapenos, diced	1/2 cup fresh cilantro
1 tbsp. tahini	

1. Add chickpeas into the instant pot and cover with vegetable stock.
2. Seal pot with lid and cook on high for 25 minutes.
3. Once done, allow to release pressure naturally. Remove lid.
4. Drain chickpeas well and transfer into the food processor along with remaining ingredients and process until smooth.
5. Serve and enjoy.

Nutrition:
425 Calories 30.4g Fat 31.8g Carbohydrates

522. Creamy Pepper Spread

Preparation Time: 10 minutes Cooking Time: 15 minutes Servings: 4

1 lb. red bell peppers, chopped and remove seeds	1 1/2 tbsp. fresh basil
1 tbsp. olive oil	1 tbsp. fresh lime juice
1 tsp garlic, minced	

1. Situate all ingredients into the inner pot of instant pot and stir well.
2. Seal pot with lid and cook on high for 15 minutes.
3. Once finish, let the pressure release naturally for 10 minutes then release the rest using quick release. Remove lid.
4. Transfer bell pepper mixture into the food processor and process until smooth.

Nutrition:
41 Calories 3.6g Fat 3.5g Carbohydrates

523. Healthy Spinach Dip

Preparation Time: 10 minutes Cooking Time: 8 minutes Servings: 4

14 oz. spinach	2 tbsp. fresh lime juice
1 tbsp. garlic, minced	2 tbsp. olive oil
2 tbsp. coconut cream	

1. Add all ingredients except coconut cream into the instant pot and stir well.
2. Seal pot with lid and cook on low pressure for 8 minutes.
3. Once done, allow to release pressure naturally for 5 minutes then release remaining using quick release. Remove lid.
4. Add coconut cream and stir well and blend spinach mixture using a blender until smooth.
5. Serve and enjoy.

Nutrition:

109 Calories 9.2g Fat 6.6g Carbohydrates

524. Spicy Chicken Dip

Preparation Time: 10 minutes Cooking Time: 15 minutes Servings: 10

1 lb. chicken breast, skinless and boneless	1/2 cup sour cream
8 oz. cheddar cheese, cream cheese	1/2 cup chicken stock
2 jalapeno pepper, sliced	

1. Add chicken, stock, jalapenos, and cream cheese into the instant pot.
2. Seal pot with lid and cook on high for 12 minutes.
3. Once done, release pressure using quick release. Remove lid.
4. Shred chicken using a fork.
5. Set pot on sauté. Put the rest of ingredients and continue cooking.
6. Serve and enjoy.

Nutrition:
248 Calories 19g Fat 1.6g Carbohydrates

525. Raisins Cinnamon Peaches

Preparation Time: 10 minutes Cooking Time: 15 minutes Servings: 4

4 peaches, cored and cut into chunks	1 tsp vanilla
1 tsp cinnamon	1/2 cup raisins
1 cup of water	

1. Mix all ingredients into the inner pot of instant pot and stir well.
2. Seal pot with lid and cook on high for 15 minutes.
3. Once cooked, release pressure naturally for 10 minutes then releases the rest by quick release. Remove lid.
4. Stir and serve.

Nutrition:
118 Calories 0.5g Fat 29g Carbohydrates

526. Lemon Pear Compote

Preparation Time: 10 minutes Cooking Time: 15 minutes Servings: 6

3 cups pears, cored and cut into chunks	1 tsp vanilla
1 tsp liquid stevia	1 tbsp. lemon zest, grated
2 tbsp. lemon juice	

1. Situate all ingredients into the inner pot of instant pot and stir well.
2. Seal pot with lid and cook on high for 15 minutes.
3. When cooked, let the pressure naturally release for 10 minutes then release remaining using quick release. Open it.
4. Stir and serve.

Nutrition:
50 Calories 0.2g Fat 12.7g Carbohydrates

527. Strawberry Stew

Preparation Time: 10 minutes Cooking Time: 15 minutes Servings: 4

12 oz. fresh strawberries, sliced	1 tsp vanilla
1 1/2 cups water	1 tsp liquid stevia
2 tbsp. lime juice	

1. Mix all ingredients into the inner pot of instant pot and stir well.
2. Seal pot with lid and cook on high for 15 minutes.
3. Once cooked, allow to release pressure naturally for 10 minutes then by using quick release, let the remaining pressure out. Remove lid.
4. Stir and serve.

Nutrition:
36 Calories 0.3g Fat 8.5g Carbohydrates

528. Brussels Sprouts and Pistachios

Preparation Time: 15 minutes Cooking Time: 15 minutes Serving: 4

1-pound Brussels sprouts, trimmed and halved lengthwise

4 shallots, peeled and quartered

1 tablespoon extra-virgin olive oil

½ cup roasted pistachios, chopped

½ lemon juice and zest

1. Pre-heat your oven to 400 degrees Fahrenheit.
2. Wrap baking sheet with aluminum foil and keep aside.
3. Take a large bowl and add Brussels sprouts, shallots with olive oil and coat well.
4. Season sea salt, pepper, spread veggies evenly on sheet.
5. Bake for 15 minutes until lightly caramelized.
6. Remove oven and transfer to a serving bowl.
7. Toss with lemon zest, pistachios, lemon juice.
8. Serve warm and enjoy!

Nutrition:
126 Calories 7g Fat 6g Protein

529. Spiced Up Kale Chips

Preparation Time: 10 minutes Cooking Time: 25 minutes Serving: 4

3 cups kale, stemmed and thoroughly washed, torn into 2-inch pieces

1 tablespoon extra-virgin olive oil

½ teaspoon chili powder

¼ teaspoon sea salt

1. Pre-heat your oven to 300 degrees Fahrenheit.
2. Cover 2 baking sheets using parchment paper and keep aside.
3. Dry kale entirely and transfer to a large bowl.
4. Add olive oil and toss.
5. Make sure each leaf is covered.
6. Season kale with chili powder and salt, toss again.
7. Divide kale between baking sheets and spread into a single layer.
8. Bake for 25 minutes.
9. Cool the chips for 5 minutes and serve.

Nutrition:
56 Calories 4g Fat 2g Protein

530. Crazy Almond Crackers

Preparation Time: 10 minutes Cooking Time: 20 minutes Serving: 20

1 cup almond flour

¼ teaspoon baking soda

3 tablespoons sesame seeds

1 egg, beaten

1. Pre-heat your oven to 350 degrees Fahrenheit.
2. Put two baking sheets with parchment paper and keep aside.
3. Mix the dry ingredients to a large bowl and add egg, mix well and form dough.
4. Divide dough into two balls.
5. Roll out the dough between two pieces of parchment paper.
6. Cut into crackers and transfer them to prepared baking sheet.
7. Bake for 15-20 minutes.
8. Do it in all the dough.
9. Leave crackers to cool and serve.

Nutrition:
302 Calories 28g Fat 9g Protein

531. Superb Stuffed Mushrooms

Preparation Time: 10 minutes Cooking Time: 15 minutes Serving: 4

4 Portobello mushrooms

1 cup crumbled blue cheese

2 teaspoons extra virgin olive oil

Salt, to taste

Fresh thyme

1. Preheat your oven to 350-degree Fahrenheit.
2. Cut out the stems from the mushrooms.
3. Chop them into small pieces.
4. Take a bowl and mix stem pieces with thyme, salt and blue cheese and mix well.
5. Fill up mushroom with the prepared cheese.
6. Top with some oil.
7. Take a baking sheet and place the mushrooms.
8. Bake for 15 minutes to 20 minutes.
9. Serve warm and enjoy!

Nutrition:
124 Calories 22.4g Fat 1.2g Protein

532. Flax and Almond Crunchies

Preparation Time: 15 minutes Cooking Time: 60 minutes Serving: 10

½ cup ground flax seeds

½ cup almond flour

1 tablespoon coconut flour

2 tablespoons shelled hemp seeds

2 tablespoons unsalted butter, melted

1. Pre-heat your oven to 300 degrees Fahrenheit.
2. Prep baking sheet using parchment paper, keep the prepared sheet on the side.
3. Add flax, coconut flour, almond, salt, hemp seed to a bowl and mix well.
4. Add 1 egg white and melted butter, mix well.
5. Transfer dough to sheet of parchment paper and cover with another sheet of paper.
6. Roll out dough.
7. Cut into crackers and bake for 60 minutes.
8. Cool and serve!

Nutrition:
47 Calories 6g Fat 0.2g Protein

533. Mashed Up Celeriac

Preparation Time: 10 minutes Cooking Time: 20 minutes Serving: 4

2 celeriac, washed, peeled and diced

2 teaspoons extra-virgin olive oil

1 tablespoon honey

½ teaspoon ground nutmeg

1. Pre-heat your oven to 400 degrees Fahrenheit.
2. Prepare the baking sheet with foil and keep it aside.
3. Take a large bowl and toss celeriac and olive oil.
4. Spread celeriac evenly on baking sheet.
5. Roast for 20 minutes until tender.
6. Transfer to large bowl.
7. Add honey and nutmeg.
8. Use a potato masher to mash the mixture until fluffy.
9. Season with salt and pepper.
10. Serve and enjoy!

Nutrition:
136 Calories 3g Fat 4g Protein

534. Easy Medi Kale

Preparation Time: 15 minutes Cooking Time: 10 minutes Serving: 6

12 cups kale, chopped

2 tablespoons lemon juice

1 tablespoon olive oil

1 tablespoon garlic, minced

1 teaspoon soy sauce

1. Add a steamer insert to your saucepan.
2. Pour water in the saucepan up to the bottom of the steamer.
3. Cover and bring water to boil (medium-high heat).
4. Add kale to the insert and steam for 7-8 minutes.
5. Take a large bowl and add lemon juice, garlic, olive oil, salt, soy sauce and pepper.
6. Mix well and add the steamed kale to the bowl.
7. Toss and serve.

Nutrition:
350 Calories 17g Fat 11g Protein

535. Black Bean Hummus

Preparation Time: 25 minutes Serving: 4

1 cup of cooked black beans	1 minced garlic clove
2 tablespoons of lemon juice	1 tablespoon of white wine vinegar
½ teaspoon of ground cumin	

1. Situate all the ingredients to your blender except ½ head of lettuce.
2. Process until everything is smooth.
3. Allow to sit for 15 minutes and serve with the iceberg lettuce.

Nutrition
81 Calories 4g Fat 4g Protein

536. Full Eggs in a Squash

Preparation Time: 10 minutes Cooking Time: 20 minutes Serving: 5

2 acorn squash	6 whole eggs
2 tablespoons extra virgin olive oil	5-6 pitted dates
8 walnut halves	

1. Pre-heat your oven to 375 degrees Fahrenheit.
2. Slice squash crosswise and prepare 3 slices with holes.
3. While slicing the squash, make sure that each slice has a measurement of ¾ inch thickness.
4. Remove the seeds from the slices.
5. Get baking sheet and line it with parchment paper.
6. Transfer the slices to your baking sheet and season them with salt and pepper.
7. Bake in your oven for 20 minutes.
8. Chop the walnuts and dates on your cutting board.
9. Take the baking dish out of the oven and drizzle slices with olive oil.
10. Beat egg into each of the holes in the slices and season well.
11. Sprinkle the chopped walnuts on top.
12. Bake for 10 minutes more.
13. Garnish with parsley and add maple syrup.

Nutrition:
198 Calories 12g Fat 8g Protein

537. Simple Coconut Porridge

Preparation Time: 15 minutes Serving: 6

Powdered erythritol as needed	1 ½ cups almond milk, unsweetened
2 tablespoons vanilla protein powder	3 tablespoons Golden Flaxseed meal
2 tablespoons coconut flour	

1. Take a bowl and mix in flaxseed meal, protein powder, coconut flour and mix well.
2. Add mix to saucepan (placed over medium heat).
3. Add almond milk and stir, let the mixture thicken.
4. Add your desired amount of sweetener and serve.

Nutrition:
259 Calories 13g Fat 16g Protein

538. Authentic Yogurt and Cucumber Salad

Preparation Time: 10 minutes Serving: 4

5-6 small cucumbers, peeled and diced	1 (8 ounces) container plain Greek yogurt
2 garlic cloves, minced	1 tablespoon fresh mint, minced
1 teaspoon dried oregano	

1. Take a large bowl and add cucumbers, garlic, yogurt, mint, and oregano.
2. Season with salt and pepper.
3. Refrigerate the salad for 1 hour and serve.

Nutrition:

74 Calories 0.7g Fat2g Protein

539. Almond and Chocolate Butter Dip

Preparation Time: 15 minutes Cooking Time: 10 minutes Serving: 14

1 cup Plain Greek Yogurt	½ cup almond butter
1/3 cup chocolate hazelnut spread	1 tablespoon honey
1 teaspoon vanilla	

1. Take a medium-sized bowl and add the first five listed ingredients.
2. With an immersion blender, blend well until you have a smooth dip.
3. Serve with your favorite sliced fruit.

Nutrition:
115 Calories 8g Fat 4g Protein

540. Cherry and Olive Bites

Preparation Time: 15 minutes Serving: 30

24 cherry tomatoes, halved	24 black olives, pitted
24 feta cheese cubes	24 toothpick/decorative skewers

1. Use a toothpick or skewer and thread feta cheese, black olives, and cherry tomato halves in that order.
2. Repeat until all the ingredients are used.
3. Arrange in a serving platter.

Nutrition:
57 Calories: 5g Fa2g Protein

541. Mouthwatering Panna Cotta with Mixed Berry Compote

Preparation Time: 5 minutes Cooking Time: 10 minutes Serving: 4

2 cups of freshly divided mixed berries	1 package of plain gelatin powder
1 cup of milk	1 2/3 cup of heavy cream
¾ cup of divided sugar	

1. Puree 1 cup of raspberries into a food processor.
2. Take a small saucepan and transfer the puree to that saucepan.
3. Add about ¼ cup of sugar and the remaining raspberries.
4. Cook over medium heat for 10 minutes, making sure to stir from time to time.
5. Remove the heat after 10 minutes and let cool.
6. Cover and chill in your fridge.
7. Take another saucepan and combine your milk and gelatin and wait until the gelatin softens.
8. Simmer over medium heat and keep stirring frequently to fully dissolve the gelatin.
9. Stir in the heavy cream alongside the rest of the sugar and cook for another 3-5 minutes.
10. Pour the mixture into 4 ramekins.
11. Chill them for 8 hours or overnight.
12. Invert the mold and place on a serving plate.
13. Once the Panna Cotta comes out, top it with your berry compote.

Nutrition:
191 Calories 15g Fat 6g Carbohydrates

542. Lemon Mousse

Preparation Time: 10 minutes Cooking Time: 10 minutes Serving: 4

1 cup coconut cream	8 ounces cream cheese, soft
¼ cup fresh lemon juice	3 pinches salt
1 teaspoon lemon liquid stevia	

1. Pre-heat your oven to 350 degrees Fahrenheit.
2. Grease a ramekin with butter.
3. Beat cream, cream cheese, fresh lemon juice, salt and lemon liquid stevia in a mixer.
4. Pour batter into ramekin.

5. Bake for 10 minutes, then transfer mouse to serving glass.
6. Let chill for 2 hours and serve.

Nutrition:
395 Calories 31g Fat 3g Carbohydrates

543.   Minty Watermelon Salad

Preparation Time: 10 minutes Serving: 6

1 medium watermelon	1 c. fresh blueberries
2 tbsp. fresh mint leaves	2 tbsp. lemon juice
1/3 c. honey	

1. Cut the watermelon into 1-inch cubes. Put them in a bowl.
2. Evenly distribute the blueberries over the watermelon.
3. Next, finely chop the mint leaves and put them into a separate bowl.
4. Add the lemon juice and honey to the mint and whisk together.
5. Drizzle the mint dressing over the watermelon and blueberries. Serve cold.

Nutrition:
296 calories 23g fat 3.3g fiber

544.   Mascarpone and Fig Crostini

Preparation Time: 8 minutes Cooking Time: 15 minutes Serving: 6

1 long French baguette	4 tbsp. (½ stick) salted butter, melted
1 (8 oz.) tub mascarpone cheese	1 (12 oz.) jar fig jam or preserves
1 tbsp. sugar	

1. Preheat the oven to 350°F.
2. Portion the bread to ¼-inch-thick slices.
3. Arrange the sliced bread on a sheet and rub each slice with the melted butter and small amount of sugar.
4. Next, put the baking sheet into your oven and toast the bread for 5 to 7 minutes, just until it turns to golden brown.
5. Let the bread cool slightly. Then, spread about a teaspoon or so of the mascarpone cheese on each piece of bread.
6. Lastly, put a teaspoon or so of the jam on top. Serve immediately.

Nutrition:
281 calories 18g fat 4g fiber

545.   Crunchy Sesame Cookies

Preparation Time: 7 minutes Cooking Time: 15 minutes Serving: 6

1 c. sesame seeds, hulled	1 c. sugar
8 tbsp. (1 stick) salted butter, softened	2 eggs
1¼ c. flour	

1. Preheat the oven to 350°F firstly. Then, toast the sesame seeds on a baking sheet for 3 minutes. Set aside and let cool.
2. Mix the sugar and the butter using the mixer.
3. Put the eggs slowly until well-blended.
4. Add the flour and toasted sesame seeds and mix until well-blended.
5. Drop spoonful of cookie dough onto your baking sheet and form them into round balls, about 1-inch in diameter, similar to a walnut.
6. Put in the oven. Then, bake approximately for 5 to 7 minutes or until golden brown.
7. Let the cookies cool and enjoy.

Nutrition:
301 calories 19g fat 2g fiber

546.   Creamy Rice Pudding

Preparation Time: 11 minutes Cooking Time: 50 minutes Serving: 6

1¼ c. long-grain rice	5 c. whole milk
1 c. sugar	1 tbsp. rose water or orange blossom water
1 tsp. cinnamon	

1. First, rinse the rice under cold water for 30 seconds.
2. Put the rice, milk, and sugar in a large pot. Bring to a gentle boil while continually stirring.
3. Turn the heat down to low and let simmer for 40 to 45 minutes, stirring every 3 to 4 minutes so that the rice does not stick to the bottom of the pot.
4. Next, add the rose water at the end and simmer for 5 minutes.
5. Divide the pudding into 6 bowls. Sprinkle the top with cinnamon. Lastly, cool for at least 1 hour before serving. Store in the fridge.

Nutrition:
303 calories 21g fat 2g fiber

547.   Ricotta-Lemon Cheesecake

Preparation Time: 14 minutes Cooking Time: 1 hour Serving: 8

2 (8 oz.) packages full-fat cream cheese	1 (16 oz.) container full-fat ricotta cheese
1½ c. granulated sugar	1 tbsp. lemon zest
5 eggs	

1. Preheat the oven to 350°F.
2. Next, using a mixer, blend together the cream cheese and ricotta cheese.
3. Blend in the sugar and lemon zest.
4. Blend in the eggs; drop in 1 egg at a time, blend for 10 seconds, and repeat.
5. Line a 9-inch spring form pan with a parchment paper and nonstick spray. Bind the lower part of the pan with foil. Pour the cheesecake batter into the pan.
6. To make a water bath, get a baking or roasting pan larger than the cheesecake pan. Fill the roasting pan about 1/3 of the way up with warm water. Put the cheesecake pan into the water bath. Situate the whole thing in the oven and let the cheesecake bake for 1 hour.
7. After baking is complete, remove the cheesecake pan from the water bath and remove the foil. Let the cheesecake cool approximately for 1 hour on the countertop. Lastly, put it in the fridge to cool for at least 3 hours before serving.

Nutrition:
311 calories 20g fat 6g fiber

548.   Thyme Zucchini Chips

Preparation Time: 7 minutes Cooking Time: 2 hours Serving: 4

4 zucchinis, thinly sliced	½ tsp. dried thyme or 2 tsp. chopped fresh thyme
2 tbsp. avocado oil, divided	½ tsp. pink Himalayan salt or sea salt
½ tsp. garlic powder	

1. Spread the zucchini slices on paper towels without overlapping. Place a large baking sheet on top of the paper towels to help press out any moisture. Let sit for 15 minutes.
2. Preheat the oven to 235°F. Then, line the same baking sheet with parchment paper. Brush 1 tablespoon avocado oil on the parchment.
3. Arrange the zucchini slices on the lined baking sheet in a single layer and brush the remaining 1 tablespoon of avocado oil on top of the slices. In a small bowl, scourge the salt, garlic powder, and thyme. Sprinkle on top of the zucchini slices.
4. Bake for 1½ to 2 hours, or until crisp and golden brown. Allow the chips to cool before enjoying.

Nutrition:
314 calories 24g fat 7g fiber

549.   Collagen Protein Bars

Preparation Time: 12 minutes Cooking Time: 30 minutes Serving: 8

1 c. dried dates, pitted	1 c. dried cranberries
½ c. collagen peptides powder	¼ tsp. pink Himalayan salt or sea salt
2 tsp. coconut oil	

1. First, line an 8-by-8-inch baking pan with parchment paper, leaving an overhang for easy lifting.
2. Combine the dates and cranberries in a blender or food processor and pulse until chopped completely. Add the collagen powder, salt, and coconut oil and pulse until fully combined.

3. Next, transfer the mixture to the lined baking pan and press it down into an even layer. Place the pan in your freezer for 20 minutes, or until firm.
4. Remove from the baking pan by lifting the parchment paper. Cut into 8 bars.

Nutrition:
297 calories 21g fat 5g fiber

550. Oven-Fried Chicken Nuggets

Preparation Time: 18 minutes Cooking Time: 30 minutes Serving: 4

½ c. full-fat unsweetened coconut milk (store-bought or homemade, here)
½ tsp. pink Himalayan salt or sea salt
1½ c. crushed plain pork rinds

1 tbsp. white wine vinegar
1 lb. boneless, skinless chicken breasts, cut into 1½-inch pieces

1. Preheat the oven to 400°F. Then, line your large baking sheet with parchment paper.
2. In a large baking pan, mix together the coconut milk, vinegar, and salt. Add the chicken pieces, then let sit for 10 minutes.
3. Pour the pork rinds into a shallow bowl. One at a time, remove the chicken pieces from your baking pan, let the excess coconut milk mixture drip off, and coat in the pork rinds, firmly pressing the crumbs onto the chicken.
4. Lastly, place on the lined baking sheet in a single layer and bake for 16 to 20 minutes approximately, or until crisp and golden brown. Serve hot.

Nutrition:
298 calories 20g fat 7g fiber

551. Tropical Pineapple Smoothie

Preparation Time: 5 minutes Serving: 1

1 c. pineapple chunks, frozen
¼ c. mango chunks, frozen
½ c. full-fat unsweetened coconut milk

½ banana
½ c. orange juice

1. Combine the pineapple, banana, mango, orange juice, and coconut milk in a blender and process until smooth.
2. Pour into a glass and enjoy. Smoothies are best when you drink them right away.

Nutrition:
300 calories 18g fat 2g fiber

552. Strawberry Coconut Parfait

Preparation Time: 7 minutes Serving: 1

1 c. plain unsweetened coconut yogurt
½ tsp. vanilla powder
½ c. Granola

1 tbsp. raw honey
1 c. chopped strawberries

1. First, in your small bowl, mix together the coconut yogurt, honey, and vanilla powder until combined.
2. In a large glass, spoon one-third of the yogurt mixture into the bottom, followed by one-third of the strawberries, then one-third of the granola. Repeat the same layers twice more.
3. Serve immediately.
4. If you're making extra parfaits, store the yogurt and the granola separately and put the parfait together right before serving, so the granola will not get soggy.

Nutrition:
281 calories 16g fat 1g fiber

553. Smoked Salmon with Avocado

Preparation Time: 11 minutes Cooking Time: 5 minutes Serving: 2

1 avocado, pitted, peeled, and sliced
8 oz. smoked salmon
1 tbsp. chopped fresh dill (optional)

2 tbsp. AIP Mayo
1 tbsp. capers

1. Divide the avocado slices between two medium plates, then add a dollop of mayo and half the salmon, capers, and dill (if using) to each plate.

Nutrition:
290 calories 21g fat 4g fiber

554. Open-Face Sandwich

Preparation Time: 8 minutes Cooking Time: 25 minutes Serving: 2

6 slices bacon
2 AIP Garlic Herb Flatbreads
½ avocado, peeled, pitted, and sliced

2 tbsp. AIP Mayo
½ c. arugula

1. First, in your large skillet, cook the bacon over medium heat for 10 to 12 minutes, or until it's crisp. Then, transfer to your plate lined with paper towels.
2. Lay out the flatbreads, and spread 1 tablespoon of mayo on each one. Divide the arugula between the flatbreads, and then top with 3 bacon slices. Arrange the avocado on top of the bacon.

Nutrition:
289 calories 18g fat 5g fiber

555. Cilantro Lime Shrimp and Avocado Salad

Preparation Time: 7 minutes Cooking Time: 10 minutes Serving: 1

6 oz. shrimp, peeled and deveined
1 avocado, pitted, peeled, and diced
¼ c. Cilantro Lime Vinaigrette

2 c. mixed greens
1 scallion, finely sliced

1. First, fill a small pot with filtered water and bring to a boil. Add the shrimp and cook for 2 or 3 minutes, until they turn pink and become opaque. Using a strainer, drain the shrimp and immediately rinse under cold running water until they're cool to touch.
2. Next, put the mixed greens in a salad bowl. Top with the avocado, scallions, and cooked shrimp.
3. Drizzle the dressing onto the salad, then toss to combine. Enjoy right away.

Nutrition:
298 calories 19g fat 2g fiber

556. Pizza Margherita

Preparation Time: 11 minutes Cooking Time: 15 minutes Serving: 4

4 (6-inch) pizza crusts
8 oz. fresh mozzarella cheese, thinly sliced
½ c. thinly sliced fresh basil leaves

4 tbsp. olive oil
2 ripe tomatoes, thinly sliced

1. Preheat the oven to 400°F. Place the pizza crusts onto a rimmed baking sheet.
2. Brush the crusts with the olive oil. Then, top with the mozzarella cheese and tomato slices.
3. Bake for 10 minutes, or until the mozzarella is melted and the tomatoes are wilted.
4. Top with the fresh basil leaves.

Nutrition:
303 calories 20g fat 3g fiber

557. Fajitas

Preparation Time: 12 minutes Cooking Time: 3 hours Serving: 4

2 lb. steak, cut into strips (buy whatever is on sale)
1 medium onion, sliced
2 tbsp. fajita seasoning

2 bell peppers, sliced
15 oz. salsa (you can also use spicy diced tomatoes)

1. Put the entire ingredients into your slow cooker. Then, cook on high for 3 hours or on low for 5–6 hours.
2. Serve with tortillas or over rice for a complete meal.

Nutrition:
298 calories 21g fat 1g fiber

BREAKFAST RECIPES

558. Eggs with Zucchini Noodles

Preparation Time: 10 minutes Cooking Time: 11 minutes Servings: 2

2 tablespoons extra-virgin olive oil
4 eggs
1 tablespoon basil, chopped

3 zucchinis, cut with a spiralizer
A pinch of red pepper flakes

1. In a bowl, combine the zucchini noodles with salt, pepper and the olive oil and toss well.
2. Grease a baking sheet with cooking spray and divide the zucchini noodles into 4 nests on it.
3. Crack an egg on top of each nest, sprinkle salt, pepper and the pepper flakes on top and bake at 350 degrees F for 11 minutes.
4. Divide the mix between plates, sprinkle the basil on top and serve.

Nutrition:
296 calories 23g fat 3.3g fiber

559. Banana Oats

Preparation Time: 10 minutes Servings: 2

½ cup cold brewed coffee
2 tablespoons cocoa powder
1 and ½ tablespoons chia seeds

2 dates, pitted
1 cup rolled oats

1. In a blender, combine the 1 banana with the ¾ almond milk and the rest of the ingredients, pulse, divide into bowls and serve for breakfast.

Nutrition:
451 calories 25g fat 9.9g fiber

560. Berry Oats

Preparation Time: 5 minutes Servings: 2

½ cup rolled oats
¼ cup chia seeds
1 cup berries, pureed

1 cup almond milk
2 teaspoons honey

1. In a bowl, combine the oats with the milk and the rest of the ingredients except 1 tbsp. of yogurt, toss, divide into bowls, top with the yogurt and serve cold for breakfast.

Nutrition:
420 calories 30g fat 6.4g protein

561. Sun-dried Tomatoes Oatmeal

Preparation Time: 10 minutes Cooking Time: 25 minutes Servings: 4

3 cups water
1 tablespoon olive oil
¼ cup sun-dried tomatoes, chopped

1 cup almond milk
1 cup steel-cut oats

1. In a pan, scourge water with the milk, bring to a boil over medium heat.
2. Meanwhile, pre-heat pan with the oil over medium-high heat, add the oats, cook them for about 2 minutes and transfer m to the pan with the milk.
3. Stir the oats, add the tomatoes and simmer over medium heat for 23 minutes.
4. Divide the mix into bowls, sprinkle the red pepper flakes on top and serve for breakfast.

Nutrition:
170 calories 17.8g fat 1.5g protein

562. Quinoa Muffins

Preparation Time: 10 minutes Cooking Time: 30 minutes Servings: 12

6 eggs
1 cup Swiss cheese
1 small yellow onion
1 cup quinoa
½ cup sun-dried tomatoes

whisked
grated
chopped
white mushrooms
chopped

1. In a bowl, combine the eggs with salt, pepper and the rest of the ingredients and whisk well.
2. Divide this into a silicone muffin pan, bake at 350 degrees F for 30 minutes and serve for breakfast.

Nutrition:
123 calories 5.6g fat 7.5g protein

563. Watermelon "Pizza"

Preparation Time: 10 minutes Servings: 4

1 watermelon slice cut 1-inch thick
and then from the center cut into 4
wedges resembling pizza slices
1-ounce feta cheese, crumbled
1 teaspoon mint, chopped

6 Kalamata olives, pitted and sliced

½ tablespoon balsamic vinegar

1. Arrange the watermelon "pizza" on a plate, sprinkle the olives and the rest of the ingredients on each slice and serve right away for breakfast.

Nutrition:
90 calories 3g fat 2g protein

564. Cheesy Yogurt

Preparation Time: 4 hours and 5 minutes Servings: 4

1 cup Greek yogurt
½ cup feta cheese, crumbled

1 tablespoon honey

1. In a blender, combine the yogurt with the honey and the cheese and pulse well.
2. Divide into bowls and freeze for 4 hours before serving for breakfast.

Nutrition:
161 calories 10g fat 6.6g protein

565. Cauliflower Fritters

Preparation Time: 10 minutes Cooking Time: 50 minutes Servings: 4

30 ounces canned chickpeas, drained and rinsed
1 small yellow onion, chopped
2 tablespoons garlic, minced

2 and ½ tablespoons olive oil

2 cups cauliflower florets chopped

1. Lay out half of the chickpeas on a baking sheet lined with parchment pepper, add 1 tablespoon oil, season with salt and pepper, toss and bake at 400 degrees F for 30 minutes.
2. Transfer the chickpeas to a food processor, pulse well and put the mix into a bowl.
3. Heat up a pan with the ½ tablespoon oil over medium-high heat, add the garlic and the onion and sauté for 3 minutes.
4. Add the cauliflower, cook for 6 minutes more, transfer this to a blender, add the rest of the chickpeas, pulse, pour over the crispy chickpeas mix from the bowl, stir and shape medium fritters out of this mix.
5. Heat up a pan with the rest of the oil over medium-high heat, add the fritters, cook them for 3 minutes on each side and serve for breakfast.

Nutrition:
333 calories 12.6g fat 13.6g protein

566.   Corn and Shrimp Salad
Preparation Time: 10 minutes Cooking Time: 10 minutes Servings: 4

4 ears of sweet corn	husked
1 avocado	peeled
pitted and chopped	
½ cup basil	chopped
1-pound shrimp	peeled and deveined
1 and ½ cups cherry tomatoes	halved

1. Put the corn in a pot, boil water and cover, over medium heat for 6 minutes.
2. Drain, cool down, cut corn from the cob and put it in a bowl.
3. Thread the shrimp onto skewers and brush with some of the oil.
4. Place the skewers on the preheated grill, cook over medium heat for 2 minutes on each side, remove from skewers and add over the corn.
5. Place the rest of the ingredients to the bowl, toss, divide between plates and serve for breakfast.

Nutrition:
371 calories 22g fat 23g protein

567.   Walnuts Yogurt Mix
Preparation Time: 10 minutes Servings: 6

2 and ½ cups Greek yogurt	1 and ½ cups walnuts, chopped
1 teaspoon vanilla extract	¾ cup honey
2 teaspoons cinnamon powder	

1. In a bowl, incorporate yogurt with the walnuts and the rest of the ingredients, toss, divide into smaller bowls and keep in the fridge for 10 minutes before serving for breakfast.

Nutrition:
388 calories 24.6g fat 10.2g protein

568.   Tahini Pine Nuts Toast
Preparation Time: 5 minutes Servings: 2

2 whole wheat bread slices, toasted	1 tablespoon tahini paste
2 teaspoons feta cheese, crumbled	Juice of ½ lemon
2 teaspoons pine nuts	

1. Whisk tahini with the 1 tsp. of water and the lemon juice well and spread over the toasted bread slices.
2. Top each serving with the remaining ingredients and serve for breakfast.

Nutrition:
142 calories 7.6g fat 5.8g protein

569.   Blueberries Quinoa
Preparation Time: 5 minutes Servings: 4

2 cups quinoa, almond milk	½ teaspoon cinnamon powder
1 tablespoon honey	1 cup blueberries
¼ cup walnuts, chopped	

1. In a bowl, scourge quinoa with the milk and the rest of the ingredients, toss, divide into smaller bowls and serve for breakfast.

Nutrition: 284 calories 14.3g fat 4.4g protein

570.   Raspberries and Yogurt Smoothie
Preparation Time: 5 minutes Servings: 2

2 cups raspberries	½ cup Greek yogurt
½ cup almond milk	½ teaspoon vanilla extract

1. In your blender, combine the raspberries with the milk, vanilla and the yogurt, pulse well, divide into 2 glasses and serve for breakfast.

Nutrition:
245 calories 9.5g fat 1.6g protein

571. Cottage Cheese and Berries Omelet
Preparation Time: 5 minutes Cooking Time: 4 minutes Servings: 1

1 egg, whisked	1 teaspoon cinnamon powder
1 tablespoon almond milk	3 ounces cottage cheese
4 ounces blueberries	

1. Scourge egg with the rest of the ingredients except the oil and toss.
2. Preheat pan with the oil over medium heat, add the eggs mix, spread, cook for 2 minutes on each side, transfer to a plate and serve.

Nutrition:
190 calories 8g fat 2g protein

572.   Salmon Frittata
Preparation Time: 5 minutes Cooking Time: 27 minutes Servings: 4

1-pound gold potatoes, roughly cubed	1 tablespoon olive oil
2 salmon fillets, skinless and boneless	8 eggs, whisked
1 teaspoon mint, chopped	

1. Put the potatoes in a boiling water at medium heat, then cook for 12 minutes, drain and transfer to a bowl.
2. Arrange the salmon on a baking sheet lined with parchment paper, grease with cooking spray, and broil over medium-high heat for 5 minutes on each side, cool down, flake and put in a separate bowl.
3. Warm up a pan with the oil over medium heat, add the potatoes, salmon, and the rest of the ingredients except the eggs and toss.
4. Add the eggs on top, put the lid on and cook over medium heat for 10 minutes.
5. Divide the salmon between plates and serve.

Nutrition:
289 calories 11g fat 4g protein

573.   Avocado and Olive Paste on Toasted Rye Bread
Preparation Time: 5 minutes Serving: 4

1 avocado, halved, peeled and finely chopped	1 tbsp. green onions, finely chopped
2 tbsp. green olive paste	4 lettuce leaves
1 tbsp. lemon juice	

1. Crush avocados with a fork or potato masher until almost smooth. Add the onions, green olive paste and lemon juice. Season with salt and pepper to taste. Stir to combine.
2. Toast 4 slices of rye bread until golden. Spoon 1/4 of the avocado mixture onto each slice of bread, top with a lettuce leaf and serve.

Nutrition:
291 calories 13g fat 3g protein

574.   Avocado and Chickpea Sandwiches
Preparation Time: 4 minutes Serving: 4

1/2 cup canned chickpeas	1 small avocado
2 green onions, finely chopped	1 egg, hard boiled
1/2 tomato, cucumber	

1. Mash the avocado and chickpeas with a fork or potato masher until smooth. Add in green onions and salt and combine well. Spread this

mixture on the four slices of bread. Top each slice with tomato, cucumber and egg, and serve.

Nutrition:
309 calories 9g fat 2g protein

575.   Raisin Quinoa Breakfast
Preparation Time: 15 minutes Serving: 4

1 cup quinoa   2 cups milk
2 tbsp. walnuts, crushed   2 tbsp. raisins, cranberries
1 tbsp. chia seeds

1.   Rinse quinoa with cold water and drain. Place milk and quinoa into a saucepan and bring to a boil. Add ½ tsp. of vanilla. Reduce heat to low and simmer for about 15 minutes stirring from time to time.
2.   Set aside to cool then serve in a bowl, topped with honey, chia seeds, raisins, cranberries and crushed walnuts.

Nutrition:
299 calories 7g fat 1g protein

576.   Banana Cinnamon Fritters
Preparation Time: 15 minutes Cooking Time: 6 minutes Serving: 4

1 cup self-rising flour   1 egg, beaten
3/4 cup sparkling water   2 tsp ground cinnamon
2-3 bananas, cut diagonally into 4
pieces each

1.   Sift flour and cinnamon into a bowl and make a well in the center. Add egg and enough sparkling water to mix to a smooth batter.
2.   Heat sunflower oil in a saucepan, enough to cover the base by 1-2 inch, so when a little batter dropped into the oil sizzles and rises to the surface. Dip banana pieces into the batter, then fry for 2-3 minutes or until golden. Pull out with a slotted spoon and drain on paper towels. Sprinkle with sugar and serve hot.

Nutrition:
209 calories 10g fat 2g protein

577.   Veggie Casserole
Preparation Time: 25 minutes Cooking Time: 45 minutes Serving: 4

1 lb. okra   trimmed
3 tomatoes   cut into wedges
3 garlic cloves   chopped
1 cup fresh parsley leaves   finely cut

1.   In a deep ovenproof baking dish, combine okra, sliced tomatoes, olive oil and garlic. Add in salt and black pepper to taste, and toss to combine. Bake in a prepared oven at 350 F for 45 minutes. Garnish with parsley and serve.

Nutrition:
302 calories 13g fat 6g protein

578.   Ground Beef and Brussels Sprouts
Preparation Time: 20 minutes Cooking Time: 36 minutes Serving: 4

6 oz. ground beef   2 garlic cloves, crushed
½ cup grated sweet potato   1 cup grated Brussels sprouts
1 egg, boiled

1.   In a medium saucepan, cook olive oil over medium heat. Gently sauté the ½ onion and garlic until the onion is soft and translucent. Add in the beef and the sweet potato and cook until the meat is fully cooked.
2.   Stir in the Brussels sprouts and cook for about 5 minutes more. Season well and serve topped with a boiled egg.

Nutrition:
314 calories 15g fat 6g protein

579.   Italian Mini Meatballs
Preparation Time: 13 minutes Cooking Time: 20 minutes Serving: 6

1 lb. ground beef   1 onion, grated
1 egg, lightly whisked   1 tsp garlic powder
1 tsp dried basil, oregano, parsley

1.   Combine ground beef, onion, egg, parsley, garlic powder, basil and oregano. Mix very well with hands. Roll tablespoonfuls of the meat mixture into balls.
2.   Place meatballs on a lined baking tray. Bake 20 minutes or until brown. Transfer to a serving plate and serve.

Nutrition:
275 calories 9g fat 1g protein

580.   Mushroom and Olives Steaks
Preparation Time: 20 minutes Cooking Time: 9 minutes Serving: 6

1 lb. boneless beef sirloin steak   1 large onion, sliced
5-6 white mushrooms   1/2 cup green olives, coarsely
                                              chopped
1 cup parsley leaves, finely cut

1.   Cook olive oil in a heavy bottomed pan at medium-high heat. Cook the steaks until well browned on each side then keep aside.
2.   Gently sauté the onion in the same pan, for 3 minutes. Cook the mushrooms and olives until the mushrooms are done.
3.   Return the steaks to the skillet, cover, and cook for 5-6 minutes. Stir in parsley and serve.

Nutrition:
281 calories 14g fat 3g protein

581. Salmon Kebabs
Preparation Time: 30 minutes Cooking Time: 6 minutes Serving: 5

2 shallots, ends trimmed, halved   2 zucchinis, cut in 2-inch cubes
1 cup cherry tomatoes   6 skinless salmon fillets, cut into 1-
                                              inch pieces
3 limes, cut into thin wedges

1.   Preheat barbecue or char grill on medium-high. Thread fish cubes onto skewers, then zucchinis, shallots and tomatoes. Repeat to make 12 kebabs. Bake the kebabs for about 3 minutes each side for medium cooked.
2.   Situate to a plate, wrap with foil and set aside for 5 minutes to rest.

Nutrition:
268 calories 9g fat 3g protein

582.   Mediterranean Baked Salmon
Preparation Time: 35 minutes Cooking Time: 11 minutes Serving: 5

2 (6 oz.) boneless salmon fillets   1 onion, tomato
1 tbsp. capers   1 tsp dry oregano
3 tbsp. Parmesan cheese

1.   Set oven to 350 F. Place the salmon fillets in a baking dish, sprinkle with oregano, top with onion and tomato slices, drizzle with olive oil, and sprinkle with capers and Parmesan cheese.
2.   Wrap the dish with foil and bake for 30 minutes.

Nutrition:
291 calories 14g fat 2g protein

583.   Feta Cheese Baked in Foil

Preparation Time: 15 minutes Cooking Time: 16 minutes Serving: 5

14 oz. feta cheese, cut in slices
1 tbsp. paprika

4 oz. butter
1 tsp dried oregano

Directions:

1. Cut the cheese into four medium-thick slices and place on sheets of butter lined aluminum foil.
2. Place a little bit of butter on top each feta cheese piece, sprinkle with paprika and dried oregano and wrap. Place on a tray and bake in a preheated to 350 F oven for 15 minutes.

Nutrition:
279 calories 9g fat 2g protein

584.   Avocado, Roasted Mushroom and Feta Spaghetti

Preparation Time: 20 minutes Cooking Time: 17 minutes Serving: 5

12 oz. spaghetti
10-15 white mushrooms, halved
2 tbsp. green olive paste

2 avocados, peeled and diced
1 cup feta, crumbled

1. Wrap baking tray with baking paper and place mushrooms on it. Spray with olive oil and season with salt and black pepper to taste. Roast in a prepared to 375 F oven for 15 minutes.
2. In a big pot of boiling salted water, cook spaghetti following package's instructions. Drain and set aside.
3. In a blender, combine lemon juice, 2 garlic cloves, olive paste and avocados and blend until smooth.
4. Combine pasta, mushrooms and avocado sauce. Sprinkle with feta cheese and serve immediately.

Nutrition:
278 calories 10g fat 4g protein

585.   Tomato, Arugula and Feta Spaghetti

Preparation Time: 20 minutes Cooking Time: 3 minutes Serving: 6

12 oz. spaghetti
1 cup fresh basil leaves, roughly torn
1 cup feta, crumbled

2 cups grape tomatoes, halved
1 cup baby arugula leaves

1. In a huge saucepan with salted boiling water, cook spaghetti according to package directions. Drain and keep aside.
2. Return saucepan to medium heat. Add olive oil, 2 garlic cloves and tomatoes. Season with pepper and cook, tossing, for 1-2 minutes or until tomatoes are hot. Add spaghetti, basil and feta. Toss lightly for 1 minute. Sprinkle with arugula and serve.

Nutrition:
278 calories 15g fat 3g protein

586.   Zucchini Fritters

Preparation Time: 20 minutes Cooking Time: 26 minutes Serving: 6

5 zucchinis, grated
2 garlic cloves, crushed
1 cup feta cheese, crumbled

3 eggs
5 spring onions, finely chopped

1. Grate zucchinis and situate them in a colander. Sprinkle with salt and leave aside to drain. After 20 minutes, squeeze and place in a bowl. Add in all other ingredients except for 1 cup of flour and sunflower oil. Combine everything very well. Add in flour and stir to combine again.
2. Cook sunflower oil in a frying pan. Drop a few scoops of the zucchini batter and fry them on medium heat for 3-5 minutes, until golden brown. Serve with yogurt.

Nutrition:
293 calories 13g fat 6g protein

587.   Cheesy Cauliflower Florets

Preparation Time: 25 minutes Cooking Time: 16 minutes Serving: 6

1 small cauliflower, cut into florets
1 tsp paprika
1/2 cup grated Parmesan cheese

1 tbsp. garlic powder
4 tbsp. extra virgin olive oil

1. Combine olive oil, paprika, salt, pepper and garlic powder. Throw in the cauliflower florets and position in a baking dish in single layer.
2. Bake in a preheated to 350 F oven for 20 minutes. Pull out from the oven, stir, and topped with Parmesan cheese. Bake for 5 minutes more.

Nutrition:
297 calories 13g fat 6g protein

MAIN DISH RECIPES

588. Steak with Olives and Mushrooms
Preparation Time: 20 minutes Cooking Time: 9 minutes Serving: 6

lb. boneless beef sirloin steak	1 large onion, sliced
5-6 white button mushrooms	1/2 cup green olives, coarsely chopped
4 tbsp. extra virgin olive oil	

1. Heat olive oil in a heavy bottomed skillet over medium-high heat. Brown the steaks on both sides then put aside.
2. Gently sauté the onion in the same skillet, for 2-3 minutes, stirring rarely. Sauté in the mushrooms and olives.
3. Return the steaks to the skillet, cover, cook for 5-6 minutes and serve.

Nutrition:
299 calories 56g fat 16g protein

589. Spicy Mustard Chicken
Preparation Time: 32 minutes Cooking Time: 36 minutes Serving: 4

4 chicken breasts	2 garlic cloves, crushed
1/3 cup chicken broth	3 tbsp. Dijon mustard
tsp chili powder	

1. In a small bowl, mix the mustard, chicken broth, garlic and chili. Marinate the chicken for 30 minutes.
2. Bake in a preheated to 375 F oven for 35 minutes.

Nutrition:
302 calories 18g fat 49g protein

590. Walnut and Oregano Crusted Chicken
Preparation Time: 36 minutes Cooking Time: 13 minutes Serving: 4

4 skinless, boneless chicken breasts	10-12 fresh oregano leaves
1/2 cup walnuts, chopped	2 garlic cloves, chopped
2 eggs, beaten	

1. Blend the garlic, oregano and walnuts in a food processor until a rough crumb is formed. Place this mixture on a plate.
2. Whisk eggs in a deep bowl. Soak each chicken breast in the beaten egg then roll it in the walnut mixture. Place coated chicken on a baking tray and bake at 375 F for 13 minutes each side.

Nutrition:
304 calories 54g fat 14g protein

591. Chicken and Onion Casserole
Preparation Time: 16 minutes Cooking Time: 47 minutes Serving: 4

4 chicken breasts	4-5 large onions, sliced
2 leeks, cut	4 tbsp. extra virgin olive oil
1 tsp thyme	

1. Cook olive oil in a large, deep frying pan over medium-high heat. Brown chicken, turning, for 2-3 minutes each side or until golden. Set aside in a casserole dish.
2. Cut the onions and leeks and add them on and around the chicken, Add in olives, thyme, salt and black pepper to taste. Cover it using aluminum foil and bake at 375 F for 35 minutes, or until the chicken is cooked through. Uncover and return to the oven for 5 minutes or until chicken is crispy.

Nutrition:

309 calories 59g fat 18g protein

592. Chicken and Mushrooms
Preparation Time: 20 minutes Cooking Time: 7 minutes Serving: 4

4 chicken breasts, diced	2 lbs. mushrooms, chopped
onion, chopped	4 tbsp. extra virgin olive oil
salt and black, pepper to taste	

1. Heat olive oil in a deep-frying pan over medium-high heat. Brown chicken, stirring, for 2 minutes each side, or until golden. Add the chopped onion, mushrooms, salt and black pepper, and stir to combine. Reduce heat, cover and simmer for 30 minutes. Uncover and simmer for 5 more minutes.

Nutrition:
290 calories 49g fat 9g protein

593. Blue Cheese and Mushroom Chicken
Preparation Time: 25 minutes Cooking Time: 18 minutes Serving: 4

4 chicken breast halves	cup crumbled blue cheese
1 cup sour cream	salt and black pepper, to taste
1/2 cup parsley, finely cut	

1. Prep the oven to 350 degrees F. Grease a casserole with nonstick spray. Place all ingredients into it, turn chicken to coat.
2. Bake for 20 minutes or until chicken juices run clear. Sprinkle with parsley and serve.

Nutrition:
287 calories 46g fat 10g protein

594. Herb-Roasted Lamb Leg
Preparation Time: 14 minutes Cooking Time: 2 hours Serving: 4

(6-lb) boneless leg of lamb, trimmed	cups fresh spinach leaves
1/3 cup water	tbsp. Italian seasoning
tbsp. extra virgin olive oil	

1. Combine spinach, Italian seasoning and olive oil in a food processor. Process until finely minced.
2. Thoroughly coat the top and sides of the lamb with this mixture.
3. Place in the bottom of a large roasting pan. Add water and cook, covered, at 300 F for approximately two hours or until cooked through.
4. Uncover and cook for 10 minutes more.

Nutrition:
309 calories 41g fat 12g protein

595. Spring Lamb Stew
Preparation Time: 34 minutes Cooking Time: 13 minutes Serving: 4

1 lb. lamb, cubed	1 lb. white mushrooms, chopped
4 cups fresh spring onions, chopped	tbsp. extra virgin olive oil
1 tbsp. Italian seasoning	

1. Heat olive oil in a deep casserole. Gently brown lamb pieces for 2-3 minutes. Add in the mushrooms and cook for a minute more, stirring.
2. Stir in Italian seasoning, cover, and cook for an hour or until tender. Add in spring onions and simmer for 10 minutes more.
3. Uncover and cook until almost all the liquid evaporates.

Nutrition:

309 calories 41g fat 10g protein

596. Balsamic Roasted Carrots and Baby Onions

Preparation Time: 50 minutes Cooking Time: 26 minutes Serving: 4

2 bunches baby carrots, scrubbed, ends trimmed	10 small onions, peeled, halved
4 tbsp. 100% pure maple syrup (unprocessed)	1 tsp thyme
1 tbsp. extra virgin olive oil	

1. Preheat oven to 350F. Line a baking tray with baking paper.
2. Place the carrots, onion, thyme and oil in a large bowl and toss until well coated. Spread carrots and onion, in a single layer, on the baking tray. Roast for 25 minutes or until tender.
3. Sprinkle over the maple syrup and vinegar and toss to coat. Roast for 25-30 minutes more or until vegetables are tender and caramelized. Season well and serve.

Nutrition:
401 calories 49g fat 20g protein

597. Baked Cauliflower

Preparation Time: 13 minutes Cooking Time: 26 minutes Serving: 4

small cauliflower, cut into florets	1 tbsp. garlic powder
1 tsp paprika	4 tbsp. extra virgin olive oil
grated Parmesan cheese, to taste	

1. Combine olive oil, paprika and garlic powder together. Mix in the cauliflower florets and situate in a baking dish in one layer.
2. Bake in a preheated to 350 F oven for 20 minutes. Take away from the oven, and drizzle with Parmesan cheese. Cook for 5 minutes more.

Nutrition:
316 calories 53g fat 17g protein

598. Baked Bean and Rice Casserole

Preparation Time: 8 minutes Cooking Time: 22 minutes Serving: 4

can red beans, rinsed	1 cup water
2/3 cup rice	onions, chopped
tsp dried mint	

1. Cook olive oil in an ovenproof casserole dish and gently sauté the chopped onions for 1-2 minutes. Stir in the rice and cook, stirring constantly, for another minute.
2. Rinse the beans and add them to the casserole. Stir in a cup of water and the mint and bake in a preheated to 350 F oven for 20 minutes.

Nutrition:
405 calories 49g fat 12g protein

599. Okra and Tomato Casserole

Preparation Time: 25 minutes Cooking Time: 26 minutes Serving: 4

lb. okra, trimmed	tomatoes, cut into wedges
garlic cloves, chopped	1 cup fresh parsley leaves, finely cut
tbsp. extra virgin olive oil	

1. In a deep ovenproof baking dish, combine okra, sliced tomatoes, olive oil and garlic.
2. Toss to combine and bake in a preheated to 350 degrees F oven for 45 minutes. Drizzle with parsley and serve.

Nutrition:
304 calories 48g fat 13g protein

600. Spicy Baked Feta with Tomatoes

Preparation Time: 15 minutes Cooking Time: 22 minutes Serving: 4

lb. feta cheese, cut in slices	ripe tomatoes, sliced
1 onion, sliced	tbsp. extra virgin olive oil
1/2 tbsp. hot paprika	

1. Preheat the oven to 430F
2. In an ovenproof baking dish, arrange the slices of onions and tomatoes overlapping slightly but not too much. Sprinkle with olive oil.
3. Bake for 5 minutes then place the feta slices on top of the vegetables. Sprinkle with hot paprika. Bake for 15 more minutes and serve.

Nutrition:
303 calories 46g fat 12g protein

601. Baked Lemon-Butter Fish

Preparation Time: 10 minutes Cooking Time: 17 minutes Serving: 4

4 tablespoons butter, plus more for coating	2 (5-ounce) tilapia fillets
2 garlic cloves, minced	lemon, zested and juiced
tablespoons capers, rinsed and chopped	

1. Preheat the oven to 400°F. Coat an 8-inch baking dish with butter.
2. Pat dry the tilapia with paper towels, and season on both sides with pink Himalayan salt and pepper. Place in the greased baking dish.
3. In a medium skillet at medium heat, heat up butter. Add the garlic and cook for 3 to 5 minutes, until slightly browned but not burned.
4. Remove the garlic butter from the heat, and mix in the lemon zest and 2 tablespoons of lemon juice.
5. Pour the lemon-butter sauce over the fish, and sprinkle the capers around the baking pan.
6. Bake for 13 minutes and serve.

Nutrition:
299 Calories 26g Fat 1g Fiber

602. Fish Taco Bowl

Preparation Time: 10 minutes Cooking Time: 15 minutes Serving: 2

2 (5-ounce) tilapia fillets	4 teaspoons Tajin seasoning salt, divided
cups pre-sliced coleslaw cabbage mix	1 tablespoon Spicy Red Pepper Miso Mayo, plus more for serving
1 avocado, mashed	

1. Preheat the oven to 425°F. Prep baking sheet with silicone baking mat.
2. Rub the tilapia with the olive oil, and then coat it with 2 teaspoons of Tajin seasoning salt. Place the fish in the prepared pan.
3. Bake for 15 minutes, or until the fish is opaque when you pierce it with a fork. Put the fish on a cooling rack and let it sit for 4 minutes.
4. Meanwhile, in a medium bowl, gently mix to combine the coleslaw and the mayo sauce. You don't want the cabbage super wet, just enough to dress it. Add the mashed avocado and the remaining 2 teaspoons of Tajin seasoning salt to the coleslaw, and season with pink Himalayan salt and pepper. Divide the salad between two bowls.
5. Shred the fish into small pieces, and add it to the bowls.
6. Top the fish with a drizzle of mayo sauce and serve.

Nutrition:
315 Calories 24g Fat 7g Fiber

603. Scallops with Creamy Bacon Sauce

Preparation Time: 5 minutes Cooking Time: 20 minutes Serving: 2

4 bacon slices	cup heavy (whipping) cream
¼ cup grated Parmesan cheese	1 tablespoon ghee
8 large sea scallops, rinsed and patted dry	

1. In a medium skillet at medium-high heat, fry bacon on both sides for 8 minutes. Transfer the bacon to a paper towel–lined plate.

2. Lower the heat to medium. Add the cream, butter, and Parmesan cheese to the bacon grease, and season with a pinch of pink Himalayan salt and pepper. Decrease the heat to low and cook, stir constantly, for 10 minutes.
3. In a separate large skillet over medium-high heat, heat the ghee until sizzling.
4. Season the scallops with pink Himalayan salt and pepper, and add them to the skillet. Cook for just 1 minute per side. Do not crowd the scallops; if your pan isn't large enough, cook them in two batches. You want the scallops golden on each side.
5. Transfer the scallops to a paper towel–lined plate.
6. Divide the cream sauce between two plates, crumble the bacon on top of the cream sauce, and top with 4 scallops each. Serve immediately.

Nutrition:
782 Calories 73g Fat 24g Protein

604.   Shrimp and Avocado Lettuce Cups
Preparation Time: 10 minutes Cooking Time: 5 minutes Serving: 2

tablespoon ghee
½ avocado, sliced
1 tablespoon Spicy Red Pepper Miso Mayo

½ pound shrimp
4 butter lettuce leaves

1. Preheat medium skillet over medium-high heat, cook the ghee. Add the shrimp and cook. Season with pink Himalayan salt and pepper. Shrimp are cooked when they turn pink and opaque.
2. Season the tomatoes and avocado with pink Himalayan salt and pepper.
3. Divide the lettuce cups between two plates. Fill each cup with shrimp, ½ cup grape tomatoes, and avocado. Drizzle the mayo sauce on top and serve.

Nutrition:
326 Calories 11g Fat 3g Fiber

605.   Garlic Butter Shrimp
Preparation Time: 10 minutes Cooking Time: 15 minutes Serving: 2

3 tablespoons butter
lemon, halved
¼ teaspoon red pepper flakes (optional)

½ pound shrimp
garlic cloves, crushed

1. Preheat the oven to 425°F.
2. Place the butter in an 8-inch baking dish, and pop it into the oven while it is preheating, just until the butter melts.
3. Sprinkle the shrimp with pink Himalayan salt and pepper.
4. Slice one half of the lemon in thin slices, and cut the other half into 2 wedges.
5. In the baking dish, add the shrimp and garlic to the butter. The shrimp should be in a single layer. Add the lemon slices. Sprinkle the top of the fish with the red pepper flakes (if using).
6. Bake the shrimp for 15 minutes, stirring halfway through.
7. Remove the shrimp from the oven, and squeeze juice from the 2 lemon wedges over the dish. Serve hot.

Nutrition:
329 Calories 20g Fat 32g Protein

606.   Parmesan-Garlic Salmon with Asparagus
Preparation Time: 10 minutes Cooking Time: 15 minutes Serving: 2

2 (6-ounce) salmon fillets, skin on
tablespoons butter
¼ cup grated Parmesan cheese

pound fresh asparagus, ends snapped off
garlic cloves, minced

1. Preheat the oven to 400°F. Prepare baking sheet with silicone baking mat.

2. Pat dry the salmon using paper towel, and season both sides with pink Himalayan salt and pepper.
3. Situate the salmon in the middle of the prepared pan, and arrange the asparagus around the salmon.
4. In a small saucepan over medium heat, melt the butter. Add the minced garlic and stir until the garlic just begins to brown, about 3 minutes.
5. Drizzle the garlic-butter sauce over the salmon and asparagus, and top both with the Parmesan cheese.
6. Bake until the salmon is cooked and the asparagus is crisp-tender, about 12 minutes. You can switch the oven to broil at the end of cooking time for about 3 minutes to get a nice char on the asparagus.
7. Serve hot.

Nutrition:
434 Calories 26g Fat 42g Protein

607.   Seared-Salmon Shirataki Rice Bowls
Preparation Time: 40 minutes Cooking Time: 10 minutes Serving: 2

2 (6-ounce) salmon fillets, skin on
2 small Persian cucumbers or ½ large English cucumber
1 avocado, diced

4 tablespoons soy sauce (or coconut aminos), divided
1 (8-ounce) pack Miracle Shirataki Rice

1. Place the salmon in an 8-inch baking dish, and add 3 tablespoons of soy sauce. Cover and marinate in the refrigerator for 30 minutes.
2. Meanwhile, slice the cucumbers thin, put them in a small bowl, and add the remaining 1 tablespoon of soy sauce. Set aside to marinate.
3. Situate skillet over medium heat, melt the ghee. Add the salmon fillets skin-side down. Pour some of the soy sauce marinade over the salmon, and sear the fish for 3 to 4 minutes on each side.
4. Meanwhile, in a large saucepan, cook the shirataki rice per package instructions:
5. Rinse the shirataki rice in cold water in a colander.
6. In a saucepan filled with boiling water, cook the rice for 2 minutes.
7. Pour the rice into the colander. Dry out the pan.
8. Transfer the rice to the dry pan and dry roast over medium heat until dry and opaque.
9. Season the avocado with pink Himalayan salt and pepper.
10. Place the salmon fillets on a plate, and remove the skin. Cut the salmon into bite-size pieces.
11. Assemble the rice bowls: In two bowls, make a layer of the cooked Miracle Rice. Top each with the cucumbers, avocado, and salmon, and serve.

Nutrition:
328 Calories 18g Fat 36g Protein

608.   Pork Rind Salmon Cakes
Preparation Time: 10 minutes Cooking Time: 10 minutes Serving: 2

6 ounces canned Alaska wild salmon, drained
egg, lightly beaten
½ tablespoon Dijon mustard

2 tablespoons crushed pork rinds
1 tablespoon ghee

1. In a medium bowl, incorporate salmon, pork rinds, egg, and 1½ tablespoons of mayonnaise, and season with pink Himalayan salt and pepper.
2. With the salmon mixture, form patties the size of hockey pucks or smaller. Keep patting until they keep together.
3. Position the medium skillet over medium-high heat, melt the ghee. When the ghee sizzles, place the salmon patties in the pan. Cook for 6 minutes both sides. Transfer the patties to a paper towel–lined plate.
4. In a small bowl, mix together the remaining 1½ tablespoons of mayonnaise and the mustard.
5. Serve the salmon cakes with the mayo-mustard dipping sauce.

Nutrition:
362 Calories 31g Fat 24g Protein

609. Creamy Dill Salmon

Preparation Time: 10 minutes Cooking Time: 10 minutes Serving: 2

2 tablespoons ghee, melted	2 (6-ounce) salmon fillets, skin on
¼ cup mayonnaise	tablespoon Dijon mustard
tablespoons minced fresh dill	

1. Preheat the oven to 450°F. Grease 9-by-13-inch baking dish with the ghee.
2. Pat salmon dry with paper towels, season on both sides with pink Himalayan salt and pepper, and place in the prepared baking dish.
3. In a small bowl, mix to combine the mayonnaise, mustard, dill, and garlic powder.
4. Slather the mayonnaise sauce on top of both salmon fillets so that it fully covers the tops.
5. Bake depending on how you like your salmon—7 minutes for medium-rare and 9 minutes for well-done—and serve.

Nutrition:
510 Calories 41g Fat 33g Protein

610. Chicken-Basil Alfredo with Shirataki Noodles

Preparation Time: 10 minutes Cooking Time: 15 minutes Serving: 2

For noodles	(7-ounce) package Miracle Noodle Fettuccini Shirataki Noodles
For sauce	4 ounces cooked shredded chicken (I usually use a store-bought rotisserie chicken)
1 cup Alfredo Sauce, or any brand you like	¼ cup grated Parmesan cheese
tablespoons chopped fresh basil leaves	

For noodles
1. Follow the instructions on the package:
2. In a colander, rinse the noodles with cold water (shirataki noodles naturally have a smell, and rinsing with cold water will help remove this).
3. Boil water in a large saucepan over high heat. Boil noodles for 2 minutes. Drain.
4. Transfer the noodles to a dry skillet over medium-low heat to evaporate any moisture. Do not grease the skillet; it must be dry. Situate to a plate and set aside.
For sauce
5. Situate saucepan over medium heat, heat the olive oil. Add the cooked chicken. Season with pink Himalayan salt and pepper.
6. Pour the Alfredo sauce over the chicken, and cook until warm. Season with more pink Himalayan salt and pepper.
7. Add the dried noodles to the sauce mixture, and toss until combined.
8. Divide the pasta between two plates, top each with the Parmesan cheese and chopped basil, and serve.

Nutrition:
673 Calories 61g Fat 29g Protein

611. Chicken Quesadilla

Preparation Time: 5 minutes Cooking Time: 5 minutes Serving: 2

low-carbohydrate tortillas	½ cup shredded Mexican blend cheese
ounces shredded chicken (I usually use a store-bought rotisserie chicken)	1 teaspoon Tajin seasoning salt
2 tablespoons sour cream	

1. In a big skillet at medium-high heat, cook olive oil. Add a tortilla, then layer on top ¼ cup of cheese, the chicken, the Tajin seasoning, and the remaining ¼ cup of cheese. Top with the second tortilla.
2. Peek under the edge of the bottom tortilla to monitor how it is browning. Once the bottom tortilla gets golden and the cheese begins to melt, after about 2 minutes, flip the quesadilla over. The second side will cook faster, about 1 minute.

3. Once the second tortilla is crispy and golden, transfer the quesadilla to a cutting board and let sit for 2 minutes. Cut the quesadilla into 4 wedges using a pizza cutter or chef's knife.
4. Transfer half the quesadilla to each of two plates. Add 1 tablespoon of sour cream to each plate, and serve hot.

Nutrition:
414 Calories 28g Fat 17g Fiber

612. Garlic-Parmesan Chicken Wings

Preparation Time: 10 minutes Cooking Time: 3 hours Serving: 2

8 tablespoons (1 stick) butter	2 garlic cloves, minced
tablespoon dried Italian seasoning	¼ cup grated Parmesan cheese, plus ½ cup
1-pound chicken wings	

1. With the crock insert in place, preheat the slow cooker to high. Cover baking sheet with silicone baking mat.
2. Put the butter, garlic, Italian seasoning, and ¼ cup of Parmesan cheese in the slow cooker, and season with pink Himalayan salt and pepper. Heat up the butter, and stir the ingredients until well mixed.
3. Add the chicken wings and stir until coated with the butter mixture.
4. Cover the slow cooker and cook for 2 hours and 45 minutes.
5. Preheat the broiler.
6. Transfer the wings to the prepared baking sheet, sprinkle the remaining ½ cup of Parmesan cheese over the wings, and cook under the broiler until crispy, about 5 minutes.
7. Serve hot.

Nutrition:
738 Calories 66g Fat 39g Protein

613. Chicken Skewers with Peanut Sauce

Preparation Time: 70 minutes Cooking Time: 15 minutes Serving: 2

1-pound boneless skinless chicken breast, cut into chunks	3 tablespoons soy sauce (or coconut aminos), divided
½ teaspoon Sriracha sauce, plus ¼ teaspoon	3 teaspoons toasted sesame oil, divided
2 tablespoons peanut butter	

1. In a large zip-top bag, mix chicken chunks with 2 tablespoons of soy sauce, ½ teaspoon of Sriracha sauce, and 2 teaspoons of sesame oil. Seal, and marinate for an hour or so in the refrigerator or up to overnight.
2. If you are using wooden 8-inch skewers, soak them in water for 30 minutes before using.
3. Preheat your grill pan or grill to low. Oil the grill pan with ghee.
4. Thread the chicken chunks onto the skewers.
5. Cook the skewers over low heat for 10 to 15 minutes, flipping halfway through.
6. Meanwhile, mix the peanut dipping sauce. Stir together the remaining 1 tablespoon of soy sauce, ¼ teaspoon of Sriracha sauce, 1 teaspoon of sesame oil, and the peanut butter. Season with pink Himalayan salt and pepper.
7. Serve the chicken skewers with a small dish of the peanut sauce.

Nutrition:
586 Calories 29g Fat 75g Protein

614. Braised Chicken Thighs with Kalamata Olives

Preparation Time: 10 minutes Cooking Time: 40 minutes Serving: 4

4 chicken thighs, skin on	2 tablespoons ghee
½ cup chicken broth	lemon, ½ sliced and ½ juiced
½ cup pitted Kalamata olives	

1. Preheat the oven to 375 degrees F.
2. Pat the chicken thighs dry using paper towels, and season with pink Himalayan salt and pepper.

3. In a medium oven-safe skillet or high-sided baking dish over medium-high heat, melt the ghee. When the ghee has melted and is hot, add the chicken thighs, skin-side down, and leave them for about 8 minutes, or until the skin is brown and crispy.
4. Cook the other side for 2 minutes. Around the chicken thighs, pour in the chicken broth, and add the lemon slices, lemon juice, and olives.
5. Bake for 30 minutes. Add the butter to the broth mixture.
6. Divide the chicken and olives between two plates and serve.

Nutrition:
567 Calories 47g Fat 33g Protein

615. Buttery Garlic Chicken
Preparation Time: 5 minutes Cooking Time: 40 minutes Serving: 2

2 tablespoons ghee, melted
tablespoon dried Italian seasoning
¼ cup grated Parmesan cheese

2 boneless skinless chicken breasts
4 tablespoons butter

1. Preheat the oven to 375°F. Select a baking dish that fit both chicken breasts and coat it with the ghee.
2. Pat dry the chicken breasts. Season with pink Himalayan salt, pepper, and Italian seasoning. Place the chicken in the baking dish.
3. In a medium skillet over medium heat, melt the butter. Sauté minced garlic, for about 5 minutes.
4. Remove the butter-garlic mixture from the heat, and pour it over the chicken breasts.
5. Roast in the oven for 30 to 35 minutes. Sprinkle some of the Parmesan cheese on top of each chicken breast. Let the chicken rest in the baking dish for 5 minutes.
6. Divide the chicken between two plates, spoon the butter sauce over the chicken, and serve.

Nutrition:
642 Calories 45g Fat 57g Protein

616. Heart-Warming Medi Tilapia
Preparation Time: 15 minutes Cooking Time: 15 minutes Serving: 4

3 tablespoons sun-dried tomatoes
tilapia fillets

tablespoons Kalamata olives, chopped and pitted

tablespoon capers, drained
1 tablespoon oil from sun-dried tomatoes

1. Pre-heat your oven to 372 degrees Fahrenheit
2. Take a small sized bowl and add sun-dried tomatoes, olives, capers and stir well
3. Keep the mixture on the side
4. Take a baking sheet and transfer the tilapia fillets and arrange them side by side
5. Drizzle olive oil all over them
6. Bake in your oven for 10-15 minutes
7. After 10 minutes, check the fish for a "Flaky" texture
8. Once cooked properly, top the fish with tomato mixture and serve!

Nutrition:
183 Calories 8g Fat 83g Protein

617. Pistachio Sole Fish
Preparation Time: 5 minutes Cooking Time: 10 minutes Serving: 4

4 (5 ounces) boneless sole fillets
Juice of 1 lemon

½ cup pistachios, finely chopped
teaspoon extra virgin olive oil

1. Pre-heat your oven to 350 degrees Fahrenheit
2. Wrap baking sheet using parchment paper and keep it on the side
3. Pat fish dry with kitchen towels and lightly season with salt and pepper
4. Take a small bowl and stir in pistachios
5. Place sol on the prepped sheet and press 2 tablespoons of pistachio mixture on top of each fillet
6. Rub the fish with lemon juice and olive oil
7. Bake for 10 minutes until the top is golden and fish flakes with a fork

Nutrition:
166 Calories 6g Fat 2g Carbohydrates

618. Exquisite Sardines and Raisin Croquettes
Preparation Time: 5 minutes Cooking Time: 20 minutes Serving: 4

cup sardine fillets
tablespoons parmesan cheese
1 whole egg

½ cup breadcrumbs
tablespoons raisins

1. Take a blender and add fish, egg, parmesan cheese, raisins, breadcrumbs and blend until you have a creamy mixture
2. Form balls using the mixture and season balls with salt and pepper
3. Take a baking dish and line it, brush the balls with oil and bake for 20 minutes at 350 degrees F/or until the top is golden brown
4. Serve and enjoy!

Nutrition:
188 Calories 11g Fat 17g Carbohydrates

619. Grilled Chicken with Lemon and Fennel
Preparation Time: 5 minutes Cooking Time: 25 minutes Serving: 4

2 cups chicken fillets
garlic cloves
1 lemon

large fennel bulb
1 jar green olives

1. Pre-heat your grill to medium-high
2. Crush garlic cloves
3. Take a bowl and add olive oil and season with salt and pepper
4. Coat chicken skewers with the marinade
5. Transfer them under grill and grill for 20 minutes, making sure to turn them halfway through until golden
6. Zest half of the lemon and cut the other half into quarters
7. Cut the fennel bulb into similarly sized segments
8. Brush olive oil all over the garlic clove segments and cook for 3-5 minutes
9. Chop them and add them to the bowl with the marinade
10. Add lemon zest and olives
11. Once the meat is read, serve with the vegetable mix

Nutrition:
649 Calories 16g Fat 33g Carbohydrates

620. Hearty Pork Belly Casserole
Preparation Time: 5 minutes Cooking Time: 25 minutes Serving: 4

8 pork belly slices, cut into small pieces
4 tablespoon lemon
Seasoning as you needed

3 large onions, chopped
Juice of 1 lemon

1. Take a large pressure cooker and place it over medium heat
2. Add onions and sweat them for 5 minutes
3. Add pork belly slices and cook until the meat browns and onions become golden
4. Cover with water and add honey, lemon zest, salt, and pepper and close the pressure seal
5. Pressure cook for 40 minutes
6. Serve and enjoy with a garnish of fresh chopped parsley if you prefer

Nutrition:
753 Calories 41g Fat 68g Carbohydrates

621. Healthy Mediterranean Lamb Chops

Preparation Time: 10 minutes **Cooking Time:** 10 minutes **Serving:** 4

4 lamb shoulder chops, 8 ounces each	2 tablespoons Dijon mustard
2 tablespoons Balsamic vinegar	½ cup olive oil
2 tablespoons shredded fresh basil	

1. Pat your lamb chop dry using a kitchen towel and arrange them on a shallow glass baking dish
2. Take a bowl and a whisk in Dijon mustard, balsamic vinegar, pepper and mix them well
3. Whisk in the oil very slowly into the marinade until the mixture is smooth
4. Stir in basil
5. Pour the marinade over the lamb chops and stir to coat both sides well
6. Cover the chops and allow them to marinate for 1-4 hours (chilled)
7. Get the chops out and leave them for 30 minutes to allow the temperature to reach a normal level
8. Pre-heat your grill to medium heat and add oil to the grate
9. Grill the lamb chops for 5-10 minutes per side until both sides are browned
10. Once the center reads 145 degrees Fahrenheit the chops are ready, serve and enjoy!

Nutrition:
521 Calories 45g Fat 3.5g Carbohydrates

622. Amazingly Baked Chicken Breast

Preparation Time: 10 minutes **Cooking Time:** 40 minutes **Serving:** 2

2 pieces of 8 ounces skinless and boneless chicken breast	Salt and pepper as needed
¼ cup of olive oil and lemon juice (equal amount)	½ a teaspoon of dried oregano
¼ teaspoon of dried thyme	

1. Season breast by rubbing salt and pepper on all sides
2. Transfer the chicken to a bowl
3. Take another bowl and add olive oil, oregano, lemon juice, thyme and mix well
4. Pour the prepared marinade over the chicken breast and allow it to marinate for 10 minutes
5. Pre-heat your oven to 400 degrees Fahrenheit
6. Set the oven rack about 6 inches above the heat source
7. Transfer the chicken breast to a baking sheet and pour extra marinade on top
8. Bake for 40 minutes
9. Remove it and place it on the top rack
10. Broil for 5 minutes more

Nutrition:
501 Calories 32g Fat 3.5g Carbohydrates

623. Homely Tuscan Tuna Salad

Preparation Time: 8 minutes **Serving:** 4

15 ounces small white beans	6 ounces drained chunks of light tuna
10 cherry tomatoes, quartered	4 scallions, trimmed and sliced
2 tablespoons lemon juice	

Direction
1. Stir all the ingredients to a bowl
2. Season with salt and pepper accordingly, enjoy!

Nutrition:
322 Calories 8g Fat 32g Carbohydrates

624. Cool Garbanzo and Spinach Beans

Preparation Time: 9 minutes **Serving:** 4

tablespoon olive oil	½ onion, diced
10 ounces spinach, chopped	12 ounces garbanzo beans
½ teaspoon cumin	

1. Take a skillet and add olive oil, let it warm over medium-low heat
2. Add onions, garbanzo and cook for 5 minutes
3. Stir in spinach, cumin, garbanzo beans and season with salt
4. Use a spoon to smash gently
5. Cook thoroughly until heated, enjoy!

Nutrition:
90 Calories 4g Fat 11g Carbohydrates

625. Clean Eating Medi Stuffed Chicken Breasts

Preparation Time: 7 minutes **Cooking Time:** 28 minutes **Serving:** 4

8 ounces chicken breast	large red bell pepper
tablespoons Kalamata olives, chopped	¼ cup feta cheese, crumbled
1 tablespoon fresh basil	

1. Prepare your broiler to high heat
2. Slice bell pepper in half lengthwise and discard membrane and seeds.
3. Take a baking sheet and place pepper halves, skin side up, flatten with hand
4. Place pepper into the oven and broil for 15 minutes until blackened
5. Once done, place peppers in a Ziplock bag and let them sit for 15 minutes
6. Peel peppers and chop them
7. Once done, place a pan on grill over medium-high heat
8. Add cheese, olives, basil and bell pepper
9. Slice horizontal slits through the thickest part of the chicken and make a sort of pocket
10. Once done, place pepper mixture into the slits and close the pockets, secure using a wooden toothpick
11. Season with salt and pepper
12. Grill both sides for 7 minutes each until thoroughly cooked
13. Once done, let it stand for 10 minutes, enjoy!

Nutrition: 210 Calories 6g Fat 32g Protein

626. Lemony Garlic Shrimp

Preparation Time: 7 minutes **Cooking Time:** 16 minutes **Serving:** 4

1 ¼ pounds shrimp, boiled or steamed	tablespoons garlic, minced
¼ cup lemon juice	tablespoons olive oil
¼ cup parsley	

1. Preheat skillet over medium heat, add garlic and oil and stir cook for 1 minute
2. Add parsley, lemon juice and season with salt and pepper accordingly
3. Add shrimp in a large bowl and transfer the mixture from the skillet over the shrimp
4. Chill and serve

Nutrition:
130 Calories 3g Fat 2g Carbohydrates

627. Completely Herbed Up Feisty Baby Potatoes

Preparation Time: 10 minutes Cooking Time: 35 minutes Serving: 4

2 pounds new yellow potatoes, scrubbed and cut into wedges
2 teaspoons fresh rosemary, chopped
½ teaspoon freshly ground black pepper and salt
2 tablespoons extra virgin olive oil
teaspoon garlic powder

1. Pre-heat your oven to 400 degrees Fahrenheit
2. Spread the foil onto the baking sheet and set it aside
3. Take a large bowl and add potatoes, olive oil, garlic, rosemary, sea salt and pepper
4. Spread potatoes in single layer on baking sheet and bake for 35 minutes
5. Serve and enjoy!

Nutrition:
225 Calories 7g Fat: 37g Carbohydrates

628. Mediterranean Kale Dish

Preparation Time: 15 minutes Cooking Time: 10 minutes Serving: 6

12 cups kale, chopped
tablespoon olive oil
Salt and pepper as needed
2 tablespoons lemon juice
1 teaspoon soy sauce

1. Add a steamer insert to your Saucepan
2. Fill in the saucepan with water up to the bottom of the steamer
3. Cover and bring water to boil (medium-high heat)
4. Add kale to the insert and steam for 7-8 minutes
5. Take a large bowl and add lemon juice, olive oil, salt, soy sauce, and pepper
6. Mix well and add the steamed kale to the bowl
7. Toss and serve

Nutrition:
350 Calories 17g Fat 41g Carbohydrates

629. Yogurt Marinated Tenderloin

Preparation Time: 8 minutes Cooking Time: 30 minutes Serving: 6

2 Pork Tenderloins, 10-12 Ounces Each
1 Tablespoon Rosemary, Fresh & Chopped
2 Tablespoons Mint, Fresh & Chopped
¼ Cup Greek Yogurt, 2%
Tzatziki Sauce

1. Start by heating the oven to 500.
2. Take huge baking sheet and line it with foil with a wire rack on top. Spray the rack down with oil.
3. Put both pieces of pork on the rack, and season with salt and pepper.
4. Get out a bowl and mix your yogurt and rosemary together and coat on all sides.
5. Roast for ten minutes.
6. Remove it from the oven, and then turn it over.
7. Roast for ten to twelve more minutes.
8. Remove the pork from the rack and cut. Allow it to rest for five minutes before slicing.
9. Serve with tzatziki and mint leaves.

Nutrition:
183 Calories 22g Protein 10g Fat

630. Buttery Herb Lamb Chops

Preparation Time: 11 minutes Cooking Time: 20 minutes Serving: 4

8 Lamb Chops
1 Tablespoon Butter
1 Lemon, Cut into Wedges
1 Tablespoon Olive Oil
4 Ounces Herb Butter

1. Season your lamb chops well, and then get out a pan.
2. Heat up butter in a pan over medium-high heat and then fry your chops for four minutes per side.
3. Arrange on a serving plate with herb butter on each one. Serve with a lemon wedge.

Nutrition:
729 Calories 43g Protein 62g Fat

631. Lemon Fruit and Nut Bars

Preparation Time: 15 minutes Servings: 10

½ Cup Raw Almonds
1 Cup Deglet Noor Dates

¾ Cup Raw Cashews
1 Lemon – Juice and Zest

1. Ground cashews and almonds in a nourishment processor until they are finely cut. Add dates, lemon juice, and lemon pieces. Beat until all ingredients are mixed.
2. Pour blend between two sheets of cling wrap. Utilize your hands to press and frame the blend into a minimized rectangular shape.
3. Fold the saran wrap over it and refrigerate for 2 hours. This will enable it to solidify and make it simpler to cut into bars.
4. Remove from the cooler and cut into 10 bars. Envelop the bars with cling wrap and store them in the ice chest.

Nutrition:
132 Calories 6.5g Fat 3.2g Protein

632. Cauliflower Fried Rice with Bacon

Preparation Time: 5 minutes Cooking Time: 10 minutes Servings: 4

4 slices bacon
1 head cauliflower
1 tsp Bragg's Liquid Amino

1 small onion
1 cup frozen mixed vegetables

1. In a wok or enormous sauté container over medium flame, cook bacon.
2. Add the onions and pan-fried food until translucent.
3. Set heat to high. Add the shredded cauliflower and pan-fried food for 1 moment. Add water and mixed vegetables, mix well, spread the dish and let the cauliflower blend steam for an additional 3 minutes or until tender.
4. Add Bragg's Liquid Amino. Taste and add salt for extra flavoring as wanted.

Nutrition:
315 Calories 25g Fat 19g Protein

633. Halloumi Cheese with Butter-Fried Eggplant

Preparation Time: 5 minutes Cooking Time: 10 minutes Serving: 2

1 eggplant
10 oz. halloumi cheese
salt and pepper

3 oz. butter
10 black olives

1. Cut the eggplant down the middle, longwise, and cut into pieces which are a big portion and an inch thick.
2. Heat up a healthful dab of butter in an enormous pan.
3. Add the cheese on one side of the dish and eggplant on the other. Season eggplant with salt and pepper
4. Fry over medium-high heat for 5-7mins. Flip the cheese after three minutes, with the aim that it's darker on the 2 sides.
5. Mix the eggplant now.
6. Present with olives.

Nutrition:
829 Calories 72g Fat 32g Protein

634. White Lasagna Stuffed Peppers

Preparation Time: 5 minutes Cooking Time: 1 hour Serving: 4

2 large sweet peppers
12 oz. ground turkey
1 cup mozzarella

1 tsp garlic salt
3/4 cup ricotta cheese

1. Preheat stove to 400.
2. Put the cut peppers in a heating dish. Sprinkle with 1/4 tsp garlic salt. Gap the ground turkey between the peppers. Sprinkle with another 1/4 tsp garlic salt. Cook for 30 minutes.
3. Partition the ricotta cheese between the peppers. Sprinkle with 1/2 tsp garlic salt. Sprinkle the mozzarella on top. Put the cherry tomatoes in the middle of the peppers, if utilizing.
4. Cook for an extra 30 minutes until the meat is cooked, and the cheese is golden.

Nutrition:
281 Calories 14g Fat 32g Protein

635. Boiled Eggs with Butter and Thyme

Preparation Time: 10 minutes Cooking Time: 6 minutes Servings: 1

3 large eggs
Freshly ground black pepper
1/4 tsp thyme leaves

1 tbsp. good quality unsalted butter
Salt

1. Fill a medium pan most of the way with water and heat until boiling.
2. When water is bubbling, tenderly put eggs in water and flip using a large spoon.
3. While your eggs are cooking, place one tsp of margarine in a microwave-safe bowl and microwave until dissolved, for around 20 seconds.
4. In the meantime, take the pan and cautiously spill out the excessive water carefully.
5. Cautiously remove shell from every egg, wash to remove any shell parts, and add in the softened margarine.
6. Add the thyme leaves as well as the salt and pepper for flavor.

Nutrition:
159 Calories 18g Fat 8g Protein

636. Fluffy Microwave Scrambled Eggs

Preparation Time: 5 minutes Cooking Time: 5 minutes Serving: 2

4 eggs
1/8 teaspoon salt

1/4 cup milk

1. Break the eggs into a microwavable bowl. Add milk and salt; blend well.
2. Pop the bowl into the microwave and cook on high for 30 seconds. Remove the bowl, beat eggs well overall, scratching down the sides of the bowl, and place back into the microwave for an additional 30 seconds.
3. Repeat this example, blending like clockwork for up to 2 1/2 minutes. Stop when eggs have the consistency you want.

Nutrition:
141 Calories 9.3g Fat 12.3g Protein

637. Caesar Salad Deviled Eggs

Preparation Time: 120 minutes Cooking Time: 10 minutes Serving: 4

6 large pastured eggs
1/2 cup Parmesan cheese
1 romaine lettuce leaf

1/3 cup creamy Caesar dressing
Cracked black pepper

1. In a blending bowl, crush the egg yolks with a fork. Add Caesar dressing, 1/4 cup of the Parmesan cheddar and half of the chopped lettuce, then mix.
2. Utilize a baked good sack to pipe the blend into the egg whites.
3. Top each egg with a little Parmesan cheddar, shredded lettuce and black pepper.

Nutrition:
254 Calories 22g Fat 13.5g Protein

638. Caesar Egg Salad Lettuce Wraps
Preparation Time: 10 minutes Cooking Time: 10 minutes Serving: 4

6 large hard-boiled eggs	3 tbsp. creamy Caesar and 3 tbsp. mayonnaise
1/2 cup Parmesan cheese	Cracked black pepper
4 large romaine lettuce leaves	

1. In a blending bowl, mix eggs, velvety Caesar dressing, mayonnaise, 1/4 cup Parmesan cheddar and black pepper.
2. Spoon blend into a mixture of romaine leaves and top with residual Parmesan cheddar.

Nutrition:
254 Calories 22g Fat 13.5g Protein

639. Sour Cream and Chive Egg Clouds
Preparation Time: 10 minutes Cooking Time: 6 minutes Serving: 4

8 large pastured eggs	1/4 cup sharp white cheddar cheese
1/4 cup sour cream	1 tsp garlic powder
2 chives and 2 tsp salted butter	

1. Preheat stove to 450°. Line an oven tray with parchment paper.
2. Separate the eggs, emptying the whites into an enormous blending bowl, and the yolks into singular ramekins.
3. Utilizing an electric blender, whip the egg whites until they are fleecy and solid pinnacles have begun to frame.
4. Utilizing an elastic spatula, delicately overlap in cheddar, cream, garlic powder, and half of the chives.
5. Spoon blend into 8 separate hills on the parchment paper. Make a hole in the focal point of each cloud.
6. Heat for 6 minutes or until the mists are golden on top and the yolks are set.
7. Put a modest quantity of margarine over every yolk. Top with chives.
8. Serve and Enjoy

Nutrition:
117 Calories 10g Fat 6g Protein

640. Turkey and Cheese Rolls
Preparation Time: 15 minutes Cooking Time: 15 minutes Serving: 3

6 slices of all	natural turkey breast
3 slices all	natural Colby jack cheese

1. Lay turkey breast level on a plate then lay a portion of the Colby jack over each bit of turkey.
2. Roll.
3. Pack them up in a compartment as quick snacks for work the following day.

Nutrition:
104 Calories 3g Fat 7g Protein

641. Bacon-Wrapped Avocado Fries
Preparation Time: 10 minutes Cooking Time: 10 minutes Servings: 20

20 strips of pre	cooked packaged bacon
1 large avocado sliced into thin fry	size pieces

1. Preheat stove to 425°F. Take one strip of precooked bacon and attempt to tenderly stretch somewhat longer without it breaking.
2. Cautiously fold-over avocado, beginning toward one side and attempting to the opposite end.
3. Repeat with remaining ingredients and put onto an oven tray. Heat for 5-10 minutes and serve.

Nutrition:

65 Calories 5.1g Fat 4g Protein

642. Crispy Sweet Potato Fries
Preparation Time: 15 minutes Cooking Time: 10 minutes Serving: 4

1 1/2 lbs. sweet potatoes	Sea salt
Garlic powder	Onion powder

1. In a cast-iron skillet over medium-high to high heat, add 1/2 to 1 inch of oil.
2. When the oil is hot and you can begin to see little air pockets forming, add the sweet potato fries to the container.
3. Fry until they are brilliant darker and marginally firm, around 10 minutes.
4. Remove from oil and move to a paper towel to absorb excess oil.
5. Add sea salt, garlic powder and onion powder in a little bowl. Sprinkle flavoring over top of the sweet potato fries.

Nutrition:
102 Calories 8g Fat 4g Protein

643. Baked Eggs and Asparagus with Parmesan
Preparation Time: 7 minutes Cooking Time: 18 minutes Serving: 2

thick asparagus spears	4- eggs
2- tsp. olive oil	salt and black pepper
2- T Parmesan cheese	

1. Preheat the stove to 400F/200C and shower two gratin dishes with a spray of olive oil.
2. Break each egg into a little dish and give eggs a chance to come to room temperature while you cook the asparagus.
3. Remove the base of every asparagus and dispose of it. Cut the remainder of asparagus into short pieces under 2 inches in length.
4. Put a large portion of the asparagus pieces into each gratin dish and put dishes into the stove to cook the asparagus, setting a clock for 10 minutes.
5. Once the timer goes off, remove gratin dishes from the stove and cautiously slide two eggs over the asparagus in each dish. Set back in the stove and set the clock for 5 minutes.
6. Following 5 minutes, remove gratin dishes and sprinkle each with a tablespoon of coarsely-ground Parmesan.

Nutrition:
248 Calories 19g Fat 20g Protein

644. Cauliflower-Spinach Side Dish
Preparation Time: 10 minutes Cooking Time: 5 minutes Serving: 7

2 3/4 cups cauliflower florets	2 cups spinach leaves
2 tablespoons butter	1 teaspoon of sea salt
2 spreadable cheese wedges	

1. Run cauliflower through a nourishment processor to get 2 cups of shredded cauliflower just bigger than the consistency of cornmeal.
2. Add cauliflower, spinach, margarine, and salt in a huge pot over low heat.
3. Cover and cook until cauliflower is delicate and spinach has withered, 5 to 7 minutes. Mix in cheddar wedges until the cauliflower and spinach are covered and no cheddar bunches remain.

Nutrition:
180 Calories 14g Fat 3.2g Protein

645. Savory Salmon Fat Bombs
Preparation Time: 2 hours Serving: 6

1/2 cup full-fat cream cheese	1/3 cup butter
1/2 package smoked salmon	1 tbsp fresh lemon juice
1-2 tbsp freshly chopped dill	

1. Put the cream cheese, butter and smoked salmon into a nourishment processor.
2. Add lemon juice and dill and beat until smooth.
3. Line a plate with parchment paper and make little fat bombs utilizing around 2 1/2 tablespoons of the blend per piece.
4. Trimming with more dill and put in the cooler for 1-2 hours or until firm

Nutrition:
300 Calories 30g Fat 3g Protein

646.   Pistachio Arugula Salad

Preparation Time: 20 minutes Serving: 6

6 Cups Kale, Chopped Rough	2 Cups arugula
½ Teaspoon Smoked Paprika	1/3 Cup Pistachios, Unsalted & Shelled
6 Tablespoons Parmesan, Grated	

1. Get out a large bowl and combine your oil, 2 tbsp. of lemon juice, kale and smoked paprika. Massage it into the leaves for about fifteen seconds. You then need to allow it to sit for ten minutes.
2. Mix everything together before serving with grated cheese on top.

Nutrition:
150 Calories 5g Protein 12g Fat

647.   Potato Salad

Preparation Time: 9 minutes Cooking Time: 12 minutes Serving: 6

2 lbs. Golden Potatoes	Cubed in 1 Inch Pieces
¼ Teaspoon Sea Salt	Fine
½ Cup Olives	Sliced
1 Cup Celery	Sliced
2 Tablespoons Oregano	mint leaves

1. Take a medium pot and put your potatoes in cold water. Set it over high heat and bring it to a boil before turning the heat down. You want to turn it down to medium-low. Allow it to cook for twelve to fifteen more minutes. The potatoes should be tender when you pierce them with a fork.
2. Get out a small bowl and whisk your oil, 3 tbsp. lemon juice, 1 tbsp. olive brine and salt together.
3. Drain your potatoes using a colander and transfer it to a serving bowl. Pour in three tablespoons of dressing over your potatoes, and mix well with oregano, and min along with the remaining dressing.

Nutrition:
175 Calories 3g Protein 7g Fat

648.   Flavorful Braised Kale

Preparation Time: 9 minutes Cooking Time: 23 minutes Serving: 6

1 lb. Kale, Stems Removed & Chopped Roughly	1 Cup Cherry Tomatoes, Halved
4 Cloves Garlic, Sliced Thin	½ Cup Vegetable Stock
1 Tablespoon Lemon Juice, Fresh	

1. Warm up olive oil in a frying pan using medium heat, and add in your garlic. Sauté for a minute or two until lightly golden.
2. Mix your kale and vegetable stock with your garlic, adding it to your pan.
3. Cover the pan and then turn the heat down to medium-low.
4. Allow it to cook until your kale wilts and part of your vegetable stock should be dissolved. It should take roughly five minutes.
5. Stir in your tomatoes and cook without a lid until your kale is tender, and then remove it from heat.
6. Mix in your salt, pepper and lemon juice before serving warm.

Nutrition:
70 Calories 4g Protein 0.5g Fat

649.   Bean Salad

Preparation Time: 15 minutes Serving: 6

1 Can Garbanzo Beans, Rinsed & Drained	1/3 Cup Parsley, Fresh & Chopped
1 Red Onion, Diced	6 Lettuce Leaves
½ Cup Celery, Chopped Fine/Black Pepper to Taste	

1. Make the vinaigrette dressing by whipping together your 4 garlic cloves, parsley, 2 tbsp. vinegar and pepper in a bowl.
2. Add the olive oil to this mixture and whisk before setting it aside.
3. Add in your onion and beans, and then pour your dressing on top. Toss until it's coated together and then cover it. Chill until it's time to serve.
4. Place a lettuce leaf on the plate when serving and spoon the mixture in. garnish with celery.

Nutrition:
218 Calories 7g Protein 0.4g Fat

650.   Basil Tomato Skewers

Preparation Time: 6 minutes Serving: 2

16 Mozzarella Balls, Fresh & Small	16 Basil Leaves, Fresh
16 Cherry Tomatoes	Olive Oil to Drizzle
Sea Salt & Black Pepper to Taste	

1. Start by threading your basil, cheese and tomatoes together on small skewers.
2. Dash with oil before seasoning with salt and pepper. Serve immediately.

Nutrition:
46 Calories 7.6g Protein0.9g Fat

651. Olives with Feta

Preparation Time: 5 minutes Serving: 4

½ Cup Feta Cheese	Diced
1 Cup Kalamata Olives	Sliced & Pitted
2 Cloves Garlic	Sliced
1 Lemon	Zested & Juiced
1 Teaspoon Rosemary	Fresh & Chopped

1. Mix everything together and serve over crackers.

Nutrition:
71 Calories 4g Protein 2.6g Fat

652.   Black Bean Medley

Preparation Time: 5 minutes Serving: 4

4 Plum Tomatoes	Chopped
14.5 Ounces Black Beans	Canned & Drained
½ Red Onion	Sliced
¼ Cup Dill	Feta Cheese
1 Lemon	Juiced

1. Mix everything in a bowl except for your feta and salt. Top the beans with salt and feta.

Nutrition:
121 Calories 6g Protein5g Fat

653.   Grilled Fish with Lemons

Preparation Time: 12 minutes Cooking Time: 22 minutes Serving: 4

3-4 Lemons	1 Tablespoon Olive Oil
4 Catfish Fillets, 4 Ounces Each	

1. Pat your fillets dry using a paper towel and let them come to room temperature. This may take ten minutes. Coat the cooking grate of your grill with nonstick cooking spray while it's cold. Once it's coated preheat it to 400 degrees.
2. Cut one lemon in half, setting it to the side. Slice your remaining half of the lemon into ¼ inch slices. Get out a bowl and squeeze a tablespoon of juice from your reserved half. Add your oil to the bowl, mixing well.
3. Brush your fish down with the oil and lemon mixture.
4. Place your lemon slices on the grill and then put our fillets on top. Grill with your lid closed. Turn the fish halfway through if they're more than a half an inch thick.

Nutrition:
147 Calories 22g Protein1g Fat

654. Lemon Faro Bowl

Preparation Time: 6 minutes Cooking Time: 20 minutes Serving: 6

1 Carrot	2 Cups Vegetable Broth, Low Sodium
1 Cup Onion, Pearled Faro	2 Avocados, Peeled, Pitted & Sliced
1 Lemon, Small	

1. Preheat saucepan over medium-high heat. Add in a tablespoon of oil and then throw in your onion once the oil is hot. Cook for about five minutes, stirring frequently to keep it from burning.
2. Add in your carrot and 2 garlic cloves. Allow it to cook for about another minute while you continue to stir.
3. Add in your broth and faro. Let it boil and adjust your heat to high to help. Once it boils, lower it to medium-low and cover your saucepan. Let it simmer for twenty minutes. The faro should be al dente and plump.
4. Pour the faro into a bowl and add in your avocado and zest. Drizzle with your remaining oil and add in your lemon wedges.

Nutrition:
279 Calories 7g Protein 14g Fat

655. Chickpea & Red Pepper Delight

Preparation Time: 26 minutes Cooking Time: 8 minutes Serving: 3

1 Red Bell Pepper, Diced	2 Cups Water
¼ Cup Red Wine Vinegar	2 Cloves Garlic, Chopped
29 Ounces Chickpeas, Canned, Drained & Rinsed	

1. In a baking sheet, put your red bell pepper on it with the skin side up.
2. Bake for eight minutes. The skin should bubble, and then place it in a bag to seal it.
3. Remove your bell peppers in about ten minutes, and then slice it into thin slices.
4. Get out two cups of water and pour it in a bowl. Microwave for four minutes and add in 4 sundried tomatoes, letting them sit for ten minutes.
5. Drain them before slicing into thin strips. Mix your red wine vinegar and garlic with your olive oil. Season roasted red bell pepper with parsley, sun dried tomatoes, and chickpeas. Season with salt before serving.

Nutrition:
195 Calories 9.3g Protein 8.5g Fat

656. Pesto Pasta

Preparation Time: 10 minutes Serving: 4

3 Cloves Garlic, Minced Fine	1/2 Cup Basil Leaves, Fresh
¼ Cup Parmesan Cheese Grated	¼ Cup Pine Nuts
8 Ounces Whole Wheat Pasta	

1. Start by cooking your pasta per package instructions.
2. In a blender combine all remaining ingredients to make your pesto.
3. Serve with hot pasta.

Nutrition:
405 Calories 13g Protein 21g Fat

657. Eggplant Rolls

Preparation Time: 11 minutes Cooking Time: 8 minutes Serving: 6

1 Eggplant, ½ Inch Sliced Lengthwise	1/3 Cup Cream Cheese
½ Cup Tomatoes, Chopped	1 Clove Garlic, Minced
2 Tablespoons Dill, Chopped	

1. Slice your eggplant before brushing it down with olive oil. Sprinkle eggplant slices with salt and pepper.
2. Grill the eggplants for three minutes per side.
3. Get out a bowl and mix cream cheese, garlic, dill and tomatoes in a different bowl.
4. Allow your eggplant slices to cool and then spread the mixture over each one. Roll them and pin them with a toothpick to serve.

Nutrition:
91 Calories 2.1g Protein 7g Fat

658. Heavenly Quinoa

Preparation Time: 7 minutes Cooking Time: 17 minutes Serving: 5

1 Cup Almonds, Quinoa	1 Teaspoon Vanilla, Cinnamon
2 Cups Milk	3 Dates, Dried, Pitted & Chopped Fine
5 Apricots, Dried & Chopped Fine	

1. Get out a skillet to toast your almonds in for about five minutes.
2. Place your quinoa and cinnamon in a saucepan using medium heat. Add in your vanilla, salt and milk. Stir and then bring it to a boil. Reduce heat, and allow it to simmer for fifteen minutes.
3. Add in your dates, 2 tbsps. honey, apricots and half of the almonds.
4. Serve topped with almonds and parsley if desired.

Nutrition:
344 Calories 12.6g Protein 13.8g Fat

659. Roasted Squash Bisque

Preparation Time: 13 minutes Cooking Time: 1 hour Serving: 2

1 ½ Cups Winter Squash, Chopped	1 Clove Garlic, Minced
1 Cup Vegetable Broth, Low Sodium	¼ Teaspoon Nutmeg
1/3 Cup Almond Milk, Unsweetened / ¼ Cup Pistachios, Chopped Fine	

1. Start by heating your oven to 375F, and then spread your squash on a baking sheet. Bake for forty minutes to one hours. Allow your squash to cool, and then place it in a food processor.
2. Add in your pepper, garlic, nutmeg and broth. Mix until smooth.
3. Pour this soup mixture into a large saucepan and place it over a low heat. Stir constantly until your soup comes to a boil, which should take about five minutes.
4. Stir in your almond milk, and allow it to continue to cook and bubble for about five minutes.
5. Garnish with chopped pistachios before serving.

Nutrition:
244 Calories 6g Protein 13g Fat

660. Red Egg Skillet

Preparation Time: 4 minutes Cooking Time: 16 minutes Serving: 6

7 Greek Olives, Pitted & Sliced	3 Tomatoes, Ripe & Diced
4 Eggs	¼ Cup Parsley, Fresh & Chopped
1/8 Teaspoon Sea Salt, Fine	

1. Get out a pan and grease it. Throw your tomatoes in and cook for ten minutes before adding in your olives. Cook for another five minutes.
2. Add your eggs into the pan, cooking over medium-heat so that your eggs are cooked all the way through.
3. Season with salt and pepper and serve topped with parsley.

Nutrition:
188 Calories 10.3g Protein 15.5g Fat

SOUP AND STEWS RECIPES

661. Meatball Soup

Preparation Time: 10 minutes Cooking Time: 30 minutes Serving: 4

1 cup ground pork
1 garlic clove, onion
3 cups chicken stock

½ teaspoon ground black pepper
1 teaspoon ground thyme

1. Heat 1 tsp. avocado oil in the saucepan.
2. Add diced onion and cook it for 3 minutes.
3. Meanwhile, mix up ground pork, ground black pepper, minced garlic, and ground thyme.
4. Make the meatballs.
5. Pour the chicken stock in the onion and bring it to boil.
6. Add meatballs and cook the soup for 10 minutes over the medium heat.

Nutrition:
141 calories 22.7g protein 3.8g carbohydrates

662. Soup with Eggs

Preparation Time: 10 minutes Cooking Time: 10 minutes Serving: 4

1 onion, diced
2 eggs, beaten
1 oz Parmesan, grated

4 cups chicken stock
2 cups snap peas, frozen

1. Heat a saucepan with 1 tbsp. olive oil over medium-high heat, add onion, stir and cook for 2 minutes.
2. Add stock and bring to a boil.
3. Add eggs and all remaining ingredients in the soup.
4. Cook it for 7 minutes more.

Nutrition:
163 calories 10g protein 14.2g carbohydrates

663. Peas Soup

Preparation Time: 10 minutes Cooking Time: 25 minutes Serving: 4

¼ cup long-grain rice
½ cup Cheddar cheese, peas
½ teaspoon Italian seasonings

4 cups chicken stock
¼ teaspoon ground black pepper

1. Heat a saucepan with the stock.
2. Add all ingredients except Cheddar cheese and bring the soup to boil.
3. Then add cheese and stir it well.
4. Cook the soup for 5 minutes over the low heat.

Nutrition:
95 calories 5.4g protein 6.1g carbohydrates

664. Red Lentil Soup

Preparation Time: 5 minutes Cooking Time: 35 minutes Serving: 5

8 cups chicken broth
1 bell pepper, onion
1 teaspoon chili powder

cup red lentils
1 tablespoon tomato paste

1. Melt 1 tsp. olive oil in the saucepan and add onion and bell pepper.
2. Roast the vegetables for 5 minutes.
3. After this, add red lentils, tomato paste, chili powder, and chicken broth. Stir the soup well.
4. Cook the soup for 30 minutes over the medium heat.

Nutrition:

225 calories 18.4g protein 29.3g carbohydrates

665. Gazpacho

Preparation Time: 10 minutes Serving: 2

cup tomatoes
1 teaspoon Italian seasonings
1 cucumber, chopped

Kalamata olives, diced
tablespoons olive oil

1. Blend the tomatoes until smooth.
2. Add olives, Italian seasonings, olive oil, and cucumber.
3. Stir the soup.

Nutrition:
171 calories 1.8g protein 9.5g carbohydrates

666. Melon Gazpacho

Preparation Time: 10 minutes Serving: 5

1-pound cantaloupe, peeled, chopped
1 red onion, diced
1 teaspoon dried basil

1 tablespoon avocado oil
¼ cup of water

Direction
1. Incorporate all ingredients in the blender until smooth.
2. Pour the cooked gazpacho in the serving bowls.

Nutrition: 43 calories 1g protein 9.6g carbohydrates

667. Chicken Soup

Preparation Time: 10 minutes Cooking Time: 30 minutes Serving: 6

1-pound chicken breast, skinless, boneless, chopped
½ teaspoon ground black pepper
6 cups of water

½ cup fresh parsley, chopped
1 onion, diced

1. elt the 1 tsp. olive oil in the pan and add the onion.
2. Cook it until light brown.
3. Add chicken breast, parsley, and ground black pepper.
4. Add water and simmer the soup for 25 minutes.

Nutrition:
102 calories 16.4g protein 2.2g carbohydrates

668. Spicy Tomato Soup

Preparation Time: 10 minutes Cooking Time: 15 minutes - Serving: 4

2 cups tomatoes, chopped
1 teaspoon cayenne pepper, basil
1 oz Parmesan, grated

1 cup beef broth
1 teaspoon ground paprika

1. Blend the tomatoes and pour the mixture in the saucepan.
2. Add all remaining ingredients except Parmesan and bring the soup to boil.
3. Then ladle the cooked soup in the bowls and top with Parmesan.

Nutrition:
69 calories 5.9g protein 6.1g carbohydrates

669.   Chicken Strips Soup

Preparation Time: 5   Cooking Time: 30 minutes Serving: 4

8 oz. chicken fillet, cut into strips

1 cup plain yogurt

1 teaspoon chili flakes

2 tablespoons fresh cilantro, chopped

2 cups of water

1. Put all ingredients in the pan and simmer for 30 minutes on the low heat.

Nutrition:
152 calories 19.9g protein 4.4g carbohydrates

670.   Tomato Bean Soup

Preparation Time: 10 minutes Cooking Time: 40 minutes Serving: 4

5 oz. beef tenderloin, sliced

5 cups of water

tablespoons tomato paste

½ cup white beans, soaked

½ teaspoon chili flakes

1. Put all ingredients in the saucepan and stir until tomato paste is dissolved
2. Close the lid and cook the soup for 40 minutes over the medium-low heat.

Nutrition:
332 calories 28.3 g protein 47.2g carbohydrates

671.Zucchini Soup

Preparation Time: 10 minutes Cooking Time: 10 minutes Serving: 4

2 zucchinis, spiralized

1 teaspoon dried oregano

2 oz Parmesan, grated

2 tablespoons Greek yogurt

3 cups chicken stock

1. Pour chicken stock in the pan.
2. Add oregano and Greek yogurt and bring the liquid to boil.
3. Add spiralized zucchini and remove the soup from the heat.
4. Leave it for 10 minutes.
5. After this, add Parmesan and stir the soup gently.

Nutrition:
77 calories 7.3g protein 5g carbohydrates

672.   Pasta Soup

Preparation Time: 10 minutes Cooking Time: 30 minutes Serving: 4

6 oz chicken breast, skinless, boneless, chopped

5 cups of water

½ teaspoon salt

4 oz whole-grain pasta

1 teaspoon white pepper

1. Pour water in the pan and bring it to boil.
2. Add chicken breast, white pepper, and salt. Simmer the chicken for 15 minutes.
3. Then add pasta and cook the soup for 10 minutes more.

Nutrition:
260 calories 18.1g protein 39.3g carbohydrates

673.   White Mushrooms Soup

Preparation Time: 10 minutes Cooking Time: 25 minutes Serving: 2

4 oz white mushrooms, chopped

½ cup white onion, diced

2 cups of water

¼ cup Cheddar cheese, shredded

1 teaspoon cayenne pepper

1. Melt the 1 tbsp. olive oil in the pan and add onion and mushrooms.
2. Cook the vegetables for 5 minutes over the medium heat.

3. Then add cayenne pepper and water.
4. Simmer the soup for 10 minutes.
5. Add Cheddar cheese and stir the soup until the cheese is melted.
6. Remove the soup from the heat.

Nutrition:
142 calories 5.7g protein 5.2g carbohydrates

674.   Lamb Soup

Preparation Time: 10 minutes Cooking Time: 35 minutes Serving: 4

9 oz lamb sirloin, sliced

1 cup cauliflower, chopped

2 tablespoons tomato paste

5 cups of water

1 teaspoon dried dill

1. Preheat the pan well and add lamb sirloin.
2. Roast it for 1 minute per side.
3. Then add water, ½ tsp. ground black pepper, and dried dill.
4. Cook the meat for 20 minutes, covered.
5. Then add tomato paste and cauliflower. Stir the soup.
6. Cook the soup for 10 minutes.

Nutrition:
144 calories 19g protein 3.2g carbohydrates

675.   Lemon Zest Soup

Preparation Time: 10 minutes Cooking Time: 15 minutes Serving: 2

2 tablespoons lemon juice

¼ cup long-grain rice

1 celery stalk, chopped

½ teaspoon lemon zest, grated

4 cups chicken stock

1. Boil chicken stock then add rice, cook for 10 minutes.
2. Then add lemon zest and celery stalk. Cook the soup for 3 minutes more.
3. After this, add lemon juice and boil it for 2 minutes.

Nutrition:
109 calories 3.2g protein 20.6g carbohydrates

676.   Pumpkin Soup

Preparation Time: 30 minutes Cooking Time: 8 minutes - Serving: 4

1 onion, chopped

30 oz. pumpkin puree

1 teaspoon garlic powder

2 cups sweet potato, chopped

1-quart chicken stock

1. Add all the ingredients in the Instant Pot.
2. Seal the pot.
3. Press manual button.
4. Cook at high pressure for 8 minutes.
5. Release the pressure quickly.
6. Transfer the contents into a blender.
7. Pulse until smooth.
8. Season with salt and pepper.

Nutrition:
186 Calories 1.4g Fat 10.2g Fiber

677.   Lentil Soup

Preparation Time: 8 minutes Cooking Time: 13 minutes - Serving: 2

1 onion, chopped

Dried herb mixture: 1/2 teaspoon of each (cumin, coriander, sumac, parsley, mint)

3 cups vegetable broth

2 cloves garlic, chopped

1/2 cup red lentils

1. Select the sauté setting in the Instant Pot.
2. Add 2 tablespoons olive oil.
3. Sauté onion for 3 minutes.
4. Add the garlic and dried herb mixture.
5. Cook for 2 minutes, stirring frequently.

6. Add the lentils and broth.
7. Season with salt and pepper.
8. Seal the pot.
9. Choose manual mode.
10. Cook at high pressure for 8 minutes.
11. Release the pressure quickly.

Nutrition:
254 Calories 2.6g Fat 20.5g Protein

678.   Chickpea Soup
Preparation Time: 16 minutes Cooking Time: 22 minutes - Serving: 6

2 cups dry chickpeas, soaked in a bowl of water overnight	1 onion, chopped
2 carrots, chopped	4 teaspoons dried herb mixture (coriander, cumin, pepper, turmeric and all spice)
6 cups vegetable broth	

1. Drain the chickpeas and set aside.
2. Set the Instant Pot to sauté.
3. Add 2 tablespoons olive oil.
4. Add the onion and carrots.
5. Season with salt.
6. Cook for 5 minutes, stirring frequently.
7. Add the chickpeas and broth.
8. Lock the lid in place.
9. Cook at high pressure for 15 minutes.
10. Release the pressure quickly.

Nutrition:
297 Calories 5.4g Fat 45g Carbohydrate

679.   Chicken & Tomato Soup
Preparation Time: 30 minutes Cooking Time: 6 minutes - Serving: 6

3 cloves garlic, minced	1 lb. chicken breasts, cubed
28 oz. canned crushed tomatoes	6 cups chicken broth
1 teaspoon mixed garlic and onion powder	

1. Set the Instant Pot to sauté.
2. Add 1 tablespoon olive oil.
3. Cook the garlic until fragrant.
4. Add the chicken breast cubes.
5. Cook until brown on both sides.
6. Pour in the rest of the ingredients.
7. Seal the pot.
8. Set it to manual mode.
9. Cook at high pressure for 10 minutes.
10. Release the pressure quickly.

Nutrition:
237 Calories 7g Fat 12g Carbohydrate

680.   Chicken & Quinoa Stew
Preparation Time: 9 minutes Cooking Time: 23 minutes - Serving: 6

1 1/4 lb. chicken thigh fillet, sliced into strips	4 cups butternut squash, chopped
4 cups chicken stock	1 cup onion, chopped
½ cup uncooked quinoa	

1. Put the chicken in the Instant Pot.
2. Mix in rest of the ingredients except the quinoa.
3. Cover the pot.
4. Turn it to manual.
5. Cook at high pressure for 8 minutes.
6. Release the pressure naturally.
7. Stir the quinoa into the stew.
8. Set it to sauté.
9. Cook for 15 minutes.

Nutrition:
251 Calories 4.2g Fat 22g Carbohydrate

681. Vegetable & Lentil Soup
Preparation Time: 13 minutes Cooking Time: 18 minutes

6 cloves garlic, minced	4 cups mixed vegetables (cabbage, carrots, bell pepper, potatoes), chopped
5 tablespoons mixed spices (cumin, coriander, curry powder, turmeric, all spice)	6 cups chicken stock
1 1/4 cup green lentils	

1. Fill in 2 tablespoons olive oil into the Instant Pot.
2. Cook the garlic for 2 minutes.
3. Add the vegetables and spices.
4. Season with salt.
5. Cook for 5 minutes.
6. Pour in the stock and add the lentils.
7. Seal the pot.
8. Choose manual mode.
9. Cook at high pressure for 12 minutes.
10. Release the pressure naturally.

Nutrition:
257 Calories 1.7g Fat 44.9g Carbohydrate

682.   Carrot Soup
Preparation Time: 27 minutes Cooking Time: 7 minutes - Serving: 3

1 onion, chopped	1 lb. carrots, cubed
1/4 teaspoon cumin powder	1/4 teaspoon smoked paprika
3 cups vegetable broth	

1. Choose the sauté setting in the Instant Pot.
2. Pour in 2 tablespoons olive oil.
3. Cook onion for 2 minutes.
4. Add the rest of the ingredients.
5. Secure the lid.
6. Hit manual button.
7. Cook at high pressure for 5 minutes.
8. Release the pressure naturally.
9. Transfer the contents to a blender.
10. Blend until smooth.
11. Season with salt and pepper.

Nutrition:
116 Calories 1.5g Fat 6.6g Protein

683.   Lentil & Spinach Soup
Preparation time: 20 minutes Cooking Time: 16 minutes Serving: 4

1 cup onion, diced	4 teaspoons spice mixture (cumin, turmeric, thyme)
1 cup dry brown lentils	4 cups vegetable broth
6 cups baby spinach	

1. Choose the sauté function in the Instant Pot.
2. Pour in 1 tablespoon of olive oil.
3. Cook the onion for 2 minutes.
4. Add the spice mixture.
5. Season with salt and pepper.
6. Add the lentils and broth.
7. Secure the lid.
8. Select manual setting.
9. Cook at high pressure for 12 minutes.
10. Release the pressure quickly.
11. Mix in the spinach and wait for it to wilt.
12. Season with salt and pepper.

Nutrition:
230 Calories 2.1g Fat 19g Protein

684. Greek Veggie Soup

Preparation Time: 19 minutes Cooking Time: 17 minutes Serving: 4

1 clove garlic, minced
2 carrots, minced
15 oz. canned roasted tomatoes
3 cups cabbage, shredded
4 cups vegetable broth

1. Stir in 2 tablespoons of olive oil into the Instant Pot.
2. Add the garlic and cabbage.
3. Cook for 5 minutes.
4. Add the carrots and cook for 2 more minutes.
5. Pour in the broth and tomatoes.
6. Season with salt and pepper.
7. Seal the pot.
8. Set it to soup mode and adjust time to 10 minutes.
9. Release the pressure naturally.

Nutrition:
94 Calories 1.4g Fat 6.8g Protein

685. Veggie Stew

Preparation Time: 19 minutes Cooking Time: 23 minutes -Serving: 4

1 onion, minced

4 cups vegetable broth
2 tsp. Italian seasoning

1 package mixed frozen vegetables (carrots, potatoes, beans, broccoli)
20 oz. tomato sauce

1. Set the Instant Pot to sauté.
2. Add 1 tablespoon of olive oil.
3. Cook the onion for 1 minute.
4. Add the frozen vegetables.
5. Cook for 3 to 5 minutes.
6. Add the rest of the ingredients.
7. Cover the pot and set it to manual.
8. Cook at high pressure for 15 minutes.
9. Release the pressure naturally.
10. Season with salt and pepper.

Nutrition:
138 Calories 2.5g Fat 8.7g Protein

686. Carrot & Mushroom Soup

Preparation Time: 17 minutes Cooking Time: 16 minutes - Serving: 4

1 onion, diced
2 carrots, sliced
4 cups chicken stock
2 stalks celery, sliced
1/4 cup mushroom

1. Stir in 1 tablespoon olive oil to the pot.
2. Cook the onion, celery, carrots and mushroom for 5 minutes.
3. Cover the pot.
4. Choose manual function.
5. Pour in the stock.
6. Close the pot.
7. Select manual mode.
8. Cook at high pressure for 10 minutes.
9. Release the pressure naturally.

Nutrition:
71 Calories 1.2g Fat 2.9g Protein

687. White Bean & Swiss Chard Stew

Preparation Time: 17 minutes Cooking Time: 4 minutes - Serving: 8

1 lb. dried Great Northern beans, rinsed and soaked overnight
28 oz. canned roasted tomatoes

4 cups vegetable stock

2 teaspoons dried herbs (rosemary, oregano)
1 bunch Swiss chard, chopped into ribbons

1. Pour 1 tablespoon olive oil into the Instant Pot.
2. Add the beans, dried herbs and tomatoes.
3. Season with salt and pepper.
4. Cook for 1 minute.
5. Pour in the broth.
6. Seal the pot.
7. Choose bean/chili function.
8. Release the pressure quickly.
9. Select the sauté button.
10. Add the Swiss chard and cook for 3 minutes.

Nutrition:
241 Calories 0.8g Fat 15g Protein

688. White Bean & Kale Soup

Preparation Time: 18 minutes Cooking Time: 13 minutes - Serving: 10

1 white onion, chopped
28 oz. canned diced tomatoes
4 cups kale
4 cups vegetable stock
30 oz. white cannellini beans

1. Pour 3 tablespoons olive oil to the Instant Pot.
2. Sauté the white onion for 3 minutes.
3. Add the rest of the ingredients.
4. Switch it to manual setting.
5. Cover the pot and cook at high pressure for 10 minutes.
6. Release the pressure naturally.
7. Stir in the kale.
8. Cover the pot and wait for the kale to wilt before serving.

Nutrition:
206 Calories 0.5g Fat12.5g Protein

689. Bacon & Potato Soup

Preparation Time: 36 minutes Cooking Time: 12 minutes - Serving: 6

4 slices bacon, sliced in half
1 1/2 lb. potatoes, diced
1/2 cup sour cream
1/2 cup onion, chopped
2 cups chicken stock

1. Pour 1 tablespoon olive oil into the Instant Pot.
2. Add the bacon and cook until crispy.
3. Drain in paper towel and then chop.
4. Add the onion and cook for 2 minutes.
5. Add the potatoes and stock.
6. Cover the pot.
7. Set it to manual.
8. Cook at high pressure for 10 minutes.
9. Release the pressure naturally.
10. Transfer the contents to a blender.
11. Puree until smooth.
12. Stir in the sour cream.
13. Top with the crispy bacon bits.

Nutrition:
195 Calories 9.6g Fat 7.6g Protein

690. Lemon Chicken Soup

Preparation time: 18 minutes Cooking Time: 11 minutes - Serving: 4

3 chicken breast fillets
1 teaspoon garlic powder
6 cups chicken stock
1 onion, diced
2 tablespoons lemon juice

1. Situate all the ingredients except the lemon juice in the Instant Pot.
2. Mix well.
3. Choose manual setting.
4. Cook at high pressure for 10 minutes.
5. Release the pressure naturally.
6. Remove the chicken and shred.
7. Put it back to the pot and press sauté.
8. Stir in the lemon juice.
9. Season with salt and pepper.

Nutrition:

238	Calories	9.1g	Fat33g	Protein

VEGETARIAN RECIPES

691. Mediterranean Veggie Bowl

Preparation Time: 10 minutes Cooking Time: 20 minutes Serving: 4

1 cup quinoa, rinsed
2 cups cherry tomatoes, cut in half
1 cup Kalamata olives

1½ teaspoons salt, divided
1 large bell pepper, cucumber

1. Using medium pot over medium heat, boil 2 cups of water. Add the bulgur (or quinoa) and 1 teaspoon of salt. Cover and cook for 15 to 20 minutes.
2. To arrange the veggies in your 4 bowls, visually divide each bowl into 5 sections. Place the cooked bulgur in one section. Follow with the tomatoes, bell pepper, cucumbers, and olives.
3. Scourge ½ cup of lemon juice, olive oil, remaining ½ teaspoon salt, and black pepper.
4. Evenly spoon the dressing over the 4 bowls.
5. Serve immediately or cover and refrigerate for later.

Nutrition:
772 Calories 6g Protein 41g Carbohydrates

692. Grilled Veggie and Hummus Wrap

Preparation Time: 15 minutes Cooking Time: 10 minutes Serving: 6

1 large eggplant
½ cup extra-virgin olive oil
1 cup Creamy Traditional Hummus

1 large onion
6 lavash wraps or large pita bread

1. Preheat a grill, large grill pan, or lightly oiled large skillet on medium heat.
2. Slice the eggplant and onion into circles. Rub the vegetables with olive oil and sprinkle with salt.
3. Cook the vegetables on both sides, about 3 to 4 minutes each side.
4. To make the wrap, lay the lavash or pita flat. Spread about 2 tablespoons of hummus on the wrap.
5. Evenly divide the vegetables among the wraps, layering them along one side of the wrap. Gently fold over the side of the wrap with the vegetables, tucking them in and making a tight wrap.
6. Lay the wrap seam side-down and cut in half or thirds.
7. You can also wrap each sandwich with plastic wrap to help it hold its shape and eat it later.

Nutrition:
362 Calories 15g Protein 28g Carbohydrates

693. Spanish Green Beans

Preparation Time: 10 minutes Cooking Time: 20 minutes Serving: 4

1 large onion, chopped
1-pound green beans, fresh or frozen, trimmed

4 cloves garlic, finely chopped
1 (15-ounce) can diced tomatoes

1. In a huge pot over medium heat, cook olive oil, onion, and garlic; cook for 1 minute.
2. Cut the green beans into 2-inch pieces.
3. Add the green beans and 1 teaspoon of salt to the pot and toss everything together; cook for 3 minutes.
4. Add the diced tomatoes, remaining ½ teaspoon of salt, and black pepper to the pot; continue to cook for another 12 minutes, stirring occasionally.
5. Serve warm.

Nutrition:
200 Calories 4g Protein 18g Carbohydrates

694. Rustic Cauliflower and Carrot Hash

Preparation Time: 10 minutes Cooking Time: 10 minutes Serving: 4

1 large onion, chopped
2 cups carrots, diced
½ teaspoon ground cumin

1 tablespoon garlic, minced
4 cups cauliflower pieces, washed

1. In a big skillet over medium heat, heat up 3 tbsps. of olive oil, onion, garlic, and carrots for 3 minutes.
2. Cut the cauliflower into 1-inch or bite-size pieces. Add the cauliflower, salt, and cumin to the skillet and toss to combine with the carrots and onions.
3. Cover and cook for 3 minutes.
4. Throw the vegetables and continue to cook uncovered for an additional 3 to 4 minutes.
5. Serve warm.

Nutrition:
159 Calories 3g Protein 15g Carbohydrates

695. Roasted Cauliflower and Tomatoes

Preparation Time: 5 minutes Cooking Time: 25 minutes Serving: 4

4 cups cauliflower, cut into 1-inch pieces
4 cups cherry tomatoes
½ cup grated Parmesan cheese

6 tablespoons extra-virgin olive oil, divided
½ teaspoon freshly ground black pepper

1. Preheat the oven to 425°F.
2. Add the cauliflower, 3 tablespoons of olive oil, and ½ teaspoon of salt to a large bowl and toss to evenly coat. Pour onto a baking sheet and spread the cauliflower out in an even layer.
3. In another large bowl, add the tomatoes, remaining 3 tablespoons of olive oil, and ½ teaspoon of salt, and toss to coat evenly. Pour onto a different baking sheet.
4. Put the sheet of cauliflower and the sheet of tomatoes in the oven to roast for 17 to 20 minutes until the cauliflower is lightly browned and tomatoes are plump.
5. Using a spatula, spoon the cauliflower into a serving dish, and top with tomatoes, black pepper, and Parmesan cheese. Serve warm.

Nutrition:
294 Calories 9g Protein 13g Carbohydrates

696. Roasted Acorn Squash

Preparation Time: 10 minutes Cooking Time: 35 minutes Serving: 6

2 acorn squash, medium to large
5 tablespoons unsalted butter
2 tablespoons fresh thyme leaves

2 tablespoons extra-virgin olive oil
¼ cup chopped sage leaves

1. Preheat the oven to 400°F.
2. Cut the acorn squash in half lengthwise. Scoop out the seeds and cut it horizontally into ¾-inch-thick slices.
3. In a large bowl, drizzle the squash with the olive oil, sprinkle with salt, and toss together to coat.
4. Lay the acorn squash flat on a baking sheet.
5. Put the baking sheet in the oven and bake the squash for 20 minutes. Flip squash over with a spatula and bake for another 15 minutes.
6. Melt the butter in a medium saucepan over medium heat.
7. Add the sage and thyme to the melted butter and let them cook for 30 seconds.

8. Transfer the cooked squash slices to a plate. Spoon the butter/herb mixture over the squash. Season with salt and black pepper. Serve warm.

Nutrition:
188 Calories 1g Protein 16g Carbohydrates

697.   Sautéed Garlic Spinach

Preparation Time: 5 minutes Cooking Time: 10 minutes Serving: 4

¼ cup extra-virgin olive oil   1 large onion, thinly sliced
3 cloves garlic, minced   6 (1-pound) bags of baby spinach, washed
1 lemon, cut into wedges

1. Cook the olive oil, onion, and garlic in a large skillet for 2 minutes over medium heat.
2. Add one bag of spinach and ½ teaspoon of salt. Cover the skillet and let the spinach wilt for 30 seconds. Repeat (omitting the salt), adding 1 bag of spinach at a time.
3. Once all the spinach has been added, remove the cover and cook for 3 minutes, letting some of the moisture evaporate.
4. Serve warm with lemon juice over the top.

Nutrition:
301 Calories 17g Protein 29g Carbohydrates

698.   Garlicky Sautéed Zucchini with Mint

Preparation Time: 5 minutes Cooking Time: 10 minutes Serving: 4

3 large green zucchinis   3 tablespoons extra-virgin olive oil
1 large onion, chopped   3 cloves garlic, minced
1 teaspoon dried mint

1. Cut the zucchini into ½-inch cubes.
2. Using huge skillet, place over medium heat, cook the olive oil, onions, and garlic for 3 minutes, stirring constantly.
3. Add the zucchini and salt to the skillet and toss to combine with the onions and garlic, cooking for 5 minutes.
4. Add the mint to the skillet, tossing to combine. Cook for another 2 minutes. Serve warm.

Nutrition:
147 Calories 4g Protein 12g Carbohydrates

699.   Stewed Okra

Preparation Time: 5 minutes Cooking Time: 25 minutes Serving: 4

4 cloves garlic, finely chopped   1 pound fresh or frozen okra, cleaned
1 (15-ounce) can plain tomato sauce   2 cups water
½ cup fresh cilantro, finely chopped

1. In a big pot at medium heat, stir and cook ¼ cup of olive oil, 1 onion, garlic, and salt for 1 minute.
2. Stir in the okra and cook for 3 minutes.
3. Add the tomato sauce, water, cilantro, and black pepper; stir, cover, and let cook for 15 minutes, stirring occasionally.

Nutrition:
201 Calories 4g Protein 18g Carbohydrates

700.   Sweet Veggie-Stuffed Peppers

Preparation Time: 20 minutes Cooking Time: 30 minutes Serving: 6

6 large bell peppers, different colors 3 cloves garlic, minced
1 carrot, chopped   1 (16-ounce) can garbanzo beans
3 cups cooked rice

1. Preheat the oven to 350°F.
2. Make sure to choose peppers that can stand upright. Cut off the pepper cap and remove the seeds, reserving the cap for later. Stand the peppers in a baking dish.

3. In a skillet over medium heat, cook up olive oil, 1 onion, garlic, and carrots for 3 minutes.
4. Stir in the garbanzo beans. Cook for another 3 minutes.
5. Remove the pan from the heat and spoon the cooked ingredients to a large bowl.
6. Add the rice, salt, and pepper; toss to combine.
7. Stuff each pepper to the top and then put the pepper caps back on.
8. Cover the baking dish with aluminum foil and bake for 25 minutes.
9. Remove the foil and bake for another 5 minutes.
10. Serve warm.

Nutrition:
301 Calories 8g Protein 50g Carbohydrates

701. Vegetable-Stuffed Grape Leaves

Preparation Time: 50 minutes Cooking Time: 45 minutes Serving: 7

2 cups white rice, rinsed   2 large tomatoes, finely diced
1 (16-ounce) jar grape leaves   1 cup lemon juice
4 to 6 cups water

1. Incorporate rice, tomatoes, 1 onion, 1 green onion, 1 cup of parsley, 3 garlic cloves, salt, and black pepper.
2. Drain and rinse the grape leaves.
3. Prepare a large pot by placing a layer of grape leaves on the bottom. Lay each leaf flat and trim off any stems.
4. Place 2 tablespoons of the rice mixture at the base of each leaf. Fold over the sides, then roll as tight as possible. Place the rolled grape leaves in the pot, lining up each rolled grape leaf. Continue to layer in the rolled grape leaves.
5. Gently pour the lemon juice and olive oil over the grape leaves, and add enough water to just cover the grape leaves by 1 inch.
6. Lay a heavy plate that is smaller than the opening of the pot upside down over the grape leaves. Cover the pot and cook the leaves over medium-low heat for 45 minutes. Let stand for 20 minutes before serving.
7. Serve warm or cold.

Nutrition:
532 Calories 12g Protein 80g Carbohydrates

702.   Grilled Eggplant Rolls

Preparation Time: 30 minutes Cooking Time: 10 minutes Serving: 5

2 large eggplants   4 ounces goat cheese
1 cup ricotta   ¼ cup fresh basil, finely chopped

1. Slice the tops of the eggplants off and cut the eggplants lengthwise into ¼-inch-thick slices. Sprinkle the slices with the salt and place the eggplant in a colander for 15 to 20 minutes. The salt will draw out excess water from the eggplant.
2. In a large bowl, combine the goat cheese, ricotta, basil, and pepper.
3. Preheat a grill, grill pan, or lightly oiled skillet on medium heat. Pat the eggplant slices dry using paper towel and lightly spray with olive oil spray. Place the eggplant on the grill, grill pan, or skillet and cook for 3 minutes on each side.
4. Remove the eggplant from the heat and let cool for 5 minutes.
5. To roll, lay one eggplant slice flat, place a tablespoon of the cheese mixture at the base of the slice, and roll up. Serve immediately or chill until serving.

Nutrition:
255 Calories 15g Protein 19g Carbohydrates

703.   Crispy Zucchini Fritters

Preparation Time: 15 minutes Cooking Time: 20 minutes Serving: 6

2 large green zucchinis   1 cup flour
1 large egg, beaten   ½ cup water
1 teaspoon baking powder

1. Grate the zucchini into a large bowl.

2. Add the 2 tbsps. of parsley, 3 garlic cloves, salt, flour, egg, water, and baking powder to the bowl and stir to combine.
3. In a large pot or fryer over medium heat, heat oil to 365°F.
4. Drop the fritter batter into 3 cups of vegetable oil. Turn the fritters over using a slotted spoon and fry until they are golden brown, about 2 to 3 minutes.
5. Strain fritters from the oil and place on a plate lined with paper towels.
6. Serve warm with Creamy Tzatziki or Creamy Traditional Hummus as a dip.

Nutrition:
446 Calories 5g Protein 19g Carbohydrates

704.   Cheesy Spinach Pies

Preparation Time: 20 minutes Cooking Time: 40 minutes Serving: 5

2 tablespoons extra-virgin olive oil   3 (1-pound) bags of baby spinach, washed

1 cup feta cheese   1 large egg, beaten

Puff pastry sheets

1. Preheat the oven to 375°F.
2. In a large skillet over medium heat, cook the olive oil, 1 onion, and 2 garlic cloves for 3 minutes.
3. Add the spinach to the skillet one bag at a time, letting it wilt in between each bag. Toss using tongs. Cook for 4 minutes. Once the spinach is cooked, drain any excess liquid from the pan.
4. Mix feta cheese, egg, and cooked spinach.
5. Lay the puff pastry flat on a counter. Cut the pastry into 3-inch squares.
6. Place a tablespoon of the spinach mixture in the center of a puff-pastry square. Fold over one corner of the square to the diagonal corner, forming a triangle. Crimp the edges of the pie by pressing down with the tines of a fork to seal them together. Repeat until all squares are filled.
7. Situate the pies on a parchment-lined baking sheet and bake for 25 to 30 minutes or until golden brown. Serve warm or at room temperature.

Nutrition:
503 Calories 16g Protein 38g Carbohydrates

705.   Instant Pot Black Eyed Peas

Preparation Time: 6 minutes Cooking Time: 25 minutes Servings: 4

2 cups black-eyed peas (dried)   1 cup parsley, dill

2 slices oranges, 2 tbsp. tomato paste   4 green onions

2 carrots, bay leaves

1. Clean the dill thoroughly with water removing stones.
2. Add all the ingredients in the instant pot and stir well to combine.
3. Lid the instant pot and set the vent to sealing.
4. Set time for twenty-five minutes. When the time has elapsed release pressure naturally.
5. Serve and enjoy the black-eyed peas.

Nutrition:
506 Calories 14g Protein 33g Carbohydrates

706.   Green Beans and Potatoes in Olive Oil

Preparation Time: 12 minutes Cooking Time: 17 minutes Serving: 4

15 oz. tomatoes (diced)   2 potatoes

1 lb. green beans (fresh)   1 bunch dill, parsley, zucchini

1 tbsp. dried oregano

1. Turn on the sauté function on your instant pot.
2. Pour tomatoes, a cup of water and olive oil. Add the rest of the ingredients and stir through.
3. Lid the instant pot and set the valve to seal. Set time for fifteen minutes.

4. When the time has elapsed release pressure. Remove the Fasolakia from the instant pot. Serve and enjoy.

Nutrition:
510 Calories 20g Protein 28g Carbohydrates

707.   Nutritious Vegan Cabbage

Preparation Time: 35 minutes Cooking Time: 15 minutes Serving: 6

3 cups green cabbage   1 can tomatoes, onion

Cups vegetable broth   3 stalks celery, carrots

2 tbsp. vinegar, sage

1. Mix 1 tbsp. of lemon juice. 2 garlic cloves and the rest of ingredients in the instant pot and. Lid and set time for fifteen minutes on high pressure.
2. Release pressure naturally then remove the lid. Remove the soup from the instant pot.

Nutrition:
67 Calories 0.4g Fat 3.8g Fiber

708.   Instant Pot Horta and Potatoes

Preparation Time: 12 minutes Cooking Time: 17 minutes Serving: 4

2 heads of washed and chopped greens (spinach, Dandelion, kale, mustard green, Swiss chard)   6 potatoes (washed and cut in pieces)

1 cup virgin olive oil   1 lemon juice (reserve slices for serving)

10 garlic cloves (chopped)

1. Position all the ingredients in the instant pot and lid setting the vent to sealing.
2. Set time for fifteen minutes. When time is done release pressure.
3. Let the potatoes rest for some time. Serve and enjoy with lemon slices.

Nutrition:
499 Calories 18g Protein 41g Carbohydrates

709.   Instant Pot Jackfruit Curry

Preparation Time: 1 hour Cooking Time: 16 minutes Serving: 2

1 tbsp. oil   Cumin seeds, Mustard seeds

2 tomatoes (purred)   20 oz. can green jackfruit (drained and rinsed)

1 tbsp. coriander powder, turmeric.

1. Turn the instant pot to sauté mode. Add cumin and mustard seeds, and allow them to sizzle.
2. Add other ingredients, and a cup of water then lid the instant pot. Set time for seven minutes on high pressure.
3. When the time has elapsed release pressure naturally, shred the jackfruit and serve.

Nutrition:
369 Calories 3g Fat 6g Fiber

710. Instant Pot Collard Greens with Tomatoes

Preparation Time: 18 minutes Cooking Time: 8 minutes Serving: 4

1 white onion (diced)   3tbsp olive oil

3 garlic cloves (minced)   Cup tomatoes (sun-dried and chopped)

1 bunch collard greens (roughly cut and hard stems removed)

1. Turn on the sauté function on your instant pot.
2. Add onions and olive oil to the instant pot and let cook for three minutes or until lightly browned.
3. Add the rest of ingredients one at a time while stirring.
4. Add salt and pepper to taste and a cup of water. Turn off the sauté function and set to manual. Set time for five minutes at high pressure.

5. When the time has elapsed, release pressure naturally.
6. Open the lid and drizzle a half lemon juice.
7. Serve and enjoy.

Nutrition:
498 Calories 19g Protein 32g Carbohydrates

711. Instant Pot Artichokes with Mediterranean Aioli

Preparation Time: 7 minutes Cooking Time: 10 minutes Serving: 3

3 medium artichokes (stems cut off)   1 cup vegetable broth
Mediterranean aioli

1. Place wire trivet in place in the instant pot then place the artichokes on the wire.
2. Pour vegetable broth over artichokes.
3. Lid the instant pot and put steam mode on. Set timer for 10 minutes. When the time has elapsed allow pressure to release.
4. Remove the artichokes from the instant pot and reserve the remaining broth, about a quarter cup.
5. Half the artichokes and place them on serving bowls. Drizzle broth.
6. Serve with aioli and enjoy.

Nutrition:
30 Calories 0.1g Fat 3.5g Fiber

712. Instant Pot Millet Pilaf

Preparation Time: 23 minutes Cooking Time: 11 minutes Serving: 4

1 cup millet   Cup apricot and shelled pistachios
                                     (roughly chopped)
1 lemon juice and zest   tbsp olive oil
Cup parsley (fresh)

1. Pour one and three-quarter cup of water in your instant pot. Place the millet and lid the instant pot.
2. Adjust time for 10 minutes on high pressure. When the time has elapsed, release pressure naturally.
3. Remove the lid and add all other ingredients. Stir while adjusting the seasonings.
4. Serve and enjoy

Nutrition:
308 Calories 11g Fat 6g Fiber

713. Instant Pot Stuffed Sweet Potatoes

Preparation Time: 13 minutes Cooking Time: 22 minutes Serving: 2

2 sweet potatoes (washed   cup chickpeas, onions
thoroughly)
2 spring onions   1 avocado
cooked couscous

1. Pour a cup and half of water in your instant pot then place steam rack in place.
2. Place the sweet potatoes on the rack. Set the valve to sealing and time for seventeen minutes under high pressure.
3. Meanwhile, roast the chickpeas on your pan with olive oil.
4. Add salt and pepper to taste then paprika. Stir until chickpeas are coated evenly.
5. Cook for a minute then put off the heat.
6. When the instant pot time elapses, release pressure naturally for five minutes. Let the sweet potatoes cool then remove them from the instant pot.
7. Cut the sweet potatoes lengthwise and use a fork to mash the inside creating a space for toppings.
8. Add the pre-prepared toppings then serve with feta cheese lemon wedges.

Nutrition:
776 Calories 26g Fat 23g Protein

714. Instant Pot Couscous and Vegetable Medley

Preparation Time: 9 minutes Cooking Time: 17 minutes Serving: 3

Onion (chopped)   1 red bell pepper and carrot
                                     (chopped)
1 cup couscous Israeli,   Garam masala, cilantro, lemon juice,
2 bays leave

1. Put on sauté function on your instant pot then add olive oil.
2. Add bay leaves followed by chopped onions the sauté for two minutes.
3. Add pepper and carrots then continue to sauté for one more minute.
4. Stir in couscous, Garam masala, salt to taste and a cup and three-quarter of water.
5. Switch the sauté function to manual and set for two minutes. When the time has elapsed naturally release pressure for ten minutes.
6. Fluff the couscous then mix in lemon juice and garnish with cilantro.
7. Remove from instant pot and serve when hot

Nutrition:
460 Calories 5g Fat 13g Protein

DESSERT RECIPES

715. Chocolate Ganache

Preparation Time: 10 minutes Cooking Time: 3 minutes Servings: 16

9 ounces bittersweet chocolate, cup heavy cream
chopped
1 tablespoon dark rum (optional)

1. Put the chocolate in a medium bowl. Heat the cream in a small saucepan over medium heat.
2. Bring to a boil. When the cream has reached a boiling point, pour the chopped chocolate over it and beat until smooth. Stir the rum if desired.
3. Allow the ganache to cool slightly before you pour it on a cake. Begin in the middle of the cake and work outside. For a fluffy icing or chocolate filling, let it cool until thick and beat with a whisk until light and fluffy.

Nutrition:
142 calories 10.8g fat 1.4g protein

716. Chocolate Covered Strawberries

Preparation Time: 15 minutes Cooking Time: 4 minutes Servings: 24

16 ounces milk chocolate chips   2 tablespoons shortening
1-pound fresh strawberries with
leaves

1. n a bain-marie, melt chocolate and shortening, occasionally stirring until smooth. Pierce the tops of the strawberries with toothpicks and immerse them in the chocolate mixture.
2. Turn the strawberries and put the toothpick in Styrofoam so that the chocolate cools.

Nutrition:
115 calories 7.3g fat 12.7g carbohydrates

717. Strawberry Angel Food Dessert

Preparation Time: 15 minutes Servings: 18

angel cake (10 inches)   packages of softened cream cheese
1 container (8 oz) of frozen fluff, 1 liter of fresh strawberries, sliced
thawed
1 jar of strawberry icing

1. Crumble the cake in a 9 x 13-inch dish.
2. Beat the cream cheese and 1 cup sugar in a medium bowl until the mixture is light and fluffy. Stir in the whipped topping. Crush the cake with your hands, and spread the cream cheese mixture over the cake.
3. Combine the strawberries and the frosting in a bowl until the strawberries are well covered. Spread over the layer of cream cheese. Cool until ready to serve.

Nutrition:
261 calories 11g fat 3.2g protein

718. Key Lime Pie

Preparation Time: 8 minutes Cooking Time: 9 minutes Servings: 8

(9-inch) prepared graham cracker   cups of sweetened condensed milk
crust
1/2 cup sour cream   3/4 cup lime juice
1 tablespoon grated lime zest

1. Preheat the oven to 175 ° C (350 ° F).

2. Combine the condensed milk, sour cream, lime juice, and lime zest in a medium bowl. Mix well and pour into the graham cracker crust.
3. Bake in the preheated oven for 5 to 8 minutes until small bubbles burst on the surface of the cake.
4. Cool the cake well before serving. Decorate with lime slices and whipped cream if desired.

Nutrition:
553 calories 20.5g fat 10.9g protein

719. Ice Cream Sandwich Dessert

Preparation Time: 20 minutes Servings: 12

22 ice cream sandwiches   Frozen whipped topping in 16 oz
                                 container, thawed
jar (12 oz) Caramel ice cream   1 1/2 cups of salted peanuts

1. Cut a sandwich in two. Place a whole sandwich and a half sandwich on a short side of a 9 x 13-inch baking dish. Repeat this until the bottom is covered, alternate the full sandwich, and the half sandwich.
2. Spread half of the whipped topping. Pour the caramel over it. Sprinkle with half the peanuts. Repeat the layers with the rest of the ice cream sandwiches, whipped cream, and peanuts.
3. Cover and freeze for up to 2 months. Remove from the freezer 20 minutes before serving. Cut into squares.

Nutrition:
559 calories 28.8g fat 10g protein

720.   Bananas Foster

Preparation Time: 5 minutes Cooking Time: 5 minutes Servings: 4

2/3 cup dark brown sugar   1/2 teaspoons vanilla extract
1/2 teaspoon of ground cinnamon bananas, peeled and cut lengthwise
                                 and broad
1/4 cup chopped nuts, butter

1. Melt the butter in a deep-frying pan over medium heat. Stir in sugar, 3 ½ tbsp. of rum, vanilla, and cinnamon.
2. When the mixture starts to bubble, place the bananas and nuts in the pan. Bake until the bananas are hot, 1 to 2 minutes. Serve immediately with vanilla ice cream.

Nutrition:
534 calories 23.8g fat 4.6g protein

721. Rhubarb Strawberry Crunch

Preparation Time: 15 minutes Cooking Time: 45 minutes Servings: 18

3 tablespoons all-purpose flour   3 cups of fresh strawberries, sliced
3 cups of rhubarb, cut into cubes 1/2 cup flour
1 cup butter

1. Preheat the oven to 190 ° C.
2. Combine 1 cup of white sugar, 3 tablespoons flour, strawberries and rhubarb in a large bowl. Place the mixture in a 9 x 13-inch baking dish.
3. Mix 1 1/2 cups of flour, 1 cup of brown sugar, butter, and oats until a crumbly texture is obtained. You may want to use a blender for this. Crumble the mixture of rhubarb and strawberry.
4. Bake in the preheated oven for 45 minutes or until crispy and light brown.

Nutrition:
253 calories 10.8g fat 2.3g protein

722.   Frosty Strawberry Dessert

Preparation Time: 5 minutes Cooking Time: 21 minutes Servings: 16

cup flour, white sugar, whipped cream

cups of sliced strawberries

1/4 cup brown sugar

1/2 cup chopped walnuts, butter

tablespoons lemon juice

1. Preheat the oven to 175 ° C (350 ° F).
2. Mix the flour, brown sugar, nuts, and melted butter in a bowl. Spread on a baking sheet and bake for 20 minutes in the preheated oven until crispy. Remove from the oven and let cool completely.
3. Beat the egg whites to snow. Keep beating until you get firm spikes while slowly adding sugar. Mix the strawberries in the lemon juice and stir in the egg whites until the mixture turns slightly pink. Stir in the whipped cream until it is absorbed.
4. Crumble the walnut mixture and spread 2/3 evenly over the bottom of a 9-inch by 13-inch dish. Place the strawberry mixture on the crumbs and sprinkle the rest of the crumbs. Place in the freezer for two hours. Take them out of the freezer a few minutes before serving to facilitate cutting.

Nutrition:
184 calories 9.2g fat 2.2g protein

723.   Dessert Pie

Preparation Time: 16 minutes Cooking Time: 18 minutes Servings: 12

cup all-purpose flour

8 oz whipped cream topping

1/2 cup butter, white sugar

1 package of cream cheese

1 (4-oz) package of instant chocolate pudding

1. Preheat the oven to 175 ° C (350 ° F).
2. In a large bowl, mix butter, flour and 1/4 cup sugar until the mixture looks like coarse breadcrumbs. Push the mixture into the bottom of a 9 x 13-inch baking dish. Bake in the preheated oven for 15 to 18 minutes or until lightly browned to allow cooling to room temperature.
3. In a large bowl, beat cream cheese and 1/2 cup sugar until smooth. Stir in half of the whipped topping. Spread the mixture over the cooled crust.
4. Mix the pudding in the same bowl according to the instructions on the package. Spread over the cream cheese mixture.
5. Garnish with the remaining whipped cream. Cool in the fridge.

Nutrition:
376 calories 23g fat 3.6g protein

724.   Sugar-Coated Pecans

Preparation Time: 15 minutes Cooking Time: 1 hour Servings: 12

egg white

1-pound pecan halves

1/2 teaspoon ground cinnamon

1 tablespoon water

1 cup white sugar

1. Preheat the oven to 120 ° C (250 ° F). Grease a baking tray.
2. In a bowl, whisk the egg whites and water until frothy. Combine the sugar, ¾ tsp. salt, and cinnamon in another bowl.
3. Add the pecans to the egg whites and stir to cover the nuts. Remove the nuts and mix them with the sugar until well covered. Spread the nuts on the prepared baking sheet.
4. Bake for 1 hour at 250 ° F (120 ° C). Stir every 15 minutes.

Nutrition:
328 calories 27.2g fat 3.8g protein

725.   Jalapeño Popper Spread

Preparation Time: 10 minutes Cooking Time: 3 minutes Servings: 32

2 packets of cream cheese, softened

1 (4-gram) can chopped green peppers, drained

1 cup grated Parmesan cheese

cup mayonnaise

grams diced jalapeño peppers, canned, drained

1. In a large bowl, mix cream cheese and mayonnaise until smooth. Stir the bell peppers and jalapeño peppers.
2. Pour the mixture into a microwave oven and sprinkle with Parmesan cheese.
3. Microwave on maximum power, about 3 minutes.

Nutrition:
110 calories 11.1g fat 2.1g protein

726.   Brown Sugar Smokies

Preparation Time: 10 minutes Cooking Time: 4 minutes Servings: 12

1-pound bacon

1 cup brown sugar, or to taste

(16 ounces) package little smokie sausages

1. Preheat the oven to 175 ° C (350 ° F).
2. Cut the bacon in three and wrap each strip around a little sausage. Place sausages wrapped on wooden skewers, several to one place the kebabs on a baking sheet and sprinkle generously with brown sugar.
3. Bake until the bacon is crispy, and the brown sugar has melted.

Nutrition:
356 calories 27.2g fat 9g protein

727.   Fruit Dip

Preparation Time: 5 minutes Servings: 12

(8 oz) package cream cheese, softened

1 (7 oz) jar marshmallow creme

1. Use an electric mixer to combine the cream cheese and marshmallow
2. Beat until everything is well mixed.

Nutrition:
118 calories 6.6g fat 13.4g carbohydrates

728.   Banana & Tortilla Snacks

Preparation Time: 5 minutes Servings: 1

flour tortilla (6 inches)

1 tablespoon honey

tablespoons raisins

tablespoons peanut butter

1 banana

1. Lay the tortilla flat. Spread peanut butter and honey on the tortilla. Place the banana in the middle and sprinkle the raisins. Wrap and serve.

Nutrition:
520 calories 19.3g fat 12.8g protein

729.   Caramel Popcorn

Preparation Time: 30 minutes Cooking Time: 1 hour Servings: 20

2 cups brown sugar

1/2 teaspoon baking powder

5 cups of popcorn

1/2 cup of corn syrup

teaspoon vanilla extract

1. Preheat the oven to 95° C (250° F). Put the popcorn in a large bowl.
2. Melt 1 cup of butter in a medium-sized pan over medium heat. Stir in brown sugar, 1 tsp. of salt, and corn syrup. Bring to a boil, constantly stirring — Cook without stirring for 4 minutes. Then remove from heat and stir in the soda and vanilla. Pour in a thin layer on the popcorn and stir well.
3. Place in two large shallow baking tins and bake in the preheated oven, stirring every 15 minutes for an hour. Remove from the oven and let cool completely before breaking into pieces.

Nutrition:
14g fat 253 calories 32.8g carbohydrates

730. Apple and Berries Ambrosia

Preparation Time: 15 minutes Serves 4

2 cups unsweetened coconut milk, chilled	2 tablespoons raw honey
1 apple, peeled, cored, and chopped	2 cups fresh raspberries
2 cups fresh blueberries	

1. Spoon the chilled milk in a large bowl, then mix in the honey. Stir to mix well.
2. Then mix in the remaining ingredients. Stir to coat the fruits well and serve immediately.

Nutrition:
386 calories 21.1g fat 4.2g protein

731. Chocolate, Almond, and Cherry Clusters

Preparation Time: 15 minutes Cooking Time: 3 minutes Serving: 5

1 cup dark chocolate (60% cocoa or higher), chopped	1 tablespoon coconut oil
½ cup dried cherries	1 cup roasted salted almonds

1. Line a baking sheet with parchment paper.
2. Melt the chocolate and coconut oil in a saucepan for 3 minutes. Stir constantly.
3. Turn off the heat and mix in the cherries and almonds.
4. Drop the mixture on the baking sheet with a spoon. Place the sheet in the refrigerator and chill for at least 1 hour or until firm.
5. Serve chilled.

Nutrition:
197 calories 13.2g fat 4.1g protein

732. Chocolate and Avocado Mousse

Preparation Time: 40 minutes Cooking Time: 5 minutes Serving: 5

8 ounces (227 g) dark chocolate (60% cocoa or higher), chopped	¼ cup unsweetened coconut milk
2 tablespoons coconut oil	2 ripe avocados, deseeded
¼ cup raw honey	

1. Put the chocolate in a saucepan. Pour in the coconut milk and add the coconut oil.
2. Cook for 3 minutes or until the chocolate and coconut oil melt. Stir constantly.
3. Put the avocado in a food processor, then drizzle with honey and melted chocolate. Pulse to combine until smooth.
4. Pour the mixture in a serving bowl, then sprinkle with salt. Refrigerate to chill for 30 minutes and serve.

Nutrition:
654 calories 46.8g fat 7.2g protein

733. Coconut Blueberries with Brown Rice

Preparation Time: 55 minutes Cooking Time: 10 minutes Serving: 4

1 cup fresh blueberries	2 cups unsweetened coconut milk
1 teaspoon ground ginger	¼ cup maple syrup
2 cups cooked brown rice	

1. Put all the ingredients, except for the brown rice, in a pot. Stir to combine well.
2. Cook over medium-high heat for 7 minutes or until the blueberries are tender.
3. Pour in the brown rice and cook for 3 more minute or until the rice is soft. Stir constantly.
4. Serve immediately.

Nutrition:
470 calories 24.8g fat 6.2g protein

734. Glazed Pears with Hazelnuts

Preparation Time: 10 minutes Cooking Time: 20 minutes Serving: 4

4 pears, peeled, cored, and quartered lengthwise	1 cup apple juice
1 tablespoon grated fresh ginger	½ cup pure maple syrup
¼ cup chopped hazelnuts	

1. Put the pears in a pot, then pour in the apple juice. Bring to a boil over medium-high heat, then reduce the heat to medium-low. Stir constantly.
2. Cover and simmer for an additional 15 minutes or until the pears are tender.
3. Meanwhile, combine the ginger and maple syrup in a saucepan. Bring to a boil over medium-high heat. Stir frequently. Turn off the heat and transfer the syrup to a small bowl and let sit until ready to use.
4. Transfer the pears in a large serving bowl with a slotted spoon, then top the pears with syrup.
5. Spread the hazelnuts over the pears and serve immediately.

Nutrition:
287 calories 3.1g fat 2.2g protein

735. Lemony Blackberry Granita

Preparation Time: 10 minutes Serving: 4

1 pound (454 g) fresh blackberries	1 teaspoon chopped fresh thyme
¼ cup freshly squeezed lemon juice	½ cup raw honey
½ cup water	

1. Put all the ingredients in a food processor, then pulse to purée.
2. Pour the mixture through a sieve into a baking dish. Discard the seeds that remain in the sieve.
3. Put the baking dish in the freezer for 2 hours. Remove the dish from the refrigerator and stir to break any frozen parts.
4. Return the dish back to the freezer for an hour, then stir to break any frozen parts again.
5. Return the dish to the freezer for 4 hours until the granita is completely frozen.
6. Remove it from the freezer and mash to serve.

Nutrition:
183 calories 1.1g fat 2.2g protein

736. Lemony Tea and Chia Pudding

Preparation Time: 30 minutes Serving: 4

2 teaspoons Matcha green tea powder (optional)	2 tablespoons ground chia seeds
1 to 2 dates	2 cups unsweetened coconut milk
Zest and juice of 1 lime	

1. Put all the ingredients in a food processor and pulse until creamy and smooth.
2. Pour the mixture in a bowl, then wrap in plastic. Store in the refrigerator for at least 20 minutes, then serve chilled.

Nutrition:
225 calories 20.1g fat 3.2g protein

737. Mint Banana Chocolate Sorbet

Preparation Time: 4 hours 5 minutes Serves 1

- 1 frozen banana
- 1 tablespoon almond butter
- 2 tablespoons minced fresh mint
- 2 to 3 tablespoons dark chocolate chips (60% cocoa or higher)
- 2 to 3 tablespoons goji (optional)

Direction
1. Put the banana, butter, and mint in a food processor. Pulse to purée until creamy and smooth.

2. Add the chocolate and goji, then pulse for several more times to combine well.
3. Pour the mixture in a bowl or a ramekin, then freeze for at least 4 hours before serving chilled.
Nutrition: 213 calories 9.8g fat 3.1g protein

738. Raspberry Yogurt Basted Cantaloupe

Preparation Time: 15 minutes Serving: 6
Ingredients:
- 2 cups fresh raspberries, mashed
- 1 cup plain coconut yogurt
- ½ teaspoon vanilla extract
- 1 cantaloupe, peeled and sliced
- ½ cup toasted coconut flakes

Direction
1. Combine the mashed raspberries with yogurt and vanilla extract in a small bowl. Stir to mix well.
2. Place the cantaloupe slices on a platter, then top with raspberry mixture and spread with toasted coconut.
3. Serve immediately.
Nutrition: 75 calories 4.1g fat 1.2g protein

739. Simple Apple Compote

Preparation Time: 15 minutes Cooking Time: 10 minutes Serving: 4
Ingredients:
- 6 apples, peeled, cored, and chopped
- ¼ cup raw honey
- 1 teaspoon ground cinnamon
- ¼ cup apple juice

Direction
1. Put all the ingredients in a stockpot. Stir to mix well, then cook over medium-high heat for 10 minutes or until the apples are glazed by honey and lightly saucy. Stir constantly.
2. Serve immediately.
Nutrition: 246 calories 0.9g fat 1.2g protein

740. Simple Peanut Butter and Chocolate Balls

Preparation Time: 45 minutes Serving: 15
Ingredients:
- ¾ cup creamy peanut butter
- ¼ cup unsweetened cocoa powder
- 2 tablespoons softened almond butter
- ½ teaspoon vanilla extract
- 1¾ cups maple sugar

Direction
1. Line a baking sheet with parchment paper.
2. Combine all the ingredients in a bowl. Stir to mix well.
3. Divide the mixture into 15 parts and shape each part into a 1-inch ball.
4. Arrange the balls on the baking sheet and refrigerate for at least 30 minutes, then serve chilled.
Nutrition: 146 calories 8.1g fat 4.2g protein

741. Simple Spiced Sweet Pecans

Preparation Time: 4 minutes Cooking Time: 17 minutes Serving: 4

1 cup pecan halves	3 tablespoons almond butter
1 teaspoon ground cinnamon	½ teaspoon ground nutmeg
¼ cup raw honey	

1. Preheat the oven to 350°F (180°C). Line a baking sheet with parchment paper.
2. Combine all the ingredients in a bowl. Stir to mix well, then spread the mixture in the single layer on the baking sheet with a spatula.
3. Bake in the preheated oven for 16 minutes or until the pecan halves are well browned.
4. Serve immediately.

Nutrition:
324 calories 29.8g fat 3.2g protein

742. Overnight Oats with Raspberries

Preparation Time: 5 minutes Serving: 2

2/3 cup unsweetened almond milk	¼ cup raspberries
1/3 cup rolled oats	1 teaspoon honey
¼ teaspoon turmeric	

1. Place the almond milk, raspberries, rolled oats, honey, turmeric, 1/8 tsp. cinnamon, and a pinch of ground cloves in a mason jar. Cover and shake to combine.
2. Transfer to the refrigerator for at least 8 hours, preferably 24 hours.
3. Serve chilled.

Nutrition:
81 calories 1.9g fat 2.1g protein

743. Yogurt Sundae

Preparation Time: 5 minutes Serving: 1

¾ cup plain Greek yogurt	¼ cup fresh mixed berries (blueberries, strawberries, blackberries)
2 tablespoons walnut pieces	1 tablespoon ground flaxseed
2 fresh mint leaves, shredded	

1. Pour the yogurt into a tall parfait glass and sprinkle with the mixed berries, walnut pieces, and flaxseed.
2. Garnish with the shredded mint leaves and serve immediately.

Nutrition:
236 calories 10.8g fat 21.1g protein

744. Blackberry-Yogurt Green

Preparation Time: 5 minutes Serves 2

1 cup plain Greek yogurt	1 cup baby spinach
½ cup frozen blackberries	½ cup unsweetened almond milk
¼ cup chopped pecans	

1. Process the yogurt, baby spinach, blackberries, almond milk, and ½ tsp. ginger in a food processor until smoothly blended.
2. Divide the mixture into two bowls and serve topped with the chopped pecans.

Nutrition: 201 calories 14.5g fat 7.1g protein

745. Moroccan Stuffed Dates

Preparation Time: 16 minutes Serving: 30

1 lb. dates	1 cup blanched almonds
1/4 cup sugar	1 1/2 tbsp orange flower water
1/4 teaspoon cinnamon	

1. Process the almonds, sugar and cinnamon in a food processor. Add 1 tbsp. butter and orange flower water and process until a smooth paste is formed.
2. Roll small pieces of almond paste the same length as a date. Take one date, make a vertical cut and discard the pit. Insert a piece of the almond paste and press the sides of the date firmly around. Repeat with all the remaining dates and almond paste.

Nutrition:
208 calories 12g fat 6g protein

746. Almond Cookies

Preparation Time: 13 minutes Cooking Time: 10 minutes Serving: 30

1 cup almonds, blanched, toasted and finely chopped

1 cup powdered sugar

4 egg whites

2 tbsp flour

1/2 tsp vanilla extract

1. Preheat oven to 320 F. Blend the almonds in a food processor until finely chopped.
2. Beat egg whites and sugar until thick. Add in vanilla extract and a pinch of cinnamon. Gently stir in almonds and flour. Place tablespoonfuls of mixture on two lined baking trays.
3. Bake for 10 minutes, or until firm. Turn oven off, leave the door open and leave cookies to cool. Dust with powdered sugar.

Nutrition:
219 calories 16g fat 8g protein

747. Watermelon Cream

Preparation Time: 15 minutes Servings: 2

1pound watermelon, peeled and chopped

1teaspoon vanilla extract

1 cup heavy cream tablespoons stevia

1 teaspoon lime juice

1. In a blender, combine the watermelon with the cream and the rest of the ingredients, pulse well, divide into cups and keep in the fridge for 15 minutes before serving.

Nutrition:
Calories 122 Fat 5.7 Fiber 3.2 Carbs 5.3 Protein 0.4

748. Grapes Stew

Preparation Time: 10 minutes Cooking Time: 10 minutes Servings: 4

2/3 cup stevia

tablespoon olive oil

1/3 cup coconut water

teaspoon vanilla extract

1 teaspoon lemon zest, grated

cup red grapes, halved

1. Heat up a pan with the water over medium heat, add the oil, stevia and the rest of the ingredients, toss, simmer for 10 minutes, divide into cups and serve.

Nutrition:
Calories 122 Fat 3.7 Fiber 1.2 Carbs 2.3 Protein 0.4

749. Cocoa Sweet Cherry Cream

Preparation Time: 2 hours Servings: 4

½ cup cocoa powder

¾ cup red cherry jam

¼ cup stevia

2 cups water

pound cherries, pitted and halved

1. In a blender, mix the cherries with the water and the rest of the ingredients, pulse well, divide into cups and keep in the fridge for 2 hours before serving.

Nutrition:
Calories 162 Fat 3.4 Fiber 2.4 Carbs 5

750. Spanish Nougat

Preparation Time: 17 minutes Cooking Time: 15 minutes Serving: 24

11/2 cup honey

3 egg whites

1 ¾ cup almonds, roasted and chopped

1. Pour the honey into a saucepan and bring it to a boil over medium-high heat, then set aside to cool. Beat the egg whites to a thick glossy meringue and fold them into the honey.
2. Bring the mixture back to medium-high heat and let it simmer, constantly stirring, for 15 minutes. When the color and consistency change to dark caramel, remove from heat, add the almonds and mix trough.
3. Line a 9x13 inch pan with foil and pour the hot mixture on it. Cover with another piece of foil and even out. Let cool completely. Place a wooden board weighted down with some heavy cans on it. Leave like this for 3-4 days, so it hardens and dries out. Slice into 1-inch squares.

Nutrition:
189 calories 12g fat 5g protein

751. Cinnamon Butter Cookies

Preparation Time: 12 minutes Cooking Time: 15 minutes Serving: 24

2 cups flour

1/2 cup sugar

5 tbsp butter

3 eggs

1 tbsp cinnamon

1. Cream the butter and sugar until light and fluffy. Combine the flour and the cinnamon. Beat eggs into the butter mixture. Gently add in the flour. Turn the dough onto a lightly floured surface and knead just once or twice until smooth.
2. Form a roll and divide it into 24 pieces. Line baking sheets with parchment paper or grease them. Roll each piece of cookie dough into a long thin strip, then make a circle, flatten a little and set it on the prepared baking sheet. Bake cookies, in batches, in a preheated to 350 F oven, for 12 to 15 minutes. Set aside to cool on a cooling rack.

Nutrition:
199 calories 13g fat 4g protein

752. Best French Meringues

Preparation Time: 15 minutes Cooking Time: 2 hours - Serving: 36

4 egg whites

2 1/4 cups powdered sugar

1. Preheat the oven to 200 F. and line a baking sheet.
2. In a glass bowl, beat egg whites with an electric mixer. Add in sugar a little at a time, while continuing to beat at medium speed. When the egg white mixture becomes stiff and shiny like satin, transfer to a large pastry bag. Pipe the meringue onto the lined baking sheet with the use of a large star tip.
3. Place the meringues in the oven and leave the oven door slightly ajar. Bake for 2 1/2 hours, or until the meringues are dry, and can easily be removed from the pan.

Nutrition:
210 calories 16g fat 9g protein

753. Cinnamon Palmiers

Preparation Time: 9 minutes Cooking Time: 17 minutes - Serving: 30

1/3 cup granulated sugar

2 tsp cinnamon

1/2 lb. puff pastry

1 egg, beaten (optional)

1. Stir together the sugar and cinnamon. Roll the pastry dough into a large rectangle. Spread the cinnamon sugar in an even layer over the dough.
2. Starting at the long ends of the rectangle, loosely roll each side inward until they meet in the middle. If needed, brush it with the egg to hold it together.
3. Slice the pastry roll crosswise into 1/4-inch pieces and arrange them on a lined with parchment paper baking sheet. Bake cookies in a preheated to 400 F oven for 12-15 minutes, until they puff and turn golden brown. Serve warm or at room temperature.

Nutrition:
211 calories 17g fat 6g protein

754. Baked Apples

Preparation Time: 17 minutes Cooking Time: 10 minutes Serving: 4

8 medium sized apples	1/3 cup walnuts, crushed
3/4 cup sugar	3 tbsp raisins, soaked in brandy or dark rum
2 oz butter	

1. Peel and carefully hollow the apples. Prepare stuffing by beating the butter, 3/4 cup of sugar, crushed walnuts, raisins and cinnamon.
2. Stuff the apples with this mixture and place them in an oiled dish. Sprinkle the apples with 1-2 tablespoons of water and bake in a moderate oven. Serve warm with a scoop of vanilla ice cream.

Nutrition:
219 calories 12g fat 5g protein

755. Pumpkin Baked with Dry Fruit

Preparation Time: 18 minutes Cooking Time: 15 minutes - Serving: 6

1lb. pumpkin, cut into medium pieces	1 cup dry fruit (apricots, plums, apples, raisins)
1/2 cup brown sugar	

1. Soak the dry fruit in some water, drain and discard the water. Cut the pumpkin in medium cubes. At the bottom of a pot arrange a layer of pumpkin pieces, then a layer of dry fruit and then again, some pumpkin.
2. Add a little water. Cover the pot and bring to boil. Simmer until there is no more water left. When almost ready add the sugar. Serve warm or cold.

Nutrition:
200 calories 14g fat 7g protein

756. Quick Peach Tarts

Preparation Time: 14 minutes Cooking Time: 10 minutes - Serving: 4

1 sheet frozen ready-rolled puff pastry	1/4 cup light cream cheese spread
2 tablespoons sugar	a pinch of cinnamon
4 peaches, peeled, halved, stones removed, sliced	

1. Line a baking tray with baking paper. Cut the pastry into 4 squares and place them on the prepared tray. Using a spoon, mix cream cheese, sugar, vanilla and cinnamon. Spread over pastry squares. Arrange peach slices on top.
2. Bake in a preheated to 350 F oven for 10 minutes, or until golden.

Nutrition:
205 calories 13g fat 4g protein

757. Bulgarian Rice Pudding

Preparation Time: 8 minutes Cooking Time: 15 minutes - Serving 4-5

1 cup short-grain white rice	6 tbsp sugar
1 1/2 cup whole milk, water	1 cinnamon stick
1 strip lemon zest	

1. Place the rice in a saucepan, cover with water and cook over low heat for about 15 minutes. Add milk, sugar, a cinnamon stick and lemon zest and cook over very low heat, stirring frequently, until the mixture is creamy. Do not let it boil. When ready, discard the cinnamon stick and lemon zest. Serve warm or at room temperature.

Nutrition:
187 calories 10g fat 3g protein

758. Caramel Cream

Preparation Time: 18 minutes Cooking Time: 1 hour - Serving: 8

11/2 cup sugar	4 cups cold milk
8 eggs	2 tsp vanilla powder

1. Melt 1/4 of the sugar in a non-stick pan over low heat. When the sugar has turned into caramel, pour it into 8 cup-sized ovenproof pots covering only the bottoms.
2. Whisk the eggs with the rest of the sugar and the vanilla, and slowly add the milk. Stir the mixture well and divide between the pots.
3. Place the 8 pots in a larger, deep baking dish. Pour 3-4 cups of water into the dish. Place the baking dish in a preheated to 280 F oven for about an hour and bake but do not let the water boil, as the boiling will overcook the cream and make holes in it: if necessary, add cold water to the baking dish.
4. Remove the baking dish from the oven; remove the pots from the dish. Place a shallow serving plate on top, then invert each pot so that the cream unmolds. The caramel will form a topping and sauce.

Nutrition:
213 calories 16g fat 8g protein

759. Yogurt-Strawberries Ice Pops

Preparation Time: 4 hours - Serving: 8-9

3 cups yogurt	3 tbsp honey
2 cups strawberries, quartered	

1. Strain the yogurt in a clean white dishtowel. Combine the strained yogurt with honey.
2. Blend the strawberries with a blender then gently fold the strawberry puree into the yogurt mixture until just barely combined, with streaks remaining. Divide evenly among the molds, insert the sticks and freeze for 3 to 4 hours until solid.

Nutrition:
216 calories 16g fat 8g protein

760. Fresh Strawberries in Mascarpone and Rose Water

Preparation Time: 11 minutes - Serving: 4

6 oz strawberries, washed	1 cup mascarpone cheese
1/2 teaspoon rose water	1/2 teaspoon vanilla extract
1/4 cup white sugar	

1. In a bowl, combine together the mascarpone cheese, sugar, rose water and vanilla. Divide the strawberries into 4 dessert bowls. Add two dollops of mascarpone mixture on top and serve.

Nutrition:
197 calories 10g fat 3g protein

761. Delicious French Eclairs

Preparation Time: 23 minutes Cooking Time: 43 minutes - Serving: 12

1/2 cup butter	1 cup boiling water
1 cup sifted flour	4 eggs
a pinch of salt	

1. In a medium saucepan, combine butter, salt, and boiling water. Bring to the boil, then reduce heat and add a cup of flour all at once, stirring vigorously until mixture forms a ball.
2. Remove from heat and add eggs, one at a time, whisking well to incorporate completely after each addition. Continue beating until the mixture is thick and shiny and breaks from the spoon.
3. Pipe or spoon onto a lined baking sheet then bake for 20 minutes in a preheated to 450 F oven. Reduce heat to 350 F and bake for 20 minutes more, or until golden. Set aside to cool and fill with sweetened whipped cream or custard.

Nutrition:
220 calories 17g fat 5g protein

762. Blueberry Yogurt Dessert

Preparation Time: 18 minutes - Serving: 6

1/3 cup blueberry jam
2 tbsp powdered sugar
2 cups yogurt

1 cup fresh blueberries
1 cup heavy cream

1. Strain the yogurt in a piece of cheesecloth.
2. In a large bowl, beat the cream and powdered sugar until soft peaks form. Add strained yogurt and 1 tsp. of vanilla and beat until medium peaks form and the mixture is creamy and thick.

3. Gently fold half the fresh blueberries and the blueberry jam into cream mixture until just barely combined, with streaks remaining. Divide dessert among 6 glass bowls, top with fresh blueberries and serve.

Nutrition:
208 calories 12g fat 6g protein

WEEK 1 MEAL PLAN

DAY	BREAKFAST	MAIN DISH	SIDES	DESSERT
SUNDAY	Egg with Zucchini Noodles	Steak with Olives and Mushroom	Lemon Fruit and Nut Bars	Chocolate Ganache
MONDAY	Banana Oats	Spicy Mustard Chicken	Cauliflower Fried Rice with Bacon	Chocolate Covered Strawberries
TUESDAY	Berry Oats	Walnut and Oregano Crusted Chicken	White Lasagna Stuffed Peppers	Strawberry Angel Food Dessert
WEDNESDAY	Sun-Dried Tomatoes Oatmeal	Chicken and Onion Casserole	Boiled Eggs with Butter and Thyme	Key Lime Pie
THURSDAY	Quinoa Muffins	Chicken and Mushroom	Fluffy Microwave Scrambled Eggs	Ice Cream Sandwich Dessert
FRIDAY	Watermelon Pizza	Herb-Roasted Lamb Leg	Caesar Salad Deviled Eggs	Bananas Foster
SATURDAY	Cheesy Yogurt	Spring Lamb Stew	Sour Cream and Chive Egg Clouds	Dessert Pie

WEEK 2 MEAL PLAN

DAY	BREAKFAST	MAIN DISH	SIDES	DESSERT
SUNDAY	Avocado and Chickpea Sandwiches	Baked-Lemon-Butter Fish	Pistachio Arugula Salad	Apple and Berries Ambrosia
MONDAY	Raisin Quinoa Breakfast	Fish Taco Bowl	Potato Salad	Chocolate, Almond, and Cherry Clusters
TUESDAY	Banana Cinnamon Fritters	Scallops with Creamy Bacon Sauce	Flavorful Braised Kale	Chocolate and Avocado Mousse
WEDNESDAY	Okra and Tomato Casserole	Shrimp and Avocado Lettuce Cups	Bean Salad	Coconut Blueberries with Brown Rice
THURSDAY	Ground Beef and Brussels Sprouts	Garlic Butter Shrimp	Basil Tomato Skewers	Glazed Pears with Hazelnuts
FRIDAY	Italian Mini Meatballs	Pork Rind Salmon Cakes	Olives with Feta	Lemony Blackberries Granita
SATURDAY	Salmon Kebabs	Creamy Dill Salmon	Black Bean Medley	Mint Banana Chocolate Sorbet

CONCLUSION

Changing your eating habits to follow the Mediterranean diet can be very exciting. Knowing that you're making the conscious decision to improve your diet – and your life – in a positive way and eating healthier is the first step of the Mediterranean diet. It might seem overwhelming at first, but you don't have to make all the changes in one day. The smaller changes you make, the more benefits you'll see, which will inspire you to make more beneficial changes. Those benefits will pay off big in the long run – for you and your family.

To successfully incorporate this new way of eating into your life, you should seriously consider adopting other parts of the Mediterranean lifestyle as well.

The Mediterranean diet – a well-balanced diet that includes healthy fats and complex carbohydrates – offers the best alternative to popular fad diets if you're looking to lose weight without sacrificing your health. By pairing this eating plan with lower stress and increased exercise, you can do more than just lose a few pounds; you can also reduce your blood pressure, cholesterol, and blood sugar.

One of the important influences' diets can have upon health is by merely establishing weight control. Being overweight can damage every body system and risk all our most serious, debilitating diseases. The Mediterranean diet helps one maintain a healthy weight by providing complex carbohydrates, fiber, and protein to help you feel full and slow digestion, so you feel satisfied.

One of the most critical keys to revamping your lifestyle to fit your new eating habits is stress reduction! This instruction may be a tricky one; after all, we all have periods of stress in our lives. Additionally, some of us seem destined to have more pressure in our lives than other people. Regardless, handling stress should begin with finding a realistic perspective on the factors that cause our stress and then doing what we can to change those factors. Maybe you can't follow the Mediterranean habit of taking a 2-hour midday break, but you can incorporate ways to reduce your stress throughout your day.

In the fast-paced and highly technical era we live in, it's sometimes hard to make time for your family. However, it should be a priority. Try planning dinner times so everyone can sit and eat a meal together. It helps build relationships and connections. Much research has shown that people with strong family interaction are less likely to suffer from depression.

If you don't live near any family members, you can create the same atmosphere with friends. Try planning weekly or bi-weekly get-togethers and maybe having a different friend host it each time. Making meals potlucks takes the stress off any one person preparing a big meal. When you go, take a Mediterranean diet recipe to share with your friends!

Besides reducing your stress level, getting more daily physical activity, and increasing your family time are solid guidelines that you should consider beginning to incorporate into your new way of life. Remember, no one is expecting you to make dramatic changes overnight.

THE MEDITERRANEAN SLOW COOKER COOKBOOK FOR BEGINNERS

250

QUICK AND EASY RECIPES FOR BUSY AND NOVICE THAT
COOK THEMSELVES
2-WEEK MEAL PLAN INCLUDED

BY
WILDA BUCKLEY

INTRODUCTION

The Mediterranean diet has been in practice in history for centuries.

Its origins can be traced to ancient Crete, Greece, Sicily, and southern Italy. It has always been associated with the healthy Mediterranean life style that produces long-lived people. Those who live a long fulfilling life are said to possess a little secret that gives them a longevity and serenity.

They do not suffer from such debilitating infirmities like heart problems, high blood pressure, Alzheimer's, stroke, and cancer. Their secret to longevity is the Mediterranean diet that they consume regularly.

For centuries the Mediterranean diet has kept people living a longer and healthier life style than others. The secret to long life is the diet's inclusion of ample vegetables, fruits, olive oil, and nuts. It is of the understanding that all vegetables and fruits, nuts, legumes, and fish are all rich in antioxidants that help the body combat the free radical damage that leads to inflammation and other diseases. Most importantly, they are rich in phytochemicals that help fight the various cancers in the body.

It is also observed that those who eat the Mediterranean way of life live a much healthier lifestyle. That's because of the simple fact that they do not suffer from obesity or obesity related conditions like diabetes 2 and heart diseases. They are active people and they burn off the excess calories so that they do not hoard them as fat in the body.

The Mediterranean diet is rich in foods that are good for the heart and blood vessels. They are also good for the proper function of the brain. This, therefore, aids in the brain's ability to affect the memory. This is why many people who have followed the Mediterranean way of life have lived for so long.

The diet can protect against a lot of infectious diseases, cancers, cardiovascular and neurodegenerative diseases. This being because of the high level of antioxidants in all the foods in the diet. A lack of these antioxidants in the body leads to a decreased immunity, reduced mental focus, and eventually Alzheimer's at some point in life.

Olive oil is the best source of monounsaturated fat that boost the HDL which stands for good cholesterol. Monounsaturated fat is also good as a heart lubricant. It helps protect the arteries from atherosclerosis. It also contains squalene, the anti-inflammatory and anti-cancer agent. Olive oil is also chocked full of antioxidants, crucial for a healthy body.

In addition, a common side effect of a monounsaturated fat is weight loss. That is because monounsaturated fat is better at filling the stomach than the saturated fat. The monounsaturated fat-filled stomach leads to a feeling of fullness, and this reduces the inclination to overeat. That is why people who follow the Mediterranean diet are not fat.

Among fruits, the grapefruit has a powerful compound called naringenin that was found effective in destroying one of the deadliest forms of cancer among women. Lemons are a rich source of phytochemicals that help prevent or reverse the damage caused by cancer and Alzheimer's. Strawberries are also packed with antioxidants and minerals that promote cardiovascular health.

Moreover, this diet is made for all, irrespective of age. Because of this, the diet is also beneficial for pregnant women because it helps to reduce the chances of having children that are born prematurely or underweight.

Nuts are also part of the diet as they help reduce heart disease, such as walnuts, also known to be effective in preventing colon cancer as well as some of the other cancers.

There are also fish, rich in omega-3 fatty acids. Among them is mackerel, salmon, and sardines. They are good for heart and brain health.

The diet also includes dairy and this was found to be helpful in combatting the risks of heart diseases as well as ailments like diabetes 2 and Alzheimer's.

Finally, the diet also includes wine and the right kind of alcohols. The wine traditions of the Mediterranean are many. Just like the diet itself, enjoying wine is one of the healthiest types of alcohols with a host of health benefits.

In modern times, people around the globe adopted the Mediterranean diet. In the US, the Mediterranean diet is viewed as a healthy, safe, and effective weight loss approach. It is promoted by the non-profit Oldways Preservation & Exchange Trust. The diet is based on the Mediterranean Diet Pyramid which was identified in the year 1992.

There were, however, critics of the diet. Some of them considered it to be too expensive to adhere to. Others felt that it was time-consuming when it came to cooking and preparation time.

But all and all, the Mediterranean diet is a great diet. It is tasty, delicious, and healthy at the same time.

BREAKFAST

763.   Egg and Vegetable Breakfast Casserole

Preparation time: 15 minutes | Cooking time: 4 hours | Servings: 8

8 eggs	4 egg whites
¾ cup milk (can use almond)	2 teaspoons stone-ground mustard
½ teaspoon garlic salt	1 teaspoon salt
½ teaspoon pepper	1 30-ounce bag frozen hash browns
4 strips cooked bacon (optional)	½ onion, roughly chopped
2 bell peppers, roughly chopped	1 small head of broccoli, roughly chopped
6 ounces cheddar cheese	

1. Mix the eggs, egg whites, milk, mustard, garlic salt, salt, and pepper until well combined.
2. Spray the inside of the slow cooker with olive oil.
3. Spread half of the hash browns bag across the slow cooker's bottom and then top with bacon.
4. Pour egg mixture over the bacon and potatoes. Add the onion, bell peppers, and broccoli, then top with remaining hash browns and cheese. Cook on low for 4 hours.

Nutrition:
Calories 320 Fat 13 g Carbs 29 g Protein 22 g Sodium 700 mg

764.   Breakfast Stuffed Peppers

Preparation time: 15 minutes | Cooking time: 4 hours | Servings: 4

½ pound ground breakfast sausage	4 bell peppers
6 large eggs	4 ounces Monterey Jack Cheese, shredded
4 ounces fire-roasted chopped green chilies	¼ teaspoon salt
1/8 teaspoon pepper	

1. Slice the peppers off the tops and clean out the seeds.
2. Brown the sausage in a skillet. Beat your eggs until fluffy in a mixing bowl. Then mix in the cheese and green chilies.
3. Put salt plus pepper in the egg mixture. Spray the slow cooker with olive oil and place the peppers inside.
4. Put the egg mixture on each pepper to the top. Set your slow cooker to high within 2 hours, or cook on low for 4 hours. Serve when the egg mixture is set.

Nutrition:
Calories 261 Fat 16.8 g Carbs 9.2 g Protein 17.3 g Sodium 401 mg

765.   Slow Cooker Frittata

Preparation time: 15 minutes | Cooking time: 2 hours | Servings: 6

1 (14-ounce) can small artichoke hearts, drained and cut into bite-sized pieces	1 jar roasted red peppers, bite-sized pieces
¼ cup sliced green onions	8 eggs, beaten
4 ounces crumbled Feta cheese	1 teaspoon seasoning salt
½ teaspoon pepper	¼ cup chopped cilantro

1. Spray the slow cooker with olive oil and add the artichoke hearts, red peppers, and green onions.
2. Put the beaten eggs over the top of the vegetables and stir to combine. Season the mixture with pepper and seasoning salt.
3. Mix in the chopped cilantro. Top with Feta cheese. Cook on low within 2–3 hours or until set.

Nutrition: Calories 243 Fat 14.5 g Carbs 12.7g Protein 15.4 g Sodium 364 mg

766.   Cranberry Apple Oatmeal

Preparation time: 15 minutes | Cooking time: 6 hours | Servings: 4

4 cups of water	2 cups old-fashioned oats
½ cup dried cranberries	2 apples, peeled and diced
¼ cup brown sugar	2 tablespoons butter, melted
½ teaspoon salt	1 teaspoon cinnamon

1. Grease your slow cooker using a nonstick cooking spray. Put all of the fixings in the slow cooker and stir to combine.
2. Cook on low for 3 hours. If you want to prepare this the night before, you can cook it for up to 6 hours. Serve.

Nutrition:
Calories 254 Fat 7.2 g Carbs 40.9 g Protein 6.4 g Sodium 138 mg

767.   Blueberry Banana Steel Cut Oats

Preparation time: 15 minutes | Cooking time: 8 hours | Servings: 4

1 cup steel-cut oats	2 ripe bananas, sliced or mashed
1–2 cups fresh or frozen blueberries	2 cups of water
2 cups milk (almond milk works very well in this recipe)	2 tablespoons honey or pure maple syrup
¼ teaspoon salt	1 teaspoon cinnamon
2 teaspoons vanilla	Optional add-ins: chopped nuts, nut butter, fresh or dried fruit, granola, shredded coconut, honey, additional milk

1. Grease your slow cooker using a nonstick cooking spray. Add all the fixings to the slow cooker and mix well. Cook on low overnight for 6–8 hours or cook on high for 2–3 hours.

Nutrition:
Calories 297 Fat 4.4 g Carbs 58 g Protein 8 g Sodium 81 mg

768.   Berry Breakfast Quinoa

Preparation time: 15 minutes | Cooking time: 3 hours | Servings: 5

1 large avocado, pitted and mashed (you can replace with bananas)	4 cups of water
2 cups quinoa, rinsed	2 cups fresh mixed berries
2 tablespoons pure maple syrup	2 teaspoons vanilla
1 teaspoon cinnamon	¼ teaspoon salt

1. Spray your slow cooker using a nonstick cooking spray. Put all the listed ingredients in the slow cooker and mix well.
2. Cook on low for 5 hours or high for 2–3 hours. Serve.

Nutrition:
Calories 229 Fat 2.8 g Carbs 44 g Protein 7 g Sodium 90 mg

769.   Mediterranean Crockpot Breakfast

Preparation Time: 15 minutes | Cooking Time: 7 hours | Servings: 8

Eggs - 1 dozen	Hash brown potatoes - 2 pounds
Milk - 1 cup	Shredded cheddar cheese - 3 cups
Diced onions - ½ cup	Bacon – 1 pound
Garlic powder - ¼ teaspoon	Dry mustard - ¼ teaspoon
Salt - 1 teaspoon	Pepper - ½ teaspoon
Spring onions – for garnishing	

1. Beat the eggs using a blender until they get combined well with one another

2. Now add garlic powder, milk, salt, mustard, and pepper along with the beaten eggs and continue blending. Keep aside.
3. Season the hash brown potatoes with pepper and salt. Place the hash brown potatoes in a layer by layer and diced onions into the crockpot.
4. Sprinkle a quarter portion of bacon and mix them well. Add a cup of cheese to the crockpot to make it a smooth looking texture.
5. Repeat this layering process two to three times. Now pour the blended egg mixture over the layers of hash potatoes in the crockpot.
6. Set slow cooking for 7 hours. Garnish with finely chopped spring onions while serving.

Nutrition:
Calories: 245 Carbs: 16g Fat: 8g Protein: 24g

770. Slow Cooker Mediterranean Potatoes

Preparation Time: 5 minutes | Cooking Time: 5 hours | Servings: 8

Fingerling potatoes - 3 pounds	Dried oregano - 1 tablespoon
Olive oil - 2 tablespoons	Smoked paprika - 1 teaspoon
Unsalted butter - 2 tablespoons	Ground black pepper, fresh – 1 teaspoon
Lemon juice - 1 teaspoon	Minced garlic - 4 cloves
Fresh parsley leaves, chopped - 2 tablespoons	Kosher salt - ½ teaspoon
Lemon - 1 zest	

1. Peel, wash potatoes, and cut into half. Keep aside. Slightly grease the inside of a 6-quart slow cooker with nonstick spray.
2. Add olive oil, potatoes, lemon juice, butter, paprika, and oregano in the cooker. Season by using pepper and salt
3. Close the lid. Set it to slow cook within 5 hours. Serve hot by garnishing with chopped parsley and lemon zest.

Nutrition:
Calories: 149 Carbs: 23g Fat: 5g Protein: 3g

771. Mediterranean Crockpot Quiche

Preparation Time: 15 minutes | Cooking Time: 6 hours | Servings: 9

Milk – 1 cup	Eggs – 8
Feta cheese, crumbled - 1½ cup	Bisquick mix – 1 cup
Spinach, fresh, chopped – 2 cups	Red bell pepper - ½ cup
Garlic, nicely chopped – 1 teaspoon	Basil leaves, fresh - ¼ cup
Sausage crumbles fully cooked – 9.6 ounces	Feta cheese, crumbled (for garnishing) - ¼ cup

1. Grease a 5-quart slow cooker using a cooking spray. In a large bowl, whisk eggs, Bisquick mix and milk thoroughly.
2. Add one and half crumbled feta cheese, garlic, basil, sausage, bell pepper, and thoroughly stir the entire mix.
3. Close the lid and set slow cooking for 6 hours. Cut into pieces for serving. Garnish with feta cheese sprinkling.

Nutrition:
Calories: 321 Carbs: 26g Fat: 22g Protein: 2g

772. Slow Cooker Meatloaf

Preparation Time: 15 minutes | Cooking Time: 4 hours | Servings: 4

Minced beef - ½ pound	Tomato sauce – 2 cups
Onion, diced - 1 small	Bacon unsmoked - 4
Red wine - ½ cup	Mustard - 1 teaspoon
Cheddar cheese - 1 oz.	Oregano - 1 teaspoon
Garlic puree - 1 teaspoon	Thyme - 1 teaspoon
Paprika - 1 teaspoon	Salt - ½ teaspoon
Pepper - ½ teaspoon	Parsley - 1 teaspoon
Fresh herbs – as required	

1. In a large bowl, put all the seasoning items. Add onion and minced beef to the bowl and mix well by combing with your hands.
2. Spread the mixture on a clean worktop and press it forms like a pastry, which can roll out cleanly.

3. In the middle portion of the meatloaf pastry, layer some chopped cheese. After adding the cheese as a layer, wrap the meat like a sausage roll.
4. Pour little olive oil into the slow cooker for greasing and then place the roll. Mix homemade tomato sauce and red wine in a separate bowl and pour it on the meatloaf's sides.
5. Do not pour this mixture over the meatloaf. Now, spread the bacon over the meatloaf. Slow cook it for four hours. Serve hot along with roast vegetables and potatoes.

Nutrition:
Calories: 234 Carbs: 17g Fat: 6g Protein: 27g

773. Crock Pot Chicken Noodle Soup

Preparation Time: 15 minutes | Cooking Time: 6 hours | Servings: 4

Chicken breasts, boneless and skinless, cut into ½" size – 3	Chicken broth - 5½ cup
Chopped celery stalks - 3	Chopped carrots - 3
Chopped onion - 1	Bay leaf - 1
Minced garlic cloves - 3	Peas, frozen - 1 cup
Egg noodles - 2½ cup	Fresh parsley, chopped - ¼ cup
Ground black pepper, fresh - ½ teaspoon	Salt - ½ teaspoon

1. Put and arrange the chicken breasts in the bottom of the slow cooker. On top of the chicken, put onion, celery stalks, garlic cloves, and carrots.
2. Pour in the chicken broth and put the bay leaf in. Add pepper and salt as per your taste.
3. Cook on slow cook mode for 6 hours. After six hours, add egg noodles and frozen peas to the cooker.
4. Cook further about 5-6 minutes until the egg noodles turn tender. Stir in chopped fresh parsley. Serve hot.

Nutrition:
Calories: 150 Carbs: 10g Fat: 6g Protein: 13g

774. Hash Brown & Cheddar Breakfast

Preparation Time: 30 minutes | Cooking Time: 6 hours | Servings: 12

Hash browns, frozen & shredded - 32 ounces	Onion, green, coarsely chopped - 6
Breakfast sausage, crumbled & cooked - 16 ounces	Eggs - 12
Shredded cheddar cheese - 12 ounces	Garlic powder - ¼ teaspoon
Milk - ¼ cup	Pepper - ½ teaspoon
Salt - 1 teaspoon	Pepper – 1 teaspoon for seasoning.
Salt - ½ teaspoon for seasoning.	

1. Oil a 6-quart slow cooker with nonstick cooking spray. In the slow cooker, layer 1/3 portion of hash brown.
2. Season this layer with pepper and salt. Now, layer 1/3 portion of the cooked and crumbled sausage over the first layer.
3. Again layer 1/3 portion of both cheddar cheese and green onions over the sausage. Repeat both these layers twice, ending with cheese
4. Take a large bowl and whisk milk, egg, salt, garlic powder, and pepper. Pour this egg mixture all over the sausage, hash brown and cheese layers in the slow cooker.
5. Slow cook it for about six to eight hours until the edges turn brown, and the center becomes firm. Serve hot.

Nutrition:
Calories: 150 Carbs: 17g Fat: 9g Protein: 1g

775. Slow Cooker Fava Beans

Preparation Time: 10 minutes | Cooking Time: 8 hours | Servings: 12

Fava beans (dried) - 1 pound
Uncooked rice – 3 tablespoons
Garlic, chopped – 3 cloves
Salt - ½ teaspoon
Onion, finely sliced in rings - ½
Olive oil – 2 tablespoons
Cumin seed - ¼ teaspoon

Red lentils – 3 tablespoons
Tomato, chopped - 1
Water – as required (about 2 cups)
For sausage:
Tomato – 1 small
Sausages, cut into halves – 4
Lemon juice - ½ teaspoon

1. Soak the fava beans for about 4 hours. Wash and drain the beans. Put the drained beans in a 6-quart slow cooker.
2. Wash the lentils, rice, and drain. Put the drained lentils and rice also into the slow cooker. Now add the chopped tomato and garlic into the slow cooker.
3. Add water above the ingredients level. Set the slow cooking for 8 hours. When cooking over, prepare the sausages. Pour olive oil into a nonstick pan and bring to heat at a medium-high temperature.
4. When the oil becomes hot, add chopped onions and sauté on medium heat until it becomes tender. Now add chopped garlic and continue stirring until the fragrance starts to release. Add cumin seeds and continue stirring.
5. After that, add chopped tomatoes and sausages. Continue stirring for 5 minutes. Now transfer the cooked beans over the sausages.
6. Drizzle the lemon juice over the beans. Add salt if required. Stir the mix and cook for 2-3 minutes to warm the food. Serve hot.

Nutrition:
Calories: 88 Carbs: 18g Fat: 1g Protein: 8g

776. Pork Sausage Breakfast

Preparation Time: 15 minutes | Cooking Time: 6 hours | Servings: 12

Pork sausage - 16 ounce
Milk - 1 cup
Hash brown potatoes, frozen - 26 ounces
Ground black pepper - as per the taste required
Salt - ½ teaspoon
Cooking spray – as required

Eggs - 12
Veg oil – 2 tablespoons
Ground mustard - 1 tablespoon
Cheddar cheese, shredded - 16 ounces.
Pepper - ¾ teaspoon

1. Spray some nonstick cooking oil into the bottom of your crockpot. Layer the hash brown potatoes in the crockpot.
2. Now pour vegetable oil into a large skillet and heat on medium-high temperature. When the oil becomes hot, put the sausages in, stir and continue cooking for 7 minutes until it becomes brown and crumbly.
3. Once the cooking is over, remove the sausage and discard the oil. Now, spread the sausage over the hash brown potatoes and top it with cheddar cheese.
4. Beat milk and eggs in a separate large bowl. Add ground mustard along with salt and pepper to this mixture and stir thoroughly. Pour this batter on top of the cheese layer. Set on a slow cook for six hours. Serve hot.

Nutrition:
Calories: 290 Carbs: 1g Fat: 24g Protein: 10g

LUNCH

777. Butcher Style Cabbage Rolls – Pork & Beef Version

Preparation time: 15 minutes | Cooking time: 8.5 hours - Servings: 6

1 large head of white cabbage – 3 pounds	1 ¾ cups beef, chopped into small pieces
1 ¾ cups pork, chopped into small pieces	1 sweet onion, cut into small pieces
1 red bell pepper, cubes	1 cup mushrooms, chopped small
2 Tablespoons olive oil	1 cup beef broth
½ cup cooking cream	Salt and pepper to taste
1 heaping teaspoon ground cumin	

1. Cut out the stalk of the cabbage head like a cone shape, place the cabbage in a pot with the hole up, boil some water and pour it over the cabbage. Let it soak in hot water within 10 minutes. Chop the meats into small pieces; place them in a mixing bowl.
2. In a pan, heat the olive oil. Sauté the onion, the bell pepper, and the mushrooms for 5 minutes, cool them in the pan, and add to the meats.
3. Add the seasoning, mix well with your hands. Separate 8-10 leaves of cabbage, lay each one flat, cut the thick part of the stalk, and stuff the leaf with about 2 tablespoons of meat mixture.
4. Roll and put aside until the meat mixture is used up. Finely cut the remaining cabbage and place it in the crockpot. Place the prepared cabbage rolls seam-side down, pour the broth and the cream evenly over the cabbage rolls. Cover, cook on low within 8.5 hours.

Nutrition:
Calories: 130 Carbs: 10g Fat: 6g Protein: 9g

778. One-Pot Oriental Lamb

Preparation time: 15 minutes | Cooking time: 4 hours - Servings: 4

3 cups lamb, de-boned and diced	2 Tablespoons almond flower
2 cups fresh spinach	4 small red onions, halved
2 garlic cloves, minced	¼ cup yellow turnip, diced
2 Tablespoons dry sherry	2-3 bay leaves
1 teaspoon hot mustard	¼ teaspoon ground nutmeg
1 teaspoon chopped fresh thyme	1 teaspoon chopped fresh rosemary
5-6 whole pimento berries	1 1/3 cups broth of your choice – beef, chicken, or lamb
Salt and pepper to taste	8 baby zucchinis, halved
2 Tablespoons olive oil	

1. Preheat the crockpot on high. Place the lamb in the crockpot, cover with almond flour. Add the remaining ingredients to the crockpot. Cover, cook on high for 4 hours. Serve.

Nutrition:
Calories: 356 Carbs: 9g Fat: 24g Protein: 27g

779. Zucchini Lasagna with Minced Pork

Preparation time: 15 minutes | Cooking time: 8 hoursServings: 6

4 medium-sized zucchinis	1 small onion, diced
1 garlic clove, minced	2 cups lean ground pork, minced
2 regular cans diced Italian tomatoes	2 Tablespoons olive oil
2 cups grated Mozzarella cheese	1 egg
Small bunch of fresh basil or 1 Tablespoon dry basil	Salt and pepper to taste
2 Tablespoons butter to grease crockpot	

1. Cut the zucchini lengthwise, making 6 slices from each vegetable. Salt and let drain. Discard the liquid.
2. In a pan, heat the olive oil. Sauté the onion and garlic within 5 minutes. Add minced meat and cook for another 5 minutes. Put tomatoes and simmer within 5 minutes.
3. Add seasoning and mix well. Add basil leaves. Cool slightly. Beat the egg, mix in 1 cup of cheese.
4. Grease the crockpot with butter and start layering the lasagna. First, the zucchini slices, then a layer of meat mixture, top it with cheese, and repeat. Finish with zucchini and the second cup of cheese. Cover, cook on low for 8 hours.

Nutrition:
Calories: 168 Carbs: 5g Fat: 11g Protein: 16g

780. Stuffed Bell Peppers Dolma Style

Preparation time: 15 minutes | Cooking time: 6 hours - Servings: 6

1 cup lean ground beef	1 ¾ cup lean ground pork
1 small white onion, diced	6 bell peppers in various colors
1 small head cauliflower	1 small can tomato paste – 28 ounces
4 garlic cloves, crushed	2 Tablespoons olive oil
Salt and pepper to taste	1 Tablespoon dried thyme

1. Cut off tops of the bell peppers, set aside. Clean inside the peppers. Chop the cauliflower into tiny pieces resembling rice grains, place in a mixing bowl.
2. Add the onion, crushed garlic, dried herbs. Combine thoroughly. Add the meats, tomato paste, and seasoning. Mix well with your hands.
3. Sprinkle olive oil along the bottom and sides of the crockpot. Stuff the bell peppers with the mixture and set them in the crockpot. Carefully place the top back on each pepper. Cover, cook on low for 6 hours.

Nutrition:
Calories: 200 Carbs: 26g Fat: 6g Protein: 10g

781. Slow BBQ Ribs

Preparation time: 15 minutes | Cooking time: 8 hours - Servings: 6

3 pounds pork ribs	1 Tablespoon of olive oil
1 small can ounces tomato paste – 28 ounces	½ cup hot water
½ cup vinegar	6 Tablespoons Worcestershire sauce
4 Tablespoons dry mustard	1 Tablespoon chili powder
1 heaping teaspoon ground cumin	1 teaspoon powdered Swerve (or a suitable substitute)
Salt and pepper to taste	

1. Warm-up, the olive oil in a frying pan, then brown the ribs on both sides. Add them to the crockpot.
2. Combine the rest of the fixing in a bowl, blend well. Pour over the ribs - coat all sides. Cover, cook on low for 8 hours.

Nutrition:
Calories: 243 Carbs: 8g Fat: 15g Protein: 19g

782. Steak and Salsa

Preparation time: 15 minutes | Cooking time: 8 hours - Servings: 6

2 ½ cups salsa made of:	2 big beef tomatoes, diced
1 tablespoon olive oil	1 small red onion finely diced
½ bunch of cilantros, chopped	Salt and pepper to taste
2 pounds stewing beef, sliced in strips	2 bell peppers, cut into strips
1 onion, sliced in semi-circles	4 tablespoons butter
2 tablespoons of mixed dry seasoning:	1 teaspoon ground cumin
½ teaspoon sweet paprika	½ teaspoon paprika flakes

1 teaspoon garlic salt   ½ teaspoon fresh ground black pepper

1. Cover the bottom of the crockpot with the salsa. Add remaining ingredients and mix well. Cover, cook on low for 6-8 hours. Serve.

Nutrition:
Calories: 480 Carbs: 1g Fat: 39g Protein: 31g

783.   Beef Pot Roast with Turnips
Preparation time: 15 minutes| Cooking time: 7 hours - Servings: 6

3 pounds beef, chuck shoulder roast   2 Tablespoons olive oil
1 red onion, cut into small pieces   1 cup beef broth + 2 cups hot water
4 Tablespoons butter   1 teaspoon dry rosemary
1 teaspoon dry thyme   Salt and pepper to taste
5 medium turnips, peeled, cut into strips

1. Warm-up, the olive oil in your frying pan, then brown your meat for 2 minutes on each side. Pour the broth and remaining ingredients, without the turnips, into the crockpot.
2. Cover, cook on low for 5 hours. Take the lid off and quickly add the turnip strips. Re-cover, cook for an additional 2 hours on low, until the turnips are soft.

Nutrition:
Calories: 462 Carbs: 10g Fat: 27g Protein: 6g

784.   Chili Beef Stew
Preparation time: 15 minutes| Cooking time: 8 hours - Servings: 6

3 pounds stewing beef, whole   2 cans Italian diced tomatoes
1 cup beef broth   4 Tablespoons butter
1 teaspoon Cayenne pepper   1 Tablespoon Worcestershire sauce
1 teaspoon dry oregano   1 teaspoon dry thyme
Salt and pepper to taste

1. Add all the fixing to the crockpot, mix well. Cover, cook on high for 6 hours.
2. Break up the beef with a fork, pull apart in the crockpot. Taste and adjust the seasoning, if needed. Re-cover, cook for an additional 2 hours on low.

Nutrition:
Calories: 385 Carbs: 52g Fat: 6g Protein: 29g

785.   Pork Shoulder Roast
Preparation time: 15 minutes| Cooking time: 8 hours - Servings: 6

3 pounds pork shoulder, whole   1 can Italian diced tomatoes
1 sweet onion, diced   3 garlic cloves, diced
4 Tablespoons lard   1 cup of water
1 bay leaf   ¼ teaspoon ground cloves
Salt and pepper to taste

1. Place meat in crockpot, pour water, and tomatoes over it, so the liquid covers 1/3 of the meat. Add remaining ingredients. Cover, cook on low for 8 hours. Serve.

Nutrition:
Calories: 240 Carbs: 0g Fat: 17g Protein: 18g

786.   Easy and Delicious Chicken Stew
Preparation time: 15 minutes| Cooking time: 5 hours - Servings: 6

pounds chicken thighs, de-boned and cubed   1 cup chicken broth + 1 cup hot water
3 diced celery sticks (approximately 1 ½ cups)   2 cups fresh spinach
1 red onion, diced   2 garlic cloves, minced
1 teaspoon dry oregano   1 teaspoon dry thyme
1 teaspoon dried rosemary   1 cup cooking cream
Salt and pepper to taste

1. Add all the ingredients to the crockpot. Cover, cook on low for 5 hours. Serve.

Nutrition:

Calories: 232 Carbs: 17g Fat: 9g Protein: 22g

787.   Chili Con Steak
Preparation time: 15 minutes| Cooking time: 6 hours - Servings: 6

3 pounds beef steak, cubed   1 Tablespoon paprika
½ teaspoon chili powder   1 teaspoon dried oregano
½ teaspoon ground cumin   Salt and pepper to taste
4 Tablespoons butter   ½ cup sliced leeks
2 cups Italian diced tomatoes   1 cup broth, beef

1. Place all the ingredients in the crockpot by order on the list. Stir. Cover, cook on high for 6 hours. Serve.

Nutrition:
Calories: 290 Carbs: 5g Fat: 6g Protein: 28g

788.   One-Pot Chicken and Green Beans
Preparation time: 15 minutes| Cooking time: 8 hours - Servings: 6

2 cups green beans, trimmed   2 large beef tomatoes, diced
1 red onion, diced   2 garlic cloves, minced
1 bunch chopped fresh dill (around 1/8 cup)   1 lemon, juiced
4 Tablespoons butter   1 cup chicken broth
6 chicken thighs, skin on   Salt and pepper to taste
2 Tablespoons olive oil

1. Add all the listed ingredients to the slow cooker in order on the list. Brush chicken thighs with olive oil; season with salt and pepper.
2. Cover, cook on low for 8 hours. When ready, if desired, take the chicken out and crisp it under a broiler for a few minutes.

Nutrition:
Calories: 317 Carbs: 27g Fat: 2g Protein: 30g

789.   Two-Meat Chili
Preparation time: 15 minutes Cooking: 6 hours & 30 minutes - Servings: 6

1 ½ cups lean ground pork sausage meat   1 ¾ cups stewing beef, cubed
2 Tablespoons olive oil   1 bell pepper, sliced
1 white onion, cut in semi-circles   1 cup beef broth
2 Tablespoons tomato paste   2 Tablespoons sweet paprika
1 teaspoon chili powder   1 teaspoon cumin
1 teaspoon oregano   Salt and pepper to taste

1. In a pan, heat the olive oil. Brown, the beef, transfer to the crockpot. Then, brown the sausage and transfer to crockpot.
2. In the same pan, sweat the onion and pepper slices for 4-5 minutes, pour over the meat. Add remaining ingredients to crockpot. Cover, cook on low for 6 hours. Turn to high, remove the lid and let the liquid reduce for 30 minutes.

Nutrition:
Calories: 240 Carbs: 0g Fat: 17g Protein: 21g

790.   Slightly Addictive Pork Curry
Preparation time: 15 minutes Cooking time: 8 hours - Servings: 6

pounds pork shoulder, cubed   1 Tablespoon coconut oil
1 yellow onion, diced   2 garlic cloves, minced
2 Tablespoons tomato paste   1 small can coconut milk – 12 ounces
1 cup of water   ½ cup white wine
1 teaspoon turmeric   1 teaspoon ginger powder
1 teaspoon curry powder   ½ teaspoon paprika
Salt and pepper to taste

1. In a pan, heat 1 tablespoon olive oil. Sauté the onion and garlic for 2-3 minutes. Add the pork and brown it. Finish with tomato paste.
2. In the crockpot, mix all remaining ingredients, submerge the meat in the liquid. Cover, cook on low for 8 hours.

Nutrition:
Calories: 110 Carbs: 11g Fat: 6g Protein: 2g

DINNER

791. Greek Style Lamb Shanks

Preparation time: 15 minutes | Cooking time: 6 hours | Servings: 8

3 Tablespoons butter

2 Tablespoons olive oil
5 garlic cloves, minced
¼ cup of green olives
1 sprig fresh rosemary
1 teaspoon ground cumin
¾ cup hot water
Salt and pepper to taste

4 lamb shanks, approximately 1 pound each
8-10 pearl onions
2 beef tomatoes, cubed
4 bay leaves
1 teaspoon dry thyme
1 cup fresh spinach
½ cup red wine, Merlot or Cabernet

1. In a pan, melt the butter, brown the shanks on each side. Remove from pan, add oil, onions, garlic. Cook for 3-4 minutes. Add tomatoes, olives, spices. Stir well.
2. Add liquids and return the meat. Bring to boil for 1 minute. Transfer everything to the crockpot. Cover, cook on medium-high for 6 hours.

Nutrition:
Calories: 250 Carbs: 3g Fat: 16g Protein: 22g

792. Homemade Meatballs and Spaghetti Squash

Preparation time: 15 minutes | Cooking time: 8 hours | Servings: 8

1 medium-sized spaghetti squash, washed
pounds lean ground beef
1 red onion, chopped
2 Tablespoons of dry Parmesan cheese
1 teaspoon ground cumin
4 cans diced Italian tomatoes
1 cup hot water
¼ cup chopped parsley

1 bay leaf

1 Tablespoon butter to grease crockpot
2 garlic cloves
½ cup almond flour
1 egg, beaten

Salt and pepper to taste
1 small can tomato paste, 28 ounces
1 red onion, chopped
½ teaspoon each, salt and sugar (optional)

1. Scoop out the seeds of the spaghetti squash with a spoon. Grease the crockpot, place both halves open side down in the crockpot. Mix meatball ingredients in a bowl. Form approximately 20 small meatballs.
2. In a pan, heat the olive oil. Brown the meatballs within 2-3 minutes on each side. Transfer to the crockpot.
3. In the small bowl, add the tomatoes, tomato paste, oil, water, onion, and parsley, add ½ teaspoon each of salt and sugar. Mix well. Pour the marinara sauce in the crockpot around the squash halves. Cover, cook on low for 8 hours.

Nutrition:
Calories: 409 Carbs: 31g Fat: 18g Protein: 32g

793. Beef and Cabbage Roast

Preparation time: 15 minutes | Cooking time: 8 hours | Servings: 10

1 red onion, quartered
2-3 stocks celery, diced (approximately 1 cup)
2 bay leaves
1 teaspoon chili powder
2 cups broth, beef + 2 cups hot water
1 medium cabbage (approximately 2.2 pounds), cut in half, then quartered

2 garlic cloves, minced
4-6 dry pimento berries

1 pounds beef brisket (two pieces)
1 teaspoon ground cumin
Salt and pepper to taste

1. Add all ingredients, except cabbage, to the crockpot in order of the list. Cover, cook on low for 7 hours. Uncover, add the cabbage on top of the stew. Re-cover, cook for 1 additional hour.

Nutrition:
Calories: 283 Carbs: 15g Fat: 11g Protein: 26g

794. Simple Chicken Chili

Preparation time: 15 minutes | Cooking time: 6 hours | Servings: 8

1 Tablespoon butter
1 bell pepper, sliced
3 pounds boneless chicken thighs
1 teaspoon chili powder
1 cup chicken broth
3 Tablespoons tomato paste

1 red onion, sliced
2 garlic cloves, minced
8 slices bacon, chopped
Salt and pepper to taste
¼ cup of coconut milk

1. Add all ingredients to the crockpot, starting with the butter. Cover, cook on low for 6 hours. Shred cooked the chicken using a fork in the crockpot. Serve.

Nutrition:
Calories: 230 Carbs: 17g Fat: 6g Protein: 27g

795. Beef Shoulder in BBQ Sauce

Preparation time: 15 minutes | Cooking time: 10 hours | Servings: 12

8 pounds beef shoulder, whole
1 yellow onion, diced
4 Tablespoons red wine vinegar
4 Tablespoons Swerve (or a suitable substitute)
1 teaspoon salt

1 Tablespoon butter
1 garlic bulb, peeled and minced
2 Tablespoons Worcestershire sauce
1 Tablespoon mustard

1 teaspoon fresh ground black pepper

1. In a bowl, mix seasoning, then reserve aside. Dissolve the butter in your pan, add the meat. Brown on all sides. Transfer to crockpot. Fry the onion for 2-3 minutes in the same pan pours over the meat. Pour in the seasoning.
2. Cover, cook on low for 10 hours. Remove, then place on a platter, cover with foil, let it rest for 1 hour. Turn the crockpot on high, reduce the remaining liquid by half and serve with the shredded beef.

Nutrition:
Calories: 140 Carbs: 5g Fat: 9g Protein: 8g

796. Moist and Spicy Pulled Chicken Breast

Preparation time: 15 minutes | Cooking time: 6 hours | Servings: 8

1 teaspoon dry oregano
1 teaspoon dried rosemary
1 teaspoon sweet paprika
Salt and pepper to taste
pounds of chicken breasts
2 Tablespoons of olive oil

1 teaspoon dry thyme
1 teaspoon garlic powder
½ teaspoon chili powder
4 tablespoons butter
1 ½ cups ready-made tomato salsa

1. Mix dry seasoning, sprinkle half on the bottom of crockpot. Place the chicken breasts over it, spread the rest of the spices. Pour the salsa over the chicken. Cover, cook on low for 6 hours.

Nutrition:
Calories: 184 Carbs: 0g Fat: 0g Protein: 22g

797. Whole Roasted Chicken

Preparation time: 15 minutes | Cooking time: 8 hours | Servings: 6

1 whole chicken (approximately 5.5 pounds)
6 small onions
2 teaspoons salt
1 teaspoon Cayenne pepper
1 teaspoon ground thyme

4 garlic cloves

1 Tablespoon olive oil, for rubbing
2 teaspoons sweet paprika
1 teaspoon onion powder
2 teaspoons fresh ground black pepper

4 Tablespoons butter, cut into cubes

1. Mix all dry ingredients well. Stuff the chicken belly with garlic and onions. On the bottom of the crockpot, place four balls of aluminum foil.
2. Set the chicken on top of the balls. Rub it generously with olive oil. Cover the chicken with seasoning, drop in butter pieces. Cover, cook on low for 8 hours.

Nutrition:
Calories: 240 Carbs: 0g Fat: 17g Protein: 21g

798.   Pot Roast Beef Brisket

Preparation time: 15 minutes | Cooking time: 12 hours | Servings: 10

1pounds beef brisket, whole	2 Tablespoons olive oil
2 Tablespoons apple cider vinegar	1 teaspoon dry oregano
1 teaspoon dry thyme	1 teaspoon dried rosemary
2 Tablespoons paprika	1 teaspoon Cayenne pepper
1 tablespoon salt	1 teaspoon fresh ground black pepper

1. In a bowl, mix dry seasoning, add olive oil, apple cider vinegar. Place the meat in the crockpot, generously coat with seasoning mix.
2. Cover, cook on low for 12 hours. Remove the beef brisket from the liquid, place it on a pan. Sear it under the broiler for 2-4 minutes, observe it, so the meat doesn't burn. Cover it with foil, let it rest within 1 hour. Slice and serve.

Nutrition:
Calories: 280 Carbs: 4g Fat: 20g Protein: 20g

799.   Seriously Delicious Lamb Roast

Preparation time: 15 minutes | Cooking time: 8 hours | Servings: 8

12 medium radishes, scrubbed, washed, and cut in half	Salt and pepper to taste
1 red onion, diced	2 garlic cloves, minced
1 lamb joint (approximately 4.5 pounds) at room temperature	2 Tablespoons olive oil
1 teaspoon dry oregano	1 teaspoon dry thyme
1 sprig fresh rosemary	4 cups heated broth, your choice

1. Place cut radishes along the bottom of the crockpot. Season. Add onion and garlic. Mix the herbs plus olive oil in a small bowl. Mix until a paste develops.
2. Place the meat on top of the radishes. Massage the paste over the surface of the meat. Heat the stock, pour it around the meat. Cover, cook on low for 8 hours. Let it rest for 20 minutes. Slice and serve.

Nutrition:
Calories: 206 Carbs: 4g Fat: 9g Protein: 32g

800.   Dressed Pork Leg Roast

Preparation time: 15 minutes | Cooking time: 8 hours | Servings: 14

8 pounds pork leg	1 Tablespoon butter
1 yellow onion, sliced	6 garlic cloves, peeled and minced
2 Tablespoons ground cumin	2 Tablespoons ground thyme
2 Tablespoons ground chili	1 teaspoon salt
1 teaspoon fresh ground black pepper	1 cup hot water

1. Butter the crockpot. Slice crisscrosses along the top of pork leg. Arrange onion slices and minced garlic along the bottom of the crockpot.
2. Place meat on top of vegetables. In a small bowl, mix the herbs. Rub it all over the pork leg. Add the water. Cover, cook on high for 8 hours. Remove from crockpot, place on a platter, cover with foil. Let it rest for 1 hour. Shred the meat and serve.

Nutrition:
Calories: 179 Carbs: 0g Fat: 8g Protein: 25g

801. Rabbit & Mushroom Stew

Preparation time: 15 minutes | Cooking time: 6 hours | Servings: 6

1 rabbit, in portion size pieces	2 cups spicy Spanish sausage, cut into chunks
2 Tablespoons butter, divided	1 red onion, sliced
1 cup button mushrooms, washed and dried	1 teaspoon cayenne pepper
1 teaspoon sweet paprika	1 teaspoon salt
1 teaspoon fresh ground black pepper	1 cup chicken broth+1 cup hot water

1. Butter the crockpot. In a large pan, melt the butter, add the rabbit pieces, brown on all sides. Transfer to crockpot.
2. In the same pan, sauté the onions, sausage chunks, and spices for 2-3 minutes. Put in chicken broth, heat on high for 1 minute, then pour the mixture over the rabbit.
3. Add the mushrooms. Adjust the seasoning if needed. Add the water. Cover, cook on high for 6 hours. Serve.

Nutrition:
Calories: 189 Carbs: 20g Fat: 6g Protein: 13g

802.   Italian Spicy Sausage & Bell Peppers

Preparation time: 15 minutes | Cooking time: 6 hours | Servings: 5

2 Tablespoons butter	2 red onions, sliced
4 bell peppers, sliced	2 regular cans Italian tomatoes, diced
pounds spicy Italian sausage	1 teaspoon dry oregano
1 teaspoon dry thyme	1 teaspoon dry basil
1 teaspoon sweet paprika	1 teaspoon salt
1 teaspoon fresh ground black pepper	

1. Butter the crockpot. Add the sliced onions, peppers, and salt. Pour the tomatoes over them. Toss well.
2. Add seasoning. Mix it in. Arrange sausages in the middle of the pepper and onion mixture. Add ¼ cup hot water. Cover, cook on low for 6 hours. Serve.

Nutrition:
Calories: 320 Carbs: 15g Fat: 17g Protein: 28g

803.   Chicken in Salsa Verde

Preparation time: 15 minutes Cooking time: 6 hours Servings: 4

2pounds of chicken breasts	3 bunches parsley, chopped
¾ cup olive oil	¼ cup capers, drained and chopped
3 anchovy fillets	1 lemon, juice, and zest
2 garlic cloves, minced	1 teaspoon salt
1 teaspoon fresh ground black pepper	

1. Place the chicken breasts in the crockpot. Mix the rest of the fixing in a blender, pour over the chicken. Cover, cook on low for 6 hours. Shred with a fork and serve.

Nutrition:
Calories: 145 Carbs: 5g Fat: 2g Protein: 26g

804.   Salmon Poached in White Wine and Lemon

Preparation time: 15 minutes Cooking time: 2 hours Servings: 4

2 cups of water	1 cup cooking wine, white
1 lemon, sliced thin	1 small mild onion, sliced thin
1 bay leaf	1 mixed bunch fresh tarragon, dill, and parsley
1 kg salmon fillet, skin on	1 teaspoon salt
1 teaspoon ground black pepper	

1. Add all ingredients, except salmon and seasoning, to the crockpot. Cover, cook on low for 1 hour. Season the salmon, place in the crockpot skin-side down. Cover, cook on low for another hour. Serve.

Nutrition:
Calories: 216   Carbs: 1g   Fat: 12g   Protein: 23g

MAINS

805. Beef and Onion Crock Pot
Preparation time: 15 minutes | Cooking time: 9 hours | Servings: 6

2 lbs. lean beef, cut into cubes
2-3 garlic cloves, peeled, whole

2 cups chicken broth
4 tbsp. red wine vinegar

2 lbs. shallots, peeled
3 tbsp. tomato paste, dissolved in 1/2 cup water
2 bay leaves
1 tsp salt

1. Combine all ingredients in crockpot. Cover and cook on low within 7-9 hours.

Nutrition:
Calories: 214 Carbs: 12g Fat: 6g Protein: 27g

806. Beef and Green Pea Crock Pot
Preparation time: 15 minutes | Cooking time: 9 hours | Servings: 6

2 lbs. stewing beef
1 onion, chopped
3-4 garlic cloves, cut
1 tsp salt
1/2 cup fresh dill, finely chopped

2 bags of frozen peas
2 carrots, chopped
2 cups chicken broth
1 tbsp. paprika
1 cup yogurt, to serve

1. Combine all the fixing listed in crockpot. Cover and cook on low within 7-9 hours. Serve sprinkled with dill and a dollop of yogurt.

Nutrition:
Calories: 391 Carbs: 31g Fat: 16g Protein: 29g

807. Beef and Root Vegetable Crock Pot
Preparation time: 15 minutes | Cooking time: 9 hours | Servings: 6

2 lbs. stewing beef
2 onions, sliced
1 beet, peeled and diced
2 cups beef broth
1 tbsp. paprika

2 carrots, cut
1 turnip, peeled and diced
1-2 parsnips, diced
1 tbsp. tomato paste
2 bay leaves

1. Combine all ingredients in crockpot. Cover and cook on low within 7-9 hours. Serve.

Nutrition:
Calories: 232 Carbs: 12g Fat: 15g Protein: 12g

808. Slow Cooked Mediterranean Beef
Preparation time: 15 minutes | Cooking time: 9 hours | Servings: 6

2 lbs. lean steak, cut into large pieces
2-3 garlic cloves, whole
1/2 bag frozen green beans
1/2 frozen bag okra
1 small eggplant, peeled and diced
2 tbsp. tomato paste or purée
1 tsp dried oregano

2 onions, sliced
1 green pepper, cut
1/2 bag frozen green peas
1 zucchini, peeled and cut
1 tomato, diced
1 cup chicken broth
salt and black pepper, to taste

1. Combine all ingredients in crockpot. Cover and cook on low within 7-9 hours.

Nutrition:
Calories: 156 Carbs: 8g Fat: 5g Protein: 19g

809. Slow Cooker Paprika Chicken
Preparation time: 15 minutes | Cooking time: 6 hours | Servings: 4

8 chicken drumsticks or 4 breast halves
3 slices bacon, finely chopped
1 large green pepper, chopped
1 tbsp. paprika
2 cups chicken broth
1 tbsp. sour cream

1 onion, chopped
1 large red pepper, chopped
2-3 garlic cloves, finely chopped
1 can of crushed tomatoes
1/3 cup medium-grain white rice
1 cup fresh parsley, finely cut, to serve

1. Combine all ingredients in a slow cooker. Cover and cook on low within 5-6 hours.

Nutrition:
Calories: 484 Carbs: 6g Fat: 32g Protein: 42g

810. Slow Cooked Lamb with Red Wine Sauce
Preparation time: 15 minutes | Cooking time: 7 hours | Servings: 4

4 trimmed lamb shanks
2 large carrots, roughly chopped
1 cup chicken broth
1 tsp brown sugar
½ tsp salt

1 onion, thinly sliced
2-3 parsnips, roughly chopped
2 cups dry red wine
½ tsp black pepper

1. Spray the slow cooker with nonstick spray. Place the lamb shanks in it with all other ingredients. Cover and cook on low for 6-7 hours.

Nutrition:
Calories: 736 Carbs: 4g Fat: 41g Protein: 17g

811. Pork and Mushroom Crock Pot
Preparation time: 15 minutes | Cooking time: 9 hours | Servings: 4

2 lbs. pork tenderloin, sliced

1 can cream of mushroom soup
salt and black pepper, to taste

1 lb. chopped white button mushrooms
1 cup sour cream

1. Spray the slow cooker with nonstick spray. Combine all ingredients into the slow cooker. Cover, and cook on low within 7-9 hours.

Nutrition:
Calories: 275 Carbs: 33g Fat: 7g Protein: 21g

812. Slow Cooked Pot Roast
Preparation time: 15 minutes | Cooking time: 10 hours | Servings: 4

2 lb. pot roast
1 small onion, finely cut
1/2 cup chicken broth
salt, to taste

1-2 garlic cloves, crushed
1/3 cup tomato paste
2 tbsp. Worcestershire sauce

1. Spray the slow cooker with nonstick spray. Place the roast in the slow cooker. In a bowl, combine the tomato paste, chicken broth, Worcestershire sauce, garlic, and onions. Spread this sauce over the meat. Cook on low within 8-10 hours.

Nutrition:
Calories: 340 Carbs: 46g Fat: 4g Protein: 29g

813. Slow-Cooked Mediterranean Pork Casserole

Preparation time: 15 minutes | Cooking time: 10 hours | Servings: 4

2 lbs. pork loin, cut into cubes	1 large onion, chopped
2 cups white button mushrooms, cut	1-2 garlic cloves, finely chopped
1 green pepper, cut into strips	1 red pepper, cut into strips
1 small eggplant, peeled and diced	1 zucchini, peeled and diced
2 tomatoes, diced	1 cup chicken broth
1/2 tsp cumin	1 tbsp. paprika
salt and black pepper, to taste	

1. Spray the slow cooker with nonstick spray. Place the pork in the slow cooker. Put in all other fixings and stir to combine. Cook on low within 8-10 hours.

Nutrition:
Calories: 265 Carbs: 0g Fat: 9g Protein: 0g

814. Pizza Ravioli Mix Up

Preparation time: 15 minutes | Cooking time: 3 hours | Servings: 12

1 1/2 lb. ground beef round	1 1/2 lb. bulk Italian pork sausage
2 medium onions, chopped	2 tablespoons finely chopped garlic
2 jars tomato pasta sauce	1 bag frozen cheese-filled ravioli
3 cups Cheddar-Monterey Jack cheese blend, shredded	1 package sliced pepperoni
1/4 cup sliced ripe olives	Fresh basil sprigs, if desired

1. Grease the bottom of 5- to 6-quart your slow cooker using cooking spray. Arrange side of your slow cooker with foil; spray it with cooking spray.
2. Cook sausage over medium heat within 8 to 10 minutes in a 12-inch skillet, then drain it after. Put the sausage in a bowl.
3. Cook the beef, onion plus garlic over medium heat 8 to 10 minutes in the same skillet, drain. Mix the beef mixture plus 1 jar of the pasta sauce to the bowl with sausage.
4. Spread half of the rest of the jar of pasta sauce to cover the bottom in a slow cooker. Arrange with half of the ravioli and half of the meat mixture.
5. Sprinkle with 1 1/2 cups of the cheese and half of the pepperoni. Repeat layers. Cook on low within 3 hours. Sprinkle with olives before serving. Garnish with basil.

Nutrition:
Calories: 140 Carbs: 20g Fat: 5g Protein: 4g

815. Chicken Cacciatore with Linguine

Preparation time: 15 minutes | Cooking time: 10 hours & 10 minutes | Servings: 6

2 1/2 lb. boneless skinless chicken thighs	1 jar sliced mushrooms, drained
2 cans Italian-style tomato paste	1 3/4 cups chicken broth
1/2 cup white wine, if desired	1 1/2 teaspoons dried basil leaves
1/2 teaspoon salt	1 dried bay leaf
12 oz. uncooked linguine	1/4 teaspoon dried thyme leaves
1 tablespoon cornstarch	Shredded Parmesan cheese, if desired

1. Grease 3- to 4-quart slow cooker using a cooking spray. Put the chicken in the cooker. Put the mushrooms, tomato paste, broth, wine, basil, salt, and bay leaf; gently stir to mix.
2. Cover then cook on Low heat within 8 to 10 hours. Before serving, cook then drain linguine.
3. Remove and cover to keep warm. Mix the thyme into the sauce in the cooker. Increase heat setting to High. In a small bowl, mix 1/4 cup sauce from the cooker and the cornstarch until smooth.
4. Cook 10 minutes longer, stirring frequently. Remove bay leaf before serving. Serve chicken and sauce over linguine. Sprinkle with cheese.

Nutrition:

Calories: 180 Carbs: 26g Fat: 3g Protein: 12g

816. Italian Steak Roll

Preparation time: 15 minutes | Cooking time: 6 hours | Servings: 2

3/4 lb. beef round steak (1/2-inch-thick), trimmed of fat	1/2 tsp dried Italian seasoning
1/4 tsp salt	1/4 tsp pepper
1 thin slice onion, halved	1 clove garlic, minced
1/2 cup mushrooms, sliced	1 medium sliced Italian plum tomato, cut into quarters
3/4 cup savory beef gravy	

1. Put the steak on your work surface, rub with Italian seasoning, salt plus pepper. Put the onion slice halves, then roll up the beef, with onion inside; tie with string.
2. Put the beef roll, seam side down, in 2- to 3-quart slow cooker. Sprinkle garlic, mushrooms, and tomato around the roll. Spoon gravy over the roll.
3. Cook on low within 5 to 6 hours. Remove then put it on serving platter. Remove the string, then slice the beef roll. Mix in the gravy batter in your slow cooker until blended. Serve beef roll slices with gravy.

Nutrition:
Calories: 190 Carbs: 37g Fat: 2g Protein: 6g

817. Chicken Parmesan with Penne Pasta

Preparation time: 15 minutes | Cooking time: 6 hours - Servings: 4

1 egg	1/3 cup plain bread crumbs
1/3 cup shredded Parmesan cheese	1/2 tsp Italian seasoning
1/4 tsp salt	1/4 tsp pepper
4 boneless skinless chicken breasts	1 jar tomato pasta sauce
1/2 cup shredded Italian cheese blend	2 & 2/3 cups uncooked penne pasta

1. Grease your 2- to 3-quart slow cooker using a cooking spray. Beat egg until foamy in a small shallow bowl. Mix the bread crumbs, Parmesan cheese, Italian seasoning, salt plus pepper in a separate shallow bowl.
2. Soak the chicken into egg, then to bread crumb mixture; place in cooker. Spread pasta sauce evenly over chicken. Cover; cook on Low heat within 5 to 6 hours.
3. Sprinkle it with Italian cheese blend on top. Cook on low within 10 minutes longer. Cook your pasta following what stated on the package directions. Serve chicken with pasta.

Nutrition:
Calories: 170 Carbs: 15g Fat: 5g Protein: 17g

818. Chicken Cacciatore

Preparation time: 15 minutes | Cooking time: 9 hours | Servings: 6

6 skinless, boneless chicken breast halves	1 (28 ounces) jar spaghetti sauce
2 green bell pepper, seeded and cubed	8 ounces fresh mushrooms, sliced
1 onion, finely diced	2 tablespoons minced garlic

1. Put the chicken in your slow cooker, then the spaghetti sauce, green bell peppers, mushrooms, onion, plus garlic. Cook on low within 7 to 9 hours.

Nutrition:
Calories: 210 Carbs: 9g Fat: 3g Protein: 26g

819. Lasagna

Preparation time: 15 minutes | Cooking time: 6 hours | Servings: 10

1-pound lean ground beef	1 onion, chopped
2 teaspoons minced garlic	1 (29 ounces) can tomato sauce
1 (6 ounces) can tomato paste	1 1/2 teaspoons salt
1 teaspoon dried oregano	1 package of lasagna noodles

150 | P a g e

12 oz. cottage cheese

1/2 cup grated Parmesan cheese

16 oz. shredded mozzarella cheese

1. Cook the onion, garlic, and ground beef until brown in a large skillet over medium heat. Put the tomato sauce, tomato paste, salt, and oregano and stir until well incorporated. Cook until heated through.
2. Mix the cottage cheese, grated Parmesan cheese, plus shredded mozzarella cheese in a large bowl. Put a layer of the meat batters into the bottom of your slow cooker. Put a double layer of the uncooked lasagna noodles.
3. Top it with a portion of the cheese mixture. Repeat the layering of sauce, noodles, and cheese until all the ingredients are used. Cook on LOW within 4 to 6 hours.

Nutrition:
Calories: 275 Carbs: 42g Fat: 3g Protein: 15g

820.   Cheesy Italian Tortellini

Preparation time: 15 minutes | Cooking time: 8 hours | Servings: 6

1/2-pound ground beef

1/2-pound Italian sausage

1 jar marinara sauce

1 can sliced mushrooms

1 can Italian-style diced tomatoes, undrained

1 package refrigerated or fresh cheese tortellini

1 cup mozzarella cheese, shredded

1/2 cup Cheddar cheese, shredded

1. Cook the ground beef plus Italian sausage into a large skillet over medium-high heat until browned, then drain. Mix the ground meats, marinara sauce, mushrooms, plus tomatoes in your slow cooker. Cook on LOW within 7 to 8 hours.
2. Mix in the tortellini, plus sprinkle the mozzarella, then the cheddar cheese over the top. Cook within 15 more minutes on LOW.

Nutrition:
Calories: 331 Carbs: 24g Fat: 16g Protein: 22g

821. Easy Meatballs

Preparation time: 15 minutes | Cooking time: 8 hours | Servings: 16

1 & 1/4 cups Italian seasoned bread crumbs

& 1/2-pounds ground beef

2 cloves garlic, minced

1/4 cup chopped fresh parsley

1 medium yellow onion, chopped

1 egg, beaten

1 jar spaghetti sauce

1 can of crushed tomatoes

1 can tomato puree

1. Mix the ground beef, bread crumbs, parsley, garlic, onion, and egg in a bowl. Shape the mixture into 16 meatballs.
2. In a slow cooker, mix the spaghetti sauce, crushed tomatoes, and tomato puree. Place the meatballs into the sauce mixture. Cook on low within 6 to 8 hours.

Nutrition:
Calories: 280 Carbs: 13g Fat: 15g Protein: 24g

822.   Chicken Alfredo

Preparation time: 15 minutes | Cooking time: 5 hours - Servings: 4

4 skinless, boneless chicken breast halves

1/4 cup water

1 package dry Italian-style salad dressing mix

1 clove garlic, pressed

1 package cream cheese, softened

1 can condensed cream of chicken soup

1 can chop canned mushrooms

1 package spaghetti

1 tablespoon chopped fresh parsley

Cooking spray

1. Grease the crock of your slow cooker using a nonstick cooking spray. Place chicken breasts in the crock. Mix the Italian dressing and water in a small bowl and pour over chicken. Rub the chicken with garlic, then cook on low within 4 hours.

2. Mix softened cream cheese plus cream of chicken soup in a bowl. Put on chicken, then stir in mushrooms. Cook on low within 1 additional hour.
3. Fill with lightly salted water in a large pot and boil over high heat. Stir in the spaghetti, then return to a boil.
4. Cook the pasta uncovered, occasionally stirring, within 12 minutes, then drain. Before you serve, scoop chicken plus sauce on hot cooked pasta, then sprinkle with parsley.

Nutrition:
Calories: 280 Carbs: 21g Fat: 16g Protein: 13g

823.   Pork Cacciatore

Preparation time: 15 minutes | Cooking time: 8 hours | Servings: 4

2 tbsp. olive oil

1 sliced onion

4 boneless pork chops

1 jar pasta sauce

1 can diced tomatoes

1 green bell pepper, strips

1 package fresh mushrooms, sliced

2 large cloves garlic, minced

1 tsp Italian seasoning

1/2 tsp dried basil

1/2 cup dry white wine

4 slices mozzarella cheese

1. Cook the pork chops over medium-high heat in a large skillet, then transfer it to your slow cooker. Cook onion in oil on medium heat in the same pan. Mix in mushrooms plus bell pepper until they are soft.
2. Mix in pasta sauce, diced tomatoes, plus white wine. Season with Italian seasoning, basil, and garlic. Pour over pork chops in the slow cooker. Cook on low within 7 to 8 hours. Put cheese slices on each chop and cover with sauce to serve.

Nutrition:
Calories: 252 Carbs: 23g Fat: 6g Protein: 26g

824.   Italian Beef Roast

Preparation time: 15 minutes | Cooking time: 8 hours - Servings: 8

1 beef chuck roast

1 quartered onion

1 can beef broth

1 packet dry au jus mix

1 package dry Italian salad dressing mix

1/2 teaspoon salt

1/2 teaspoon ground black pepper

1. Put the beef chuck roast into your slow cooker, then scatter onion quarters around the meat. Put the beef broth on the meat, then sprinkle the au jus mix, Italian salad dressing mix, salt, plus black pepper over the roast. Set on low within 6 to 8 hours.

Nutrition:
Calories: 60 Carbs: 1g Fat: 2g Protein: 11g

825.   Rosemary and Red Pepper Chicken

Preparation time: 15 minutes | Cooking time: 7 hours - Servings: 8

1 thinly sliced small onion

1 medium red bell pepper, thinly sliced

4 cloves garlic, minced

2 teaspoons dried rosemary

1/2 teaspoon dried oregano

8 ounces Italian turkey sausages, casings removed

8 skinless, boneless chicken breast halves

1/4 teaspoon coarsely ground pepper

1/4 cup dry vermouth

1 1/2 tablespoons cornstarch

2 tablespoons cold water

Salt to taste

1/4 cup chopped fresh parsley

1. In a 5 to 6-quart slow cooker, mix onion, bell pepper, garlic, rosemary, plus oregano. Put the sausages over the onion mixture. Rinse chicken, then pat dry; arrange in a single layer on the sausage.
2. Put pepper, then pour in vermouth. Cook on low within 5 to 7 hours. Stir cornstarch plus cold water in a small bowl. Mix into cooking liquid in your slow cooker. Adjust the heat to high, stirring within 2 to 3 times, until sauce is thickened. Serve with a sprinkle of parsley.

Nutrition:
Calories: 130 Carbs: 13g Fat: 7g Protein: 4g

826. Braciole

Preparation time: 15 minutes | Cooking time: 8 hours - Servings: 6

2 jars marinara sauce
1/2 cup dry bread crumbs
1 tsp kosher salt
5 bacon slices
2 tbsp. vegetable oil

2 beaten eggs
1 flank steak, pounded
Ground black pepper
1 cup Italian cheese blend, shredded

1. Put the marinara sauce into your slow cooker and set it on High to warm. Mix the eggs plus the breadcrumbs in a bowl. Rub each side of the meat with salt plus pepper.
2. Pat the breadcrumb batter over one side of the flank steak, leaving about a one-inch border around the edges. Top it with the bacon slices, then with shredded cheese. Beginning from one long side, roll flank steak into a log, then use toothpicks to secure the log.
3. Warm the oil in a heavy skillet. Cook the stuffed flank steak in the hot oil within 10 minutes, then transfer it to the warm sauce in your slow cooker. Put the sauce on meat to cover. Cook on low within 6 to 8 hours. Remove the toothpicks before slicing. Serve with marinara.

Nutrition:
Calories: 137 Carbs: 0g Fat: 5g Protein: 23g

827. Eggplant Parmesan

Preparation time: 15 minutes | Cooking time: 5 hours - Servings: 8

4 eggplant, sliced
1 cup extra-virgin olive oil
1/3 cup water
1/3 cup seasoned bread crumbs
1 jar prepared marinara sauce

1 tbsp. salt
2 eggs
3 tbsp. all-purpose flour
1/2 cup Parmesan cheese, grated
1 package mozzarella cheese, sliced

1. Put the eggplant slices in a bowl in layers, sprinkle it with salt. Let stand for 30 minutes to drain. Rinse and dry on paper towels.

2. Warm-up olive oil in a skillet on medium heat. Mix the eggs with water plus flour. Soak the eggplant slices in batter, then fry in the hot oil until golden brown. Mix the seasoned bread crumbs with Parmesan cheese in a bowl.
3. Put 1/4 of the eggplant slices into your crockpot, then top with 1/4 of the crumbs, 1/4 of the marinara sauce, plus 1/4 of the mozzarella cheese. Repeat layers three more times. Cook on low within 4 to 5 hours.

Nutrition:
Calories: 271 Carbs: 21g Fat: 17g Protein: 9g

828. Ravioli Lasagna

Preparation time: 15 minutes | Cooking time: 6 hours - Servings: 8

1-pound ground beef
1 tsp garlic powder
1/2 tsp ground black pepper
1 tsp Italian seasoning
1 tsp dried oregano
2 cups mozzarella cheese, shredded

1 tbsp. chopped garlic
1 tsp salt
2 jars prepared pasta sauce
1 tsp dried basil
1 package cheese ravioli

1. Warm a large skillet on medium-high heat. Cook the beef, garlic, garlic powder, salt, plus pepper in the hot skillet within 5 to 7 minutes.
2. Drain and discard all the grease, then mix in pasta sauce, Italian seasoning, basil, plus oregano into the ground beef batter.
3. Put a layer of meat sauce into your slow cooker, then put a layer of ravioli. Put another layer of meat sauce on the ravioli layer; alternate.
4. Cook on low within 3 to 5 hours. Put the ravioli mixture with mozzarella cheese and cook again within 45 minutes to 1 hour more.

Nutrition:
Calories: 240 Carbs: 23g Fat: 9g Protein: 15g

SIDES

829. Sauerkraut

Preparation time: 15 minutes | Cooking time: 8 hours | Servings: 6

2 pounds of sauerkraut, drained	2 tablespoons bacon drops
2 onion, coarsely chopped	1 1/4 cup beef broth
3 whole cloves	1 bay leaf
4 juniper berries	2 teaspoons caraway seed
salt to taste	1 tsp of white sugar, or to taste

1. Put the sauerkraut, bacon drops, and onion in a slow cooker. Put in the beef broth, then season with cloves, bay leaves, juniper berries, caraway seeds, salt, and sugar. Stir to combine. Cook on Low 8 hours.

Nutrition:
Calories 111 Fat 5.2 g Carbos 14.9 g Protein 3 g

830. Refried Beans without the Refry

Preparation time: 15 minutes | Cooking time: 8 hours | Servings: 15

1 onion, peeled and halved	3 cups of dry pinto beans, rinsed
1/2 fresh jalapeno pepper, without seeds and minced meat	2 tablespoons chopped garlic
5 teaspoons of salt	1 3/4 teaspoons of freshly ground black pepper
1/8 teaspoon ground cumin, optional	9 cups of water

1. Put the onion, rinsed beans, jalapeno, garlic, salt, pepper, and cumin in a slow cooker. Put in the water and mix to combine. Boil for 8 hours on High and add more water if necessary.
2. When the beans are done, sift them and save the liquid. Puree the beans with a potato masher and add the reserved water if necessary to achieve the desired consistency.

Nutrition:
Calories 139 Fat 0.5 g Carbo 25.4 g Protein 8.5 g

831.Spicy Black-Eyed Peas

Preparation time: 15 minutes | Cooking time: 6 hours - Servings: 10

6 cups of water	1 cube chicken broth
1 pound of dried peas with black eyes, sorted and rinsed	1 onion, diced
2 cloves of garlic, diced	1 red pepper, stemmed, seeded, and diced
1 jalapeno Chili, without seeds and minced meat	8 grams diced ham
4 slices of bacon, minced meat	1/2 teaspoon cayenne pepper
1 1/2 teaspoon of cumin	salt
1 tsp ground black pepper	

1. Put the water into your slow cooker, add the stock cube, and stir to dissolve. Combine the peas with black eyes, onion, garlic, bell pepper, jalapeno pepper, ham, bacon, cayenne pepper, cumin, salt, and pepper; stir to mix. Cover the slow cooker and cook for 6 to 8 hours on low until the beans are soft.

Nutrition:
Calories 199 Fat 2.9 g Carbo 30.2 g Protein 14.1 g

832. Sweet Potato Casserole

Preparation time: 15 minutes | Cooking time: 4 hours | Servings: 8

2 (29 ounces) cans of sweet potatoes, drained and mashed	1/3 cup butter, melted
2 tablespoons white sugar	2 tablespoons brown sugar
1 tablespoon orange juice	2 eggs, beaten
1/2 cup of milk	1/3 cup chopped pecans
1/3 cup of brown sugar	2 tablespoons all-purpose flour
2 teaspoons butter, melted	

1. Lightly grease a slow cooker. Mix sweet potatoes, 1/3 cup butter, white sugar, and 2 tablespoons brown sugar in a large bowl. Add orange juice, eggs, and milk. Transfer it to the prepared oven dish.
2. Mix the pecans, 1/3 cup brown sugar, flour plus 2 tablespoons butter in a small bowl. Spread the mixture over the sweet potatoes. Cover the slow cooker and cook for 3 to 4 hours on HIGH.

Nutrition:
Calories 406 Fat 13.8 g Carbohydrates 66.1 g Protein 6.3 g

833. Baked Potatoes

Preparation time: 15 minutes | Cooking: 4 hours & 30 minutes | Servings: 4

Bake 4 potatoes, scrubbed well	1 tablespoon extra-virgin olive oil
kosher salt to taste	4 sheets of aluminum foil

1. Prick the potatoes all over, then massage the potatoes with olive oil, sprinkle with salt, and wrap them firmly in foil. Put the potatoes in a slow cooker, cook for 4 1/2 to 5 hours on High, or 7 1/2 to 8 hours on low until cooked.

Nutrition:
Calories 254 Fat 3.6 g Carbohydrates 51.2 g Protein 6.1 g

834. Slow Cooker Stuffing

Preparation time: 15 minutes | Cooking time: 8 hours - Servings: 4

1 cup of butter or margarine	2 cups chopped onion
2 cups chopped celery	1/4 cup chopped fresh parsley
12 grams of sliced mushrooms	12 cups of dry bread cubes
1 teaspoon seasoning for poultry	1 1/2 teaspoons dried sage
1 teaspoon dried thyme	1/2 teaspoon dried marjoram
1 1/2 teaspoons of salt	1/2 teaspoon ground black pepper
4 & 1/2 cups of chicken broth	2 eggs, beaten

1. Dissolve the butter or margarine in a frying pan over medium heat. Cook onion, celery, mushroom, and parsley in butter, stirring regularly.
2. Put boiled vegetables over bread cubes in a huge mixing bowl. Season with poultry herbs, sage, thyme, marjoram, and salt and pepper.
3. Pour enough broth to moisten and mix the eggs. Transfer the mixture to the slow cooker and cover. Bake 45 minutes on High, turn the heat to low, and cook for 4 to 8 hours.

Nutrition:
Calories 197 Fat 13.1 g Carbohydrates 16.6 g Protein 3.9 g

835. Slow Cooker Mashed Potatoes

Preparation time: 15 minutes | Cooking: 3 hours & 15 minutes - Servings: 8

5 pounds of red potatoes, cut into pieces	1 tablespoon minced garlic, or to taste
3 cubes of chicken broth	1 (8 ounces) container of sour cream
1 package of cream cheese, softened	1/2 cup butter
salt and pepper to taste	

1. Boil the potatoes, garlic, and broth in a large pan with lightly salted boiling water until soft but firm, about 15 minutes.
2. Drain, reserve water. Mashed potatoes in a bowl with sour cream and cream cheese; add reserved water if necessary to achieve the desired consistency.

3. Transfer it to your slow cooker, cook for 2 to 3 hours on low. Stir in butter just before serving and season with salt and pepper.

Nutrition:
Calories 470 Fat 27.7 g Carbo 47.9 g Protein 8.8 g

836.   Scalloped Potatoes with Ham

Preparation time: 15 minutes | Cooking time: 4 hours | Servings: 8

3 pounds of potatoes, thin slices	1 cup grated Cheddar cheese
1/2 cup chopped onion	1 cup chopped cooked ham
1 can of condensed mushroom soup	1/2 cup of water
1/2 teaspoon of garlic powder	1/4 teaspoon of salt
1/4 teaspoon of black pepper	

1. Place sliced potatoes in a slow cooker. Mix the grated cheese, onion, and ham in a medium bowl. Mix with potatoes in a slow cooker.
2. Use the same bowl and mix condensed soup and water. Season with garlic powder, salt, and pepper. Pour evenly over the potato mixture. Cook on High within 4 hours.

Nutrition:
Calories 265 Fat 10.2 g Carbohydrates 33.3 g Protein 10.8 g

837.   Classic Coney Sauce

Preparation time: 15 minutes | Cooking time: 2 hours - Servings: 12

2 pounds of ground beef	1/2 cup chopped onion
1 1/2 cups of ketchup	1/4 cup of white sugar
1/4 cup white vinegar	1/4 cup prepared yellow mustard
1/2 teaspoon celery seed	3/4 teaspoon Worcestershire sauce
1/2 teaspoon ground black pepper	3/4 teaspoon of salt

1. Place the minced meat and onion in a large frying pan over medium-high heat. Cook, stirring, until the meat is brown. Drain.
2. Transfer the steak plus onion to your slow cooker, then mix in the ketchup, sugar, vinegar, plus mustard. Put the celery seed, Worcestershire sauce, pepper plus salt. Simmer on low within a few hours before you serve.

Nutrition:
Calories 186 Fat 9.2 g Carbohydrates 12.8 g Protein 13.5 g

838.   Spiced Slow Cooker Applesauce

Preparation time: 15 minutes | Cooking: 6 hours & 30 minutes - Servings: 8

8 apples - peeled, without the core and cut into thin slices	1/2 cup of water
3/4 cup packaged brown sugar	1/2 teaspoon pumpkin pie spice

1. Mix the apples plus water in your slow cooker; cook on low within 6 to 8 hours. Mix in the brown sugar plus pumpkin pie spice; continue cooking for another 30 minutes.

Nutrition:
Calories 150 Fat 0.2 g Carbohydrates 39.4 g Protein 0.4 g

839.   Homemade Beans

Preparation time: 15 minutes | Cooking time: 10 hours - Servings: 12

3 cups of dried navy beans, soaked overnight or cooked for an hour	1 1/2 cups of ketchup
1 1/2 cups of water	1/4 cup molasses
1 large onion, minced	1 tablespoon dry mustard
1 tablespoon of salt	6 thick-sliced bacon, cut into 1-inch pieces
1 cup of brown sugar	

1. Pour soaking liquid from beans and place in a slow cooker. Stir ketchup, water, molasses, onion, mustard, salt, bacon, and brown sugar through the beans until everything is well mixed. Cook on LOW within 8 to 10 hours, occasionally stirring if possible, although not necessary.

Nutrition:
Calories 296 Fat 3 g Carbohydrates 57 g Protein 12.4 g

840.   Western Omelet

Preparation time: 15 minutes | Cooking time: 12 hours - Servings: 12

1 (2 pounds) package of frozen grated hashish brown potatoes	1 pound diced cooked ham
1 onion, diced	1 green pepper, seeded and diced
1 1/2 cups grated cheddar cheese	12 eggs
1 cup of milk	salt and pepper to taste

1. Grease a slow cooker of 4 liters or larger in light. Layer 1/3 of the mashed potatoes in a layer on the bottom.
2. Layer 1/3 of the ham, onion, green pepper, and cheddar cheese. Repeat layers two more times. Whisk the eggs plus milk in a large bowl and season with salt and pepper. Put over the contents of the slow cooker. Cook on low within 10 to 12 hours.

Nutrition:
Calories 310 Fat 22.7 g Carbo 16.1 g Protein 19.9 g

841. Green Bean Casserole

Preparation time: 15 minutes | Cooking time: 5 hours – Servings: 8

2 (16 ounces) packages of frozen sliced green beans	2 tins of cream of chicken soup
2/3 cup of milk	1/2 cup grated Parmesan cheese
1/4 teaspoon of salt	1/4 teaspoon ground black pepper
1 (6 ounces) can of fried onions, divided	

1. Mix the green beans, cream of chicken soup, milk, Parmesan cheese, salt, black pepper, and half the can of fried onions in a slow cooker. Cover and cook on low for 5 to 6 hours. Top casserole with remaining French-fried onions to serve.

Nutrition:
Calories 272 Fat 16.7 g Carbohydrates 22.9 g Protein 5.9 g

842.   Texas Cowboy Baked Beans

Preparation time: 15 minutes Cooking time: 2 hours - Servings: 12

1-pound ground beef	4 cans of baked beans with pork
1 (4 ounces) can of canned chopped green chili peppers	1 small Vidalia onion, peeled and chopped
1 cup of barbecue sauce	1/2 cup of brown sugar
1 tablespoon garlic powder	1 tablespoon chili powder
3 tablespoons hot pepper sauce, to taste	

1. Fry the minced meat in a frying pan over medium heat until it is no longer pink; remove fat and set aside. In a 3 1/2 liter or larger slow cooker, combine the minced meat, baked beans, green chili, onion, and barbecue sauce.
2. Put the brown sugar, garlic powder, chili powder, plus hot pepper sauce. Bake for 2 hours on HIGH or low for 4 to 5 hours.

Nutrition:
Calories 360 Fat 12.4 g Carbo 50 g Protein 14.6 g

843.   Frijoles La Charra

Preparation time: 15 minutes Cooking time: 5 hours - Servings: 8

1 pound of dry pinto beans	5 cloves of garlic, minced
1 teaspoon of salt	1/2 pound of bacon, diced
1 onion, minced	2 fresh tomatoes, diced
1 (3.5 ounces) can of sliced jalapeno peppers	1 can of beer
1/3 cup chopped fresh coriander	

1. Cook or brown the bacon in a frying pan over medium heat until it is evenly brown but still soft. Drain about half the fat. Put the onion in the frying pan, then cook until tender.
2. Mix in the tomatoes and jalapenos and cook until everything is hot. Transfer to the slow cooker and stir into the beans. Cover the slow cooker and continue cooking on low for 4 hours. Mix the beer and coriander about 30 minutes before the end of the cooking time.

Nutrition:
Calories 353 Fat 13.8 g Carbohydrates 39.8 g Protein 16 g

SEAFOOD

844. Italian Flavored Salmon

Preparation Time: 15 minutes | Cooking: 2 hours 8 minutes | Servings: 6

For Salmon:
1 tsp garlic powder
½ tsp sweet paprika
ground black pepper
Olive oil cooking spray
1 C. low-sodium vegetable broth
For Lemon Sauce:
¼ C. white wine
1/8 tsp. lemon zest, grated finely

1 tsp. Italian seasoning
½ tsp red chili powder
Salt
2 lb. skin-on salmon fillet
1 lemon, cut into slices
2 tbsp. fresh lemon juice
2/3 C. heavy cream
3 tbsp. fresh lemon juice
2-3 tbsp. fresh parsley, chopped

1. Line a slow cooker with a large piece of parchment paper. In a small bowl, mix the spices. Spray the salmon fillet with cooking spray and rub with cooking spray evenly.
2. In the center of the prepared slow cooker, arrange the lemon slices. Put the salmon fillet on top of lemon slices and pour the broth and lemon juice around the fish. Cook on low within 2 hours.
3. Prepare to preheat the oven to 400 degrees F. Uncover the slow cooker and transfer the salmon with liquid into a baking dish. Bake for about 5-8 minutes.
4. For the sauce, add the cream, wine, and lemon juice on medium-high heat and boil, frequently stirring in a small pan. Adjust the heat to low and simmer within 8 minutes. Uncover the pan and stir in the lemon zest.
5. Adjust the heat to high setting, then cook within 2 minutes. Remove from heat and set aside. Remove, then place the salmon fillet onto a cutting board. Cut the salmon into 4 equal-sized fillets and top with sauce. Garnish with parsley and serve.

Nutrition:
Calories: 265 Carbohydrates: 1.8g Protein: 30.2g Fat: 14.6g Sugar: 0.4g Sodium: 115mg Fiber: 0.3g

845. Marvelous Salmon

Preparation Time: 15 minutes | Cooking Time: 2½ hours | Servings: 4

¾ C. fresh cilantro leaves, chopped
2-3 tbsp. fresh lime juice
Salt, to taste

2 garlic cloves, chopped finely
1 tbsp. olive oil
1 lb. salmon fillets

1. Put all the ingredients except for salmon fillets and mix well in a medium bowl. In the bottom of a greased slow cooker, place the salmon fillets and top with garlic mixture. Cook on low within 2-2½ hours. With a spoon, mix the meat with pan juices and serve.

Nutrition:
Calories: 184 Carbohydrates: 0.7g Protein: 22.2g Fat: 10.5g Sugar: 0.1g Sodium: 90mg Fiber: 0.1g

846. Nutrient-Packed Salmon

Preparation Time: 15 minutes | Cooking Time: 6 hours | Servings: 4

1 tbsp. Italian seasoning
1 tsp. garlic powder
ground black pepper
1 tbsp. olive oil
1 red bell pepper, seeded and julienned
½ of onion, sliced

1 tsp. onion powder
Salt
1 lb. salmon fillets
1 zucchini, quartered and sliced
1 tomato, chopped
3 garlic cloves, sliced

1. Generously, grease an oval as a Pyrex dish that will fit inside the slow cooker insert. Mix the Italian seasoning and spices in a small bowl.

Season the salmon fillets with half of the spice mixture evenly and then coat with half of the oil.
2. In a large bowl, add the vegetables, remaining spice mixture, and oil and toss to coat well. Put the salmon fillets into the baking dish and top with vegetables. With a piece of foil, cover the baking dish and place in the slow cooker. Cook on low within 6 hours. Serve hot.

Nutrition:
Calories: 224 Carbohydrates: 7.9g Protein: 23.5g Fat: 11.8g Sugar: 4.1g Sodium: 98mg Fiber: 4.1g

847. Highly Nutritious Meal

Preparation Time: 20 minutes | Cooking: 5 hours 55 minutes | Servings: 6

¾ C. French lentils
¼ C. celery, chopped finely
1 bay leaf
1 lb. small golden beets, scrubbed and trimmed
Salt
1 tbsp. raw honey
1 tbsp. orange zest, grated
1 tsp. lemon zest, grated
2 tbsp. fresh parsley, chopped

½ C. carrots, peeled and chopped finely
¼ C. red onion, chopped finely
2¼ C. low-sodium chicken broth
1 tbsp. olive oil
ground black pepper
3-4 tbsp. fresh orange juice
2 tbsp. fresh lemon juice, divided
6 (5-oz.) wild salmon fillets

1. In a slow cooker, add the lentils, carrots, celery, onion, bay leaf, and broth and mix well. Arrange a piece of foil onto a smooth surface. In a bowl, add the beets, oil, salt, and black pepper and toss to coat well.
2. Place the beets in the center of foil and wrap tightly. Arrange the foil packet on top of the lentil mixture. Cook on low within 5-5½ hours. For the glaze, add the honey, juices, and zest over medium heat and boil in a small pan.
3. Adjust the heat to medium, then simmer for about 1-2 minutes, stirring continuously. Uncover the slow cooker and transfer the beets packet onto a plate. Unwrap the foil and set the beets aside to cool slightly. Peel the beets and cut into wedges.
4. Place 1 parchment paper over the lentil mixture in the slow cooker. Massage the salmon fillets with salt plus black pepper and brush the tops with glaze. Arrange the salmon fillets over the parchment, skin side down. Cook on low within 25 minutes.
5. Uncover the slow cooker and transfer the salmon fillets onto a platter. Discard the bay leaf and add the parsley, salt, and black pepper into lentil mixture. Serve lentils with salmon fillets and beet slices.

Nutrition:
Calories: 407 Carbohydrates: 28g Protein: 38.4g Fat: 15.2g Sugar: 10.9g Sodium: 191mg Fiber: 9.5g

848. Super-Healthy Dinner

Preparation Time: 15 minutes | Cooking: 1 hour 15 minutes | Servings: 4

2 lb. boneless cod fillets
2 (14-oz.) cans diced tomatoes
¼ C. capers
6 garlic cloves, sliced
1 tsp. red pepper flakes, crushed
3 tbsp. olive oil, divided
1 C. couscous

Salt, to taste
½ C. Kalamata olives, pitted and sliced
½ of onion, sliced
3 tbsp. fresh parsley, chopped roughly and divided
Freshly ground black pepper, to taste
1 lemon, sliced
1 C. hot boiling water

1. Season each cod fillet with salt and set aside at room temperature for about 10-15 minutes. In a slow cooker, place the tomato, olives,

capers, onion, garlic, 1 tbsp. of parsley, red pepper flakes, black pepper, and 1½ tbsp. olive oil and mix well.

2. Place the cod fillets over the sauce in a single layer and spoon some of the tomato mixtures on top. Arrange 2 lemon slices on top. Cook on high within 1 hour. Uncover the slow cooker and, with a slotted spoon, transfer the cod fillets onto a platter.

3. Place about 2/3 of the sauce on top of cod fillets. In your slow cooker with the remaining sauce, add the couscous, boiling water, and a little salt and mix well. Cook on high within 10 minutes. Uncover the slow cooker and with a fork fluff the couscous. Stir in the remaining olive oil and serve with cod fillets.

Nutrition:
Calories: 507 Carbohydrates: 45.9g Protein: 48.7g Fat: 15.2g Sugar: 6g Sodium: 599mg Fiber: 6g

849.   Paleo-Friendly Tilapia
Preparation Time: 15 minutes | Cooking Time: 2 hours | Servings: 4

1 (15-oz.) can diced tomatoes	1 bell pepper, seeded and chopped
1 small onion, chopped	1 garlic clove, minced
1 tsp. dried rosemary	1/3 C. low-sodium chicken broth
Salt	ground black pepper
1 lb. tilapia fillets	

1. In a slow cooker, place all the ingredients except for tilapia and stir to combine. Place the tilapia on top and gently submerge in sauce. Cook on high within 2 hours. Serve hot.

Nutrition:
Calories: 132 Carbohydrates: 8.5g Protein: 22.8g Fat: 1.4g Sugar: 5.1g Sodium: 92mg Fiber: 2.2g

850.   Winner Halibut
Preparation Time: 10 minutes | Cooking Time: 2 hours | Servings: 2

12 oz. halibut fillet	Salt
ground black pepper	1 tbsp. fresh lemon juice
1 tbsp. olive oil	1½ tsp. dried dill

1. Arrange a large 18-inch piece of greased piece foil onto a smooth surface. Massage the halibut fillet with salt plus black pepper. In a small bowl, add the lemon juice, oil, and dill and mix well.

2. Put the halibut fillet in the center of foil and drizzle with oil mixture. Carefully bring up the edges of foil and crimp them, leaving plenty of air inside the foil packet.

3. Place the foil packet in the bottom of a slow cooker. Cook on high within 1½-2 hours. Uncover the slow cooker and remove the foil packet. Carefully open the foil packet and serve.

Nutrition:
Calories: 258 Carbohydrates: 1.7g Protein: 36.4g Fat: 11.2g Sugar: 0.2g Sodium: 174mg Fiber: 0.4g

851. Unique Salmon Risotto
Preparation Time: 15 minutes | Cooking: 1 hour 20 minutes | Servings: 4

2 tbsp. olive oil	2 shallots, chopped
½ of a medium cucumber, peeled, seeded, and chopped	1¼ C. Arborio rice
3 C. hot vegetable broth	½ C. white wine
1¼ lb. skinless salmon fillet, chopped	Salt
ground black pepper	1 scallion, chopped
3 tbsp. fresh dill, chopped	

1. In a pan, heat the oil over medium-high heat and sauté the shallot and cucumber for about 2-3 minutes. Cook on low within 15 minutes. Add the rice and stir to combine. Increase the heat to high and sauté for about 1 minute.

2. Remove from the heat and transfer the rice mixture into a slow cooker. Pour the hot broth and wine on top. Cook on high within 45 minutes, then stir in the salmon pieces, salt, and black pepper.

3. Cook on high within 15 minutes. Let the risotto stand, covered for about 5 minutes. Remove and stir in the scallion and dill. Serve hot.

Nutrition:
Calories: 534 Carbohydrates: 53.2g Protein: 36.1g Fat: 17.3g Sugar: 1.5g Sodium: 686mg Fiber: 2.2g

852.   Delish Dinner Shrimp
Preparation Time: 20 minutes | Cooking Time: 5 hours | Servings: 4

1 medium onion, chopped	½ of medium green bell pepper, seeded and chopped
1 can whole tomatoes, undrained and chopped roughly	1 (2½-oz.) jar sliced mushrooms
¼ C. ripe olives, pitted and sliced	2 garlic cloves, minced
1 (14½-oz.) can low-sodium chicken broth	1 (8-oz.) can tomato sauce
½ C. dry white wine	½ C. orange juice
1 tsp. dried basil leaves	2 bay leaves
¼ tsp. fennel seed, crushed	Salt
ground black pepper	1 lb. medium shrimp, peeled

1. In a slow cooker, place all the ingredients except for shrimp and mix. Cook on low within 4-4½ hours. Remove cover, then mix in the shrimp. Cook on low within 20-30 minutes. Uncover the slow cooker and discard the bay leaves. Serve hot.

Nutrition:
Calories: 217 Carbohydrates: 16.9g Protein: 28.2g Fat: 2.8g Sugar: 10.2g Sodium: 705mg Fiber: 10.2g

853.   Loveable Feta Shrimp
Preparation Time: 15 minutes | Cooking: 2 hours 25 minutes | Servings: 6

¼ C. extra-virgin olive oil	1 medium onion, chopped
1 (28-oz.) can crushed tomatoes	½ C. dry white wine
½ tsp. dried oregano	Pinch of red pepper flakes, crushed
Salt, to taste	1½ lb. medium shrimp, peeled and deveined
1 C. feta cheese, crumbled	2 tbsp. fresh parsley, chopped

1. Warm-up the oil over medium heat in a skillet and cook the onion for about 10 minutes, stirring frequently. Remove from the heat and transfer the onion into a large slow cooker. Add the tomatoes, wine, oregano, red pepper flakes, and salt and stir to combine.

2. Cook on high within 2 hours. Remove cover, then stir in the shrimp. Sprinkle with feta cheese evenly. Cook on high within 10-15 minutes. Serve hot with the garnishing of parsley.

Nutrition:
Calories: 324 Carbohydrates: 14g Protein: 31.3g Fat: 15.1g Sugar: 9.4g Sodium: 819mg Fiber: 4.7g

854.   Luncheon Party Meal
Preparation Time: 20 minutes | Cooking Time: 4½ hours | Servings: 4

1 (14½-oz.) can diced tomatoes, drained	1 C. red sweet pepper, seeded and chopped
1 C. zucchini, sliced	2 garlic cloves, minced
½ C. dry white wine	8 oz. frozen medium shrimp, thawed
8 Kalamata olives, pitted and chopped roughly	¼ C. fresh basil, chopped
1 tbsp. olive oil	1½ tsp. fresh rosemary, chopped
Salt, to taste	2 oz. feta cheese, crumbled

1. In a greased slow cooker, put the tomatoes, sweet pepper, zucchini, garlic, and wine and mix well. Cook on low within 4 hours, then remove the cover and stir in the shrimp. Cook on high within 30

minutes. Uncover, then stir in the remaining ingredients. Serve hot with the topping of feta cheese.

Nutrition:
Calories: 206 Carbohydrates: 10.8g Protein: 16.7g Fat: 8.9g Sugar: 5.5g Sodium: 423mg Fiber: 2.5g

855. Easiest Shrimp Scampi

Preparation Time: 15 minutes | Cooking Time: 1½ hours | Servings: 4

1 lb. raw shrimp, peeled and deveined	¼ C. chicken broth
2 tbsp. butter	2 tbsp. olive oil
1 tbsp. fresh lemon juice	1 tbsp. garlic, minced
1 tbsp. dried parsley	Salt
ground black pepper	

1. In a slow cooker, place all the ingredients and stir to combine. Cook on high within 1½ hours. Uncover the slow cooker and stir the mixture. Serve hot.

Nutrition:
Calories: 252 Carbohydrates: 2.6g Protein: 26.4g Fat: 14.8g Sugar: 0.2g Sodium: 406mg Fiber: 0.1g

856. Amazingly Tasty Shrimp Orzo

Preparation Time: 15 minutes | Cooking: 3 hours 16 minutes | Servings: 6

2 C. uncooked orzo pasta	2 tsp. dried basil
3 tbsp. olive oil, divided	2 tbsp. butter
1½ tbsp. shallot, chopped	1 (14½-oz.) can diced tomatoes, drained
3 garlic cloves, minced	2 tsp. dried oregano
1 lb. jumbo shrimp, peeled and deveined	1 C. oil-packed sun-dried tomatoes, chopped
1½ C. Greek olives pitted	2½ C. feta cheese, crumbled

1. Cook the orzo within 8-10 minutes or according to the package's directions in a large pan of salted boiling water. Drain, then rinse under cold running water. Transfer the orzo into a large bowl with basil and 1 tbsp. of oil and toss to coat well. Set aside. Warm-up the remaining oil and butter over medium heat and sauté the shallot for about 2-3 minutes in a large skillet.
2. Put the tomatoes, garlic, plus oregano and cook within 1-2 minutes. Add the shrimp and sun-dried tomatoes and cook for about 1 minute. Remove from the heat and place the shrimp mixture into a greased slow cooker. Add the orzo mixture, olives, and cheese and stir. Cook on low within 2-3 hours. Serve hot.

Nutrition:
Calories: 633 Carbohydrates: 57.9g Protein: 35.4g Fat: 30.2g Sugar: 8.5g Sodium: 1390mg Fiber: 5.3g

857. Delightful Shrimp Pasta

Preparation Time: 15 minutes | Cooking Time: 7¼ hours | Servings: 4

1 (14½-oz.) can peeled tomatoes, chopped	1 (6-oz.) can tomato paste
2 tbsp. fresh parsley, minced	1 garlic clove, minced
1 tsp. dried oregano	1 tsp. dried basil
1 tsp. seasoned salt	1 lb. cooked shrimp
Salt	ground black pepper
¼ C. parmesan cheese, shredded	

1. In a slow cooker, place all the ingredients except for shrimp and Parmesan and stir to combine. Cook on low within 6-7 hours, then stir in the cooked shrimp. Sprinkle with parmesan cheese. Cook on high within 15 minutes. Serve hot.

Nutrition:
Calories: 212 Carbohydrates: 14.6g Protein: 30.6g Fat: 3.8g Sugar: 7.9g Sodium: 828mg Fiber: 3.2g

858. Meltingly Tender Octopus

Preparation Time: 20 minutes | Cooking Time: 6 hours | Servings: 4

1½ lb. octopus	6 fingerlings potatoes
½ lemon, cut into slices	Salt
ground black pepper	Water, as required
3 tbsp. extra-virgin olive oil	3 tbsp. capers

1. Remove the beak, eyes, and any other parts of the octopus, then rinse carefully. Slice off the head of the octopus at its base. In a pan of boiling water, dip the octopus with a pair of for about 10-15 seconds.
2. Now, place the octopus in a slow cooker. Place the potatoes, lemon slices, salt, black pepper, and enough water to cover. Cook on high within 5-6 hours. Uncover the slow cooker and drain the octopus in a colander.
3. With a slotted spoon, transfer the potatoes onto a platter. Pat dry the potatoes and slice it into thin. Cut the octopus into thin slices. In a large bowl, add the octopus, potatoes, oil, capers, salt, and black pepper and toss to coat. Serve immediately.

Nutrition:
Calories: 308 Carbohydrates: 18.5g Protein: 30.6g Fat: 12.3g Sugar: 1.6g Sodium: 230mg Fiber: 3.3g

859. Greek Shrimp and Feta Cheese

Preparation time: 15 minutes | Cooking time: 8 hours | Servings: 8

2 Tablespoons extra virgin olive oil	1 medium onion, chopped
1 clove garlic, minced	1 (28 oz.) canned San Marzano tomatoes
1 (12 oz.) can tomato paste	1/4 cup dry white wine
2 tablespoons parsley, chopped	1 teaspoon dried oregano
1/4 teaspoon freshly ground black pepper	1 1/2-pound medium shrimp, peeled and deveined
2 oz. feta cheese, crumbled	

1. In a medium sauté pan, heat olive oil until hot but not smoking. Add onion and cook about 4-5 minutes or until onions are soft. Add garlic and cook for 1 minute, do not brown. Mix all fixing except shrimp and feta in the slow cooker.
2. Cook on low within 6-8 hours. Adjust the heat to high; add shrimp, cook within 15 minutes, or until just pink. Stir in feta cheese and serve.

Nutrition:
Calories 204 Fat: 7g Carbs: 15g Fiber: 3g Cholesterol: 136mg Protein: 21g Sodium: 689mg

860. Basque Tuna with Potatoes and Peppers

Preparation time: 15 minutes | Cooking time: 4 hours | Servings: 6

2 Tablespoons extra virgin olive oil	2 Tablespoons smoked paprika or more to taste
1 teaspoon kosher salt	1-1/2 lbs. fresh tuna, cut into 1-1/2-inch chunks
1 large sweet onion, cut into wedges	6 large cloves garlic, chopped
1 teaspoon freshly ground black pepper	1/2 cup dry white wine
2 cups San Marzano tomatoes, undrained	3 potatoes, unpeeled and cut into chunks
1 cup chicken stock	1 green bell pepper, cut into 3/4" pieces
1 red bell pepper, slice into 3/4" pieces	1/4 cup green olives, pitted
1/4 cup Kalamata olives, pitted	1 Tablespoon cornstarch
Lemon wedges, for garnish	

1. In a bowl, combine olive oil, smoked paprika, salt, and tuna chunks. Toss until fish is well coated. Cover and refrigerate.
2. "Smoosh" the tomatoes up with your fingers and add to the slow cooker along with the onion, garlic, black pepper, wine, diced tomatoes, potatoes, and chicken stock. Cook on high within 2 hours or low within 4 hours.

3. Add the bell peppers and olives, and cook on high for 1 hour. Add the tuna chunks and the marinade. Cover and cook on high within 30 minutes. Transfer the tuna and vegetables to a serving bowl and cover to keep warm. Put the liquid from the crockpot into a small saucepan, and bring to a boil.

4. Place cornstarch in a small dish or measuring cup and add 2 tablespoons of cold water. Pour into the liquid in the saucepan in a small stream, stirring continuously. When it has thickened slightly, pour over the fish and vegetables. Garnish with lemon wedges. Serve hot, over polenta, couscous, or brown rice with a green salad and a crusty loaf of bread.

Nutrition:
Calories: 317 Sodium: 630mg Carbs: 25.9g Fat: 11.9g Fiber: 4.8g Sugars: 5.5g Cholesterol: 23mg Protein: 23.2g

861. Citrus Salmon

Preparation time: 15 minutes | Cooking: 3 hours & 30 minutes | Servings: 6

1 1/2 pounds salmon fillets	Kosher salt
Freshly ground white pepper to taste	1/4 cup freshly squeezed lemon juice
1teaspoon toasted sesame oil	2 teaspoons tamari
A few drops of hot sauce	1 clove garlic, minced
1/2 cup scallions, sliced	5 Tablespoons fresh parsley, chopped
1 Tablespoon extra-virgin olive oil	2 teaspoons lemon zest
2 teaspoons orange zest	Orange and lemon slices, for garnish
Parsley, chopped, for garnish	

1. Butter slow cooker; and add lemon juice, sesame oil, tamari, hot sauce, and garlic to slow cooker. Sprinkle salmon fillets with salt and pepper. Place fish in a slow cooker.

2. Drizzle olive oil over salmon, top with scallions, parsley, orange, and lemon zest. Cook on low within 3 1/2 hours. Transfer salmon to serving platter and remove the skin. Serve garnished with orange and lemon slices and sprigs of fresh parsley.

Nutrition:
Calories: 270 Sodium: 213mg Carbs: 1.6g Fat: 17.2g Fiber: 0.5g Sugars: 0.5g Cholesterol: 71mg Protein: 25.6g

862. Salmon with Mango Avocado Salsa

Preparation time: 15 minutes | Cooking: 3 hours & 30 minutes | Servings: 6

1 1/2 lbs. salmon fillets	1/4 cup cilantro stems removed, chopped
2 cloves garlic, minced	2-3 Tablespoons freshly squeezed lime juice
2 Tablespoons extra virgin olive oil	1/4 teaspoon kosher salt
Freshly ground white pepper	Mango Avocado Salsa

1. Coat slow cooker with olive oil. Place fillets, skin side down, in the slow cooker. Top with cilantro. In a small bowl, combine garlic, lime juice, olive oil, salt, and white pepper.

2. Pour mixture over salmon. Cook on Low 3 1/2 hours. Transfer salmon to serving platter and remove the skin. Pour juices over the top and serve with Mango Avocado Salsa.

Nutrition:
Calories: 275 Cholesterol: 71mg Sodium: 167mg Fat: 18.7g Carbs: 0.4g Protein: 25.1g

863. Salmon with Asparagus

Preparation time: 15 minutes | Cooking: 3 hours & 30 minutes | Servings: 6

1/2 cup water	1/2 cup chicken broth
1 cup dry white wine	1/2 thinly sliced small onion
3 sprigs tarragon, plus 1 tsp minced tarragon leaves	1/2 teaspoon kosher salt
Freshly ground white pepper	1 1/2 lbs. salmon fillets
11/2 lbs. fresh asparagus spears, trimmed	1 Tablespoon butter
1 Tablespoon olive oil	1 large shallot, minced

2 teaspoons white wine vinegar

1. Mix the water, broth, wine, onion, tarragon sprigs, salt, and white pepper in the slow cooker. Cook on low within 30 minutes.

2. Add the salmon fillets. Cover and cook on low within 3 hours or until salmon is opaque and tender. Transfer it to a serving platter, and remove the skin. Cover loosely to keep warm.

3. Discard the braising liquid and tarragon sprigs. During the last 30 minutes of salmon cooking time, over high heat, bring a large pot of lightly salted water to a boil.

4. Add asparagus spears and cook for about 4 minutes or until crisp-tender. Put into a colander in the sink and rinse well under cold running water, then pat dry.

5. Before you serve, heat butter and oil in a large skillet over medium heat until hot but not smoking. Add the shallot and cook for 2 or 3 minutes, or until slightly softened but not browned.

6. Add asparagus spears and stir to coat and warm thoroughly, then add the vinegar and minced tarragon, tossing to incorporate. Arrange asparagus spears around salmon fillets. Serve with parslied new red potatoes.

Nutrition:
Calories: 392 Sodium: 351mg Carbs: 17.8g Fat: 18.9g Fiber: 8.9g Sugars: 8.4g Cholesterol: 77mg Protein: 34.7g

864. Shrimp Marinara

Preparation time: 15 minutes | Cooking time: 8 hours | Servings: 8

1 (28 oz.) can ground, peeled tomatoes	1 (12 oz.) can tomato paste
1/2 cup dry red wine	1/4 cup fresh parsley, minced
4 cloves garlic, minced	1 1/2 tsp. dried basil
2 teaspoon dried oregano	1 teaspoon kosher salt
1/4 teaspoon freshly ground black pepper	1/2 teaspoon seasoned salt
2 lb. medium shrimp, shelled, cooked, and thawed if frozen	Grated Parmesan cheese, for garnish

1. Combine tomatoes, tomato paste, red wine, parsley, garlic, basil, oregano, salt, pepper, and seasoned salt in a slow cooker.

2. Cover and cook on low within 7-8 hours. Adjust temperature to high, stir in cooked shrimp, cover and cook on high for about 15 minutes, or until just heated through. Serve over pasta, spaghetti squash, or polenta with a big green salad.

Nutrition:
Calories: 243 Carbs: 18.4g Fiber: 4.6g Fat: 2.1g Sugars: 9.1g Cholesterol: 297mg Protein: 35.1g Sodium: 1294 mg

865. Foil Wrapped Lemon Pepper Sole with Asparagus

Preparation time: 15 minutes | Cooking time: 4 hours | Servings: 4

1 bunch asparagus, trimmed	1 1/2 lbs. sole filets, thawed if frozen
1/2 cup freshly squeezed lemon juice	Lemon Pepper Seasoning
1/2 Tablespoon extra-virgin olive oil for each packet	

1. You will need a piece of foil for each serving large enough to wrap contents completely. Portion sole into 4 even portions, place each portion in the foil sheet center, and season with lemon pepper seasoning using approximately 1/4 teaspoon per packet. Put 2 tablespoons of lemon juice and 1/2 tablespoon of olive oil.

2. Divide asparagus into 4 equal portions. Top sole with asparagus. Fold or flip the foil's sides over the sole and fold to close the foil up to form a packet. It should form a tightly wrapped packet.

3. Repeat this process with the remaining 3 portions. Place packets in the slow cooker, stacking if necessary. Cover and cook on high within 4 hours.

Nutrition:
Calories: 213 Sodium: 125mg Carbs: 3.4g Fat: 9.0g Fiber: 1.7g Sugars: 1.8g Cholesterol: 77mg Protein: 29.2g

866. Slow Cooker Chicken and Shrimp

Preparation time: 15 minutes| Cooking: 8 hours & 20 minutes Servings: 4

1 lb. boneless, skinless chicken thighs

1/2 teaspoon kosher salt

1/8 teaspoon freshly ground black pepper

1/2 teaspoon crushed red pepper flakes

2 onions, chopped

6 cloves garlic, minced

1 (14 oz.) can season diced tomatoes, undrained

1 (8oz.) can tomato sauce

3 Tablespoons tomato paste

1 cup chicken broth

1 teaspoon dried thyme leaves

1/2 teaspoon dried basil leaves

3 Tablespoons lemon juice

1 (8 oz.) package frozen cooked shrimp, thawed

1 (12 oz.) can quarter artichoke hearts, drained

1 Tablespoon cornstarch

2/3 cup crumbled feta cheese

1. Slice the chicken into large chunks, then season with salt and pepper to taste. Place onion and garlic in the bottom slow cooker and top with chicken.
2. Mix diced tomatoes, tomato sauce, tomato paste, chicken broth, thyme, basil, and lemon juice in a medium bowl. Pour over chicken. Cook on low within 6-8 hours until chicken is tender with the juices running clear or 165°F.on a thermometer.
3. Stir in thawed and drained shrimp and artichoke hearts. Put the cornstarch in a bowl, then add 2 tablespoons of water. Stir well to blend. Pour into a slow cooker.
4. Cover and cook within 15-20 minutes or until heated through and slightly thickened. Serve with hot cooked pasta or couscous and sprinkle with feta cheese.

Nutrition:
Calories: 369 Sodium: 701mg Carbs: 29.8g Fat: 11.1g Fiber: 7.8g Sugars: 17.4 Cholesterol: 162m Protein: 39.5g

867. Poached Swordfish with Lemon-Parsley Sauce

Preparation time: 15 minutes| Cooking: 1 hour & 15 minutes - Servings: 4

1 tablespoon butter

4 thin slices of sweet onion

2 cups of water

4 (6-ounce) swordfish steaks

Kosher salt, to taste

1 lemon, thinly sliced, seeds removed

6 tablespoons extra-virgin olive oil

3 tablespoons fresh lemon juice

3/4 teaspoon Dijon mustard

Freshly ground white pepper, to taste

3 tablespoons fresh flat-leaf parsley, minced

8 cups baby salad greens

1. Butter the bottom and halfway up the side of the slow cooker. Arrange the onion slices on the slow cooker, then pour in the water. Cook on high within 30 minutes.
2. Salt and white pepper swordfish steaks to taste and place on onion slices. Top with lemon slices. Cover and cook on high within 45 minutes or until the fish is opaque. Remove from slow cooker and either wrap to keep warm or chill in the fridge.
3. In a bowl, combine oil, lemon juice, mustard, and white pepper, then mix the parsley. Split the sauce between the swordfish steaks. Toss 8 cups of salad greens with 2/3 of dressing. Arrange 2 cups of greens on each of 4 individual plates.
4. Place a hot or chilled swordfish steak on top of each plate of dressed greens. Spoon the remaining sauce over the fish.

Nutrition:
Calories: 330 Sodium: 189mg Carbs: 3.2g Fat: 22.1g Fiber: 1.8g Sugars: 1.3g Protein: 29.9g

868. Easy Cheesy Salmon Loaf

Preparation time: 15 minutes| Cookin: 3 hours & 20 minutes - Servings: 4

1 tablespoon extra-virgin olive oil

1 (8 oz.) package sliced mushrooms

1 small onion, minced

1 can salmon, drained

1 1/2 cups fresh breadcrumbs

2 eggs, beaten

1 cup grated cheddar cheese

1 tablespoon lemon juice

1/4 teaspoon dry mustard

1 teaspoon Worcestershire sauce

1/2 teaspoon kosher salt

1 (10 oz.) package frozen peas, thawed, optional

1. Cut three 24-in. x 3-inches strips of foil; crisscross. Put the strips on the bottom and up the sides of a slow cooker coated with cooking spray.
2. In a medium sauté pan, heat olive oil, add mushrooms and onion and sauté until vegetables are soft and liquid has evaporated.
3. Flake fish in the bowl, removing all bones. Add all remaining ingredients, including sautéed vegetables, excepting peas, and mix thoroughly.
4. Pour into a lightly greased crockpot or casserole dish and shape into a rounded loaf, pulling the foil strips up the side of the slow cooker so they can act as handles for removing salmon loaf.
5. Cover and cook on high within 1 hour, then reduce to low and cook for an additional 3 to 5 hours. If desired, top the salmon loaf with optional peas during the last hour of cooking.

Nutrition:
Calories: 394 Sodium: 393mg Carbs: 22.3g Fat: 21.0g Fiber: 1.9g Sugars: 3.2g Cholesterol: 122mg Protein: 28.2g

869. Slow-Cooker Halibut Stew

Preparation time: 15 minutes| Cooking time: 9 hours - Servings: 6

1 red bell pepper, slice into 3/4" pieces

1 small yellow onion, roughly chopped

2 carrots, thinly sliced

1 stalk celery, thinly sliced

1 large potato, peeled, cut into 1" pieces

1 1/2 cups clam broth or chicken stock

2 Tablespoons freshly squeezed lime juice

3 cloves garlic, minced

1/2 teaspoon freshly ground black pepper

Kosher salt to taste

1 teaspoon chili powder

1/4 cup cilantro, chopped

1/2 teaspoon cumin

1/2 teaspoon red pepper flakes

1-pound halibut fillets, thawed if frozen, rinsed, and cut into bite-size pieces

Cilantro, for garnish

Lime wedges, for garnish

1. Combine all the above ingredients in slow-cooker, except halibut and garnishes. Cover and cook on Low 8-9 hours. During the last 30 minutes, add halibut pieces, cover, and cook until halibut is opaque. Garnish with additional cilantro if desired.

Nutrition:
Calories: 148 Sodium: 296 mg Fat: 2 g Carbs: 12 g Fiber: 2 g Sugars: 4 g Cholesterol: 26 mg Protein: 18 g

870. Salmon and Green Beans

Preparation time: 15 minutes| Cooking time: 4 hours - Servings: 4

1 1/4 lbs. salmon, thawed if frozen

1 lb. fresh green beans, washed and tops removed

1/4 cup tamari

1/4 cup honey

1 clove garlic, finely minced

freshly ground white pepper, to taste

1 tablespoon fresh ginger, finely minced

1/4 cup freshly squeezed lemon juice

1/4 cup squeezed blood orange juice or substituted squeezed orange juice

1. In a small bowl, combine tamari, honey, garlic, ginger, citrus juices, and white pepper. Wash and trim green beans, place in the slow cooker. Place fish on top of green beans.
2. Pour liquid mixture over the top. Cover and cook on low within 3-4 hours. Transfer salmon and green beans to a serving platter. Remove skin from salmon and drizzle juices over the top. Serve with quinoa or brown rice.

Nutrition:
Calories: 279 Sodium: 736mg Carbs: 19.8g Fat: 11.9g Fiber: 2.9g Sugars: 14.0g Cholesterol: 60mg Protein: 23.8g

871. Vegetable Ragout with Cornmeal Crusted Halibut Nuggets

Preparation time: 15 minutes | Cooking time: 10 hours - Servings: 6

1 tablespoon extra-virgin olive oil	2 onions, finely chopped
2 carrots, peeled and finely chopped	1 teaspoon dried oregano
1 teaspoon kosher salt	1/2 teaspoon freshly ground black pepper
2 cups bottled clam juice or chicken stock	2 cups dry vermouth or dry white wine
2 cups, water	1 tablespoon freshly squeezed lime juice
2 potatoes cut into 1/2-inch dice	1 sweet potato, cut into 1" dice
1 red bell pepper, coarsely chopped	1/2 cup yellow cornmeal
1 teaspoon chili powder	1/4 teaspoon cayenne pepper
kosher salt	ground black pepper
1 1/2 pounds, halibut, cut into 1/2-inch pieces	2 tablespoons extra virgin olive oil for frying halibut
sour cream, garnish	lime wedges, garnish

1. In a large sauté pan, heat the1 Tablespoon of oil over medium heat until hot but not smoking. Add chopped onions, carrots, and celery. Cook, stirring until the carrots are softened, about 7 minutes.
2. Add oregano, salt, and pepper and cook, stirring, for 1 minute. Transfer to a slow cooker. Add clam juice or broth, vermouth, water, and lime juice. Add the potatoes and sweet potatoes and stir to combine. Cover and cook on low for 8-10 hours or on high for 4-5 hours or until vegetables are tender.
3. Stir in the bell pepper. Cover the pot once again and cook on high for 20 minutes or until the bell pepper is soft. In a zip-top plastic bag, mix the cornmeal and chili powder. Add the halibut pieces and toss gently until the pieces are evenly coated.
4. In a medium sauté pan, heat the remaining 2 tablespoons olive oil over medium-high heat until hot but not smoking. Add halibut pieces, in batches if necessary, and sauté, turning once, until the fish pieces are nicely browned.
5. Discard any excess cornmeal mixture. Put the stew into serving bowls and top with browned halibut nuggets. Top with a dollop of sour cream, add a lime wedge, and serve.

Nutrition:
Calories: 430 Sodium: 506mg Carbs: 33.9g Fat: 11.1g Fiber: 5.5g Sugars: 7.3g Cholesterol: 46mg Protein: 35.0g

872. Salmon with Lemon and Green Olive Sauce

Preparation time: 15 minutes | Cooking time: 6 hours - Servings: 6

Extra virgin olive oil for coating slow cooker	1 large lemon, thinly sliced and seeds removed
2 medium shallots, thinly sliced	1/2 cup water
1 1/2 pounds thick salmon fillet, cut into 6 pieces	2 Tablespoons extra virgin olive oil
Kosher salt and freshly ground black pepper	**Sauce:**
2 tablespoons extra virgin olive oil	1 tablespoon freshly squeezed lemon juice
1/2 teaspoon lemon zest	1/2 teaspoon dried oregano
kosher salt and freshly ground black pepper	1/2 cup pitted green olives, chopped
1 tablespoon fresh flat-leaf parsley, chopped	1 tablespoon capers, rinsed

1. Grease your slow cooker with extra virgin olive oil. Drop half of the shallots into the bottom of the slow cooker. Add half the lemon slices and water.
2. Massage the salmon with olive oil and sprinkle with salt and pepper, to taste. Place salmon skin-side down in the slow cooker. Top with remaining lemon slices and shallot.
3. Cover and cook on low for 60-75 minutes, or until the salmon is opaque and cooked through. While salmon is cooking, make the sauce:
4. Mix the olive oil, lemon juice, zest, oregano, salt, and pepper to taste in a small bowl. Stir in olives, parsley, and capers. Transfer salmon to individual plates, remove the skin and drizzle with sauce.
5. It's also excellently served at room temperature on a bed of baby greens accompanied by a loaf of crusty bread.

Nutrition:
Calories: 318 Cholesterol: 71mg Sodium: 113mg Fat: 23.4g Carbs: 0.8g Protein: 25.2g

873. Salmon with Dill and Shallots

Preparation time: 15 minutes | Cooking time: 6 hours - Servings: 6

4 large shallots, thinly sliced	1/4 cup dry white wine
1 cup of water	1 1/2 lbs. boneless salmon fillet
1 Tablespoon extra-virgin olive oil	Kosher salt
ground black pepper	2 Tablespoons freshly squeezed lemon juice
3 or 4 sprigs fresh dill, chopped or 1/2 tsp. dried dill weed	1 lemon, sliced and seeds removed

1. Rinse salmon on both sides and pat dry with paper towels. With skin side down, cut into 6 even portions. Sprinkle shallots in the bottom of the slow cooker. Pour wine and water over. Mix oil and dill and spoon over the top of salmon.
2. Rub oil in to make sure salmon is evenly coated with oil. Place salmon pieces in the slow cooker, skin side down. Put the lemon juice and season with salt and pepper.
3. Top with lemon slices and cover, and cook on low for 90 minutes. Gently remove salmon from slow cooker with a slotted spatula. Remove skin. Serve warm with thyme roasted sweet potatoes and a green salad.

Nutrition:
Calories: 341 Cholesterol: 95mg Sodium: 95mg Fat: 21.0 Carbs: 0.4g Protein: 33.5g

874. Calamari Stuffed with Sausage and Raisins

Preparation time: 15 minutes | Cooking time: 2 hours - Servings: 6

1 1/2 pounds large squid (about 10 to 12)	3 tablespoons olive oil, divided
1/4-pound bulk sweet Italian sausage	2 shallots, minced
2 garlic cloves, minced	1/2 cup cooked white rice
2 tablespoons finely chopped raisins	Salt
ground black pepper	1 cup Herbed Tomato Sauce or purchased marinara sauce
1/3 cup dry white wine	Toothpicks

1. Rinse squid inside and out, and clean if necessary. Chop the tentacles very finely, and set aside. Warm a 1 tablespoon oil in a medium skillet over medium-high heat.
2. Crumble sausage into the skillet, and cook, breaking up lumps with a fork, for 2 minutes. Put the shallots and garlic, and cook within 3 minutes, or until shallots begin to soften.
3. Put the batter into a mixing bowl, add rice, raisins, and squid tentacles, put salt and pepper and stir well. Stuff a portion of stuffing into each squid, and close each tightly with toothpicks. Warm-up the rest of the oil in the skillet over medium-high heat.
4. Add squid, and brown on both sides, turning them gently with tongs. Transfer squid to the slow cooker, and add tomato sauce and wine.
5. Cook on high within 1 hour, then reduce the heat to low, and cook for 1 to 1 1/2 hours or until the squid are tender when pierced with the tip of a parking knife. Remove squid from the slow cooker with a slotted spoon, and discard toothpicks. Season sauce to taste with salt and pepper, and serve hot.

Nutrition:
Calories: 223 Carbs: 11g Fat: 11g Protein: 19g

875. Calamari with Garbanzo Beans and Greens

Preparation time: 15 minutes | Cooking: 1 hour & 30 minutes - Servings: 6

1 large bunch of Swiss chard	1 1/2 pounds cleaned squid
1/4 cup olive oil	1 medium onion, diced
2 garlic cloves, minced	1 carrot, chopped
1 (14.5-ounce) can diced tomatoes, undrained	1/2 cup Seafood Stock or purchased stock

¹/2 cup dry white wine
1 tbsp. chopped oregano
1 can garbanzo beans, drained
ground black pepper to taste

2 tablespoons chopped fresh parsley
¹/2-1 tsp crushed red pepper flake
Salt

1. Boil a pot of salted water, and have a bowl of ice water handy. Discard tough stems from Swiss chard, and cut leaves into 1-inch slices. Boil Swiss chard for 2 minutes, then drain and plunge into ice water to stop the cooking action. Drain again, and transfer Swiss chard to the slow cooker.
2. Rinse squid inside and out, and clean if necessary. Cut bodies into rings ³/4-inch wide, and leave tentacles whole. Set aside. Warm-up oil in a medium skillet over medium-high heat. Add onion, garlic, carrot, and cook, frequently stirring, for 5 minutes, or until onions soften.
3. Add tomatoes, stock, wine, parsley, oregano, and red pepper flakes to the skillet, and bring to a boil over high heat. Pour mixture into the slow cooker. Add squid to the slow cooker, and stir well. Cook on low for 2 to 4 hours, or on high for 1 to 2 hours, or until squid is tender. If cooking on low, raise the heat to high.
4. Put the garbanzo beans, and cook within 15 minutes, or until heated through. Sea- son to taste with salt and pepper, and serve hot.

Nutrition:
Calories: 216 Carbs: 34g Fat: 4g Protein: 0g

876.   Tomato-Braised Tuna

Preparation time: 15 minutes | Cooking: 1 hour & 30 minutes - Servings: 4

1 (1¹/2 to 2 pound) tuna fillet in one thick slice
¹/2 small red onion, chopped
1¹/2 cups Herbed Tomato Sauce or purchased marinara sauce
3 tablespoons capers, drained and rinsed
1 bay leaf
ground black pepper

¹/4 cup olive oil, divided

3 garlic cloves, minced
¹/2 cup dry white wine

2 tablespoons chopped fresh parsley

Salt

1. Soak tuna in cold salted water for 10 minutes. Pat dry with paper towels. 2. Heat 2 tablespoons oil in a large skillet over medium-high heat. Put the onion plus garlic, and cook, frequently stirring, for 3 minutes.
2. Scrape mixture into the slow cooker. Add tomato sauce, wine, capers, parsley, and bay leaf to the slow cooker, and stir well. Cook on high for 1 hour.
3. Warm-up the rest of the oil in the skillet over medium-high heat. Add tuna and brown well on both sides. Add tuna to the slow cooker, and cook on high for an additional 1 to 1¹/2 hours or until tuna is cooked but still rare in the center. Remove the bay leaf, season to taste with salt and pepper, and serve hot.

Nutrition:
Calories: 101 Carbs: 3g Fat: 1g Protein: 19g

877.   Fish with Tomatoes and Fennel

Preparation time: 15 minutes | Cooking time: 3 hours - Servings: 6

2 medium fennel bulbs
1 large onion, thinly sliced
1 (28-ounce) can diced tomatoes, drained
1 tablespoon grated orange zest

1 tablespoon fennel seeds, crushed

Salt

¹/4 cup olive oil
2 garlic cloves, minced
¹/2 cup dry white wine

¹/2 cup freshly squeezed orange juice
2 pounds thick firm-fleshed white fish fillets, cut into serving-sized pieces
ground black pepper

1. Discard stalks from fennel, and save for another use. Rinse fennel, cut in half lengthwise, and discard core and the top layer of flesh. Slice fennel thinly and set aside.
2. Warm-up oil in a large skillet on medium-high heat. Put the onion and garlic, and cook, for 3 minutes, or until onion is translucent. Add fennel and cook for an additional 2 minutes. Scrape mixture into the slow cooker.

3. Add tomatoes, wine, orange zest, orange juice, and fennel seeds to the slow cooker, and stir well. Cook on low 5 to 7 hours or on high for 2¹/2 to 3 hours, or until fennel is crisp-tender.
4. If cooking on low, raise the heat to high. Massage the fish with salt plus pepper, and place it on top of vegetables. Cook within 30 to 45 minutes. Put salt and pepper, and serve hot.

Nutrition:
Calories: 317 Carbs: 0g Fat: 8g Protein: 40g

878.   Monkfish with Cabbage, Pancetta, and Rosemary

Preparation time: 15 minutes | Cooking time: 2 hours - Servings: 6

¹/2 small (1¹/2-pound) head Savoy or green cabbage
2 pounds monkfish fillets, trimmed and cut into serving pieces
1 cup Seafood Stock or purchased stock
1 tablespoon chopped fresh parsley
Salt
2 tablespoons unsalted butter

¹/4-pound pancetta, diced

2 garlic cloves, minced

2 tbsp. chopped fresh rosemary

2 teaspoons grated lemon zest
ground black pepper to taste

1. Rinse and core cabbage. Cut into wedges and then shred the cabbage. Boil a large pot of salted water. Add cabbage and boil for 4 minutes. Drain the cabbage and place it in the slow cooker.
2. Cook pancetta in a heavy skillet over medium heat for 5 to 7 minutes, or until crisp. Remove pancetta, and place it in the slow cooker. Raise the heat to high, and sear monkfish in the fat on all sides, turning the pieces gently with tongs, until browned. Refrigerate monkfish.
3. Add garlic, stock, rosemary, parsley, and lemon zest to the slow cooker, and stir well. Cook on low within 3 to 4 hours or on high for 1¹/2 to 2 hours, or until cabbage is almost tender.
4. If cooking on low, raise the heat to high. Season monkfish with salt and pepper, and place it on top of vegetables. Cook monkfish for 30 to 45 minutes, or until it is cooked through.
5. Remove monkfish from the slow cooker, and keep it warm. Add butter to cabbage, and stir to melt butter. Season to taste with salt and pepper. To serve, mound equal size portions of cabbage on each plate. Slice monkfish into medallions, and arrange on top of the cabbage.

Nutrition:
Calories: 84 Carbs: 2g Fat: 2g Protein: 14g

879.   Poached Fish with Vegetables and Herbs

Preparation time: 15 minutes Cooking time: 2 hours - Servings: 6

1-pound thick firm-fleshed white fish fillets, cut into serving pieces
Salt
1 large sweet onion, thinly sliced
¹/2 small fennel bulb, trimmed, cored, and thinly sliced
1 (14.5-ounce) can diced tomatoes, undrained
¹/2 cup chopped fresh parsley, divided
2 teaspoons grated lemon zest
¹/2-pound large shrimp, peeled and deveined

¹/4 cup olive oil, divided

ground black pepper
2 celery ribs, sliced
2 cups Seafood Stock or purchased stock
¹/2 cup dry white wine

2 tbsp. chopped fresh oregano

1 bay leaf
1 dozen littleneck clams, well-scrubbed

1. Drizzle the fish with two tablespoons of olive oil, then put salt and pepper. Refrigerate, tightly covered with plastic wrap. Warm-up oil in a large skillet over medium-high heat. Add onion, celery, and fennel, and cook, frequently stirring, for 3 minutes, or until onion is translucent. Scrape mixture into the slow cooker.
2. Add stock, tomatoes, wine, 3 tablespoons parsley, oregano, lemon zest, and bay leaf to the slow cooker, and stir well. Cook on low within 4 to 5 hours or on high for 2 to 2¹/2 hours, until vegetables are crisp-tender.
3. If cooking on low, raise the heat to high. Add fish, shrimp, and clams, and cook for 45 minutes to 1 hour. Remove the bay leaf, and put salt plus pepper. Serve hot, sprinkling each serving with remaining parsley.

Nutrition:: Calories: 223 Carbs: 2g Fat: 5g Protein: 37g

POULTRY

880. Poached Chicken Breasts

Preparation time: 15 minutes Cooking time: 8 hours Servings: 6

1 leek, sliced	1 shallot, diced
2 cloves garlic, minced	1 large carrot, peeled and diced
1 stalk celery, diced	11/2 pounds boneless, skinless chicken breasts
1/4 cup dry white wine	1 cup Roasted Chicken Broth
1/4 cup olive oil	

1. Grease a 4- to 5-quart slow cooker using a nonstick olive oil cooking spray. Place all of the fixings in the cooker. Cover and cook on low within 7–8 hours. Serve each breast with some of the cooking liquid and a drizzle of olive oil.

Nutrition:
Calories: 252 Fat: 13g Protein: 25g Sodium: 322mg Fiber: 1g Carbohydrates: 7g Sugar: 2g

881. Rosemary Chicken with Potatoes

Preparation time: 15 minutes Cooking: 4 hours & 10 minutes Servings: 6

1 tablespoon olive oil	2 pounds boneless, skinless chicken thighs
1/2 teaspoon kosher salt	1/2 teaspoon freshly ground black pepper
6 small red potatoes, halved	1 leek (white and pale green parts only), sliced into 1" pieces
6 sprigs rosemary, divided	1 garlic clove, minced
1/2 cup Roasted Chicken Broth	1/4 cup capers

1. Warm-up the olive oil in a large skillet over medium heat until hot but not smoking. Put the chicken and massage with salt and pepper. Cook within 5 minutes on one side and flip. Cook for an additional 5 minutes.
2. Place the potatoes and leek into a 4- to 5-quart slow cooker. Top with 5 sprigs of rosemary and garlic. Place chicken thighs on the rosemary. Pour broth over chicken and potatoes. Cover and cook on high within 3–4 hours. Put capers before serving, and garnish with remaining rosemary.

Nutrition:
Calories: 336 Fat: 9g Protein: 33g Sodium: 595mg Fiber: 3g Carbohydrates: 30g Sugar: 2g

882. Sage Ricotta Chicken Breasts

Preparation: 15 minutes Cooking time: 8 hours & 6 minutes Servings: 4

- 6 fresh sage leaves, chopped
- 1/2 cup part-skim ricotta cheese
- 4 (4-ounce) boneless, skinless chicken breasts
- 1/2 teaspoon kosher salt
- 1/2 teaspoon freshly ground black pepper
- 1 tablespoon olive oil
- 1/2 cup white wine
- 3/4 cup chicken broth
- 1/4 cup niçoise olives, pitted and chopped

1. Combine sage and ricotta in a small bowl. Gently slice a slit into a chicken breast to form a pocket. Stuff 2 tablespoons of filling into the chicken. Tie with kitchen twine and trim ends. Repeat with the rest of the chicken and cheese.

2. Flavor the chicken breasts with salt plus pepper. Heat olive oil in a large skillet until it's hot but not smoking. Place chicken in the skillet and sear on one side, about 3 minutes. Flip and brown on the second side, about 3 minutes.
3. Gently place chicken in a 4- to 5-quart slow cooker. Pour wine and chicken broth into the slow cooker. Cook on low for 6–8 hours. Cut twine from chicken breasts and sprinkle with olives.

Nutrition:
Calories: 168 Fat: 7g Protein: 19g Sodium: 489mg Fiber: 0g Carbohydrates: 3g Sugar: 0g

883. Sweet and Tangy Duck

Preparation: 15 minutes Cooking time: 4 hours & 4 minutes Servings: 6

1 (3-pound) duckling, skin removed	1 tablespoon olive oil
1/2 teaspoon kosher salt	1/2 teaspoon freshly ground black pepper
1/2 teaspoon red pepper flakes	2 cloves garlic, minced
1 medium apple, cut into 1" pieces	1 medium pear, peeled, slice into 1" pieces
1 tablespoon lemon juice	1 large red onion, peeled and chopped
1 large carrot, peeled and chopped	1 stalk celery, chopped
1/2 cup dry red wine	1/4 cup honey
1/4 cup cider vinegar	1 cup Roasted Chicken Broth

1. Remove any extraneous fat from the duck. Cut into serving-size portions. Warm-up the olive oil in a large skillet or Dutch oven until hot but not smoking. Add the duck and season with salt, pepper, and red pepper flakes.
2. Cook for 3 minutes on one side. Add garlic to the pan, flip the duck, and cook for 1 minute. While the duck is browning, place apple and pear pieces in a bowl of cold water with lemon juice.
3. Put the onion, carrot, and celery in the bottom of a 4- to 5-quart slow cooker. Drain the apple and pear, and top vegetables with the duck and apple and pear mixture.
4. In a small bowl, whisk the wine, honey, vinegar, and broth. Pour over the duck. Cover and cook on high within 3–4 hours.

Nutrition:
Calories: 422 Fat: 12g Protein: 46 Sodium: 516mg Fiber: 2g Carbohydrates: 26g Sugar: 19g

884. Classic Chicken Parmesan

Preparation: 15 minutes Cooking time: 4 hours & 13 minutes Servings: 4

1 large egg	1/2 cup bread crumbs
1/2 teaspoon dried basil	1/2 teaspoon dried oregano
6 (4-ounce) boneless, skinless chicken breast halves	1 tablespoon olive oil
13/4 cups Tomato Sauce	1/2 cup shredded mozzarella cheese
2 tablespoons grated Parmesan cheese	1/4 cup chopped fresh parsley

1. Mix the egg until foamy in a shallow dish. Mix the bread crumbs, basil, and oregano in another shallow dish. Soak the chicken in the egg, then into the bread crumb mixture to coat.
2. Warm-up olive oil in a large skillet until hot but not smoking. Put the chicken and brown within 3 minutes. Flip, and cook again within 3 minutes.
3. Put the chicken in a 4- to 5-quart slow cooker. Cover with tomato sauce. Cook on high for 3–4 hours. Sprinkle with cheeses, turn heat to low, and cook for 10 minutes. Remove from slow cooker and garnish with parsley.

Nutrition:
Calories: 278 Fat: 11g Protein: 32g Sodium: 732mg Fiber: 1.5g Carbohydrates: 11g Sugar: 4g

885. Lemony Roast Chicken

Preparation time: 15 minutes Cooking time: 7 hours Servings: 6

1 (31/2- to 4-pound) frying chicken	1 teaspoon kosher salt
1 teaspoon freshly ground black pepper	1 clove garlic, crushed
3 tablespoons olive oil	2 lemons, quartered
1/2 cup Roasted Chicken Broth	

1. Massage the chicken with salt, pepper, plus garlic. Brush with olive oil. Put the lemon quarters in the slow cooker. Top with the chicken. Pour the broth over the chicken. Cover and cook on high within 1 hour. Adjust the heat to low and cook for 5–6 hours.

Nutrition:
Calories: 608 Fat: 20g Protein: 96g Sodium: 825mg Fiber: 1g Carbohydrates: 3g Sugar: 0.5g

886. Cornish Game Hens

Preparation time: 15 minutes Cooking: 5 hours & 10 minutes Servings: 2

2 (11/2-pound) game hens	1 teaspoon kosher salt, divided
1 teaspoon freshly ground black pepper, divided	2 scallions, finely diced
2 fresh mint leaves, chopped	1/4 cup coarse cornmeal
2 tablespoons olive oil, divided	1/2 cup White Wine Vegetable Stock

1. Wash the hens inside and out. Pat dry. Season the inside of each with half of the salt and pepper. Combine scallions, mint, and cornmeal in a small bowl. Place 2 tablespoons of the cornmeal mixture in the cavity of each hen. Pull loose skin over the cavity and secure with kitchen string.
2. Warm-up 1 tablespoon of olive oil in a large skillet over medium heat until hot but not smoking. Massage the hens with the rest of the salt and pepper. Place hens in the pan and cook for 5 minutes. Flip and brown for 5 minutes more.
3. Grease inside of a 4-5-quart slow cooker with 2 teaspoons olive oil. Use the rest of the olive oil to brush on the hens. Place hens in the slow cooker and pour in the stock. Cover and cook on high within 4–5 hours. The stuffing temperature should read 165 F with an instant-read thermometer.

Nutrition:
Calories: 991 Fat: 34g Protein: 145g Sodium: 1,837mg Fiber: 1g Carbohydrates: 16g Sugar: 1g

887. Mediterranean Chicken Casserole

Preparation time: 15 minutes Cooking time: 6 hours Servings: 4

1 medium butternut squash, 2" cubes	1 medium bell pepper, seeded and diced
1 (141/2-ounce) can diced tomatoes, undrained	4 boneless, skinless chicken breast halves, bite-sized pieces
1/2 cup mild salsa	1/4 cup raisins
1/4 teaspoon ground cinnamon	1/4 teaspoon ground cumin
2 cups cooked white rice	1/4 cup chopped fresh parsley

1. Add squash and bell pepper to the bottom of a greased 4- to 5-quart slow cooker. Mix tomatoes, chicken, salsa, raisins, cinnamon, and cumin and pour on top of squash and peppers.
2. Cover and cook on low within 6 hours or on high for 3 hours. Remove chicken and vegetables, then serve over cooked rice. Spoon remaining sauce from slow cooker over the vegetables. Garnish with parsley.

Nutrition:
Calories: 317 Fat: 3g Protein: 28.5g Sodium: 474mg Fiber: 3g Carbohydrates: 43g Sugar: 10g

888. Chicken Pesto Polenta

Preparation: 15 minutes Cooking time: 6 hours & 45 minutes Servings: 6

4 boneless, skinless chicken breasts, bite-sized pieces	1 cup prepared pesto, divided
1 medium onion, peeled and finely diced	4 cloves garlic, minced
11/2 teaspoons dried Italian seasoning	1 (16-ounce) tube prepared polenta, cut into 1/2" slices
2 cups chopped fresh spinach	1 (141/2-ounce) can diced tomatoes
1 (8-ounce) bag shredded low-fat Italian cheese blend	

1. Mix the chicken pieces with pesto, onion, garlic, and Italian seasoning in a large bowl. Layer half of the chicken mixture, half the polenta, half the spinach, and half the tomatoes in a greased 4- to 5-quart slow cooker.
2. Continue to layer, ending with tomatoes. Cover and cook on low within 4–6 hours or on high for 2–3 hours. Top with cheese. Cover and continue to cook for 45 minutes to an hour until cheese has melted.

Nutrition:
Calories: 535 Fat: 16g Protein: 32g Sodium: 429mg Fiber: 4g Carbohydrates: 65g Sugar: 4g

889. Rotisserie-Style Chicken

Preparation: 15 minutes Cooking time: 5 hours & 15 minutes Servings: 6

1 (4-pound) whole chicken	11/2 teaspoons kosher salt
2 teaspoons paprika	1/2 teaspoon onion powder
1/2 teaspoon dried thyme	1/2 teaspoon dried basil
1/2 teaspoon ground white pepper	1/2 teaspoon ground cayenne pepper
1/2 teaspoon ground black pepper	1/2 teaspoon garlic powder
2 tablespoons olive oil	

1. In a small bowl, mix salt, paprika, onion powder, thyme, basil, white pepper, cayenne pepper, black pepper, plus garlic powder. Massage with the spice mixture the entire chicken.
2. Place the spice-rubbed chicken in a greased 6-quart slow cooker. Drizzle olive oil evenly over the chicken. Cook on high for 3–31/2 hours or on low for 4–5 hours. Remove chicken carefully from the slow cooker and place on a large plate or serving platter.

Nutrition:
Calories: 400 Fat: 14g Protein: 64g Sodium: 820mg Fiber: 0.5g Carbohydrates: 1g Sugar: 0g

890. Spicy Olive Chicken

Preparation time: 15 minutes Cooking time: 6 hours Servings: 4

1 whole chicken, slice into 8 pieces	1 teaspoon kosher salt
1/2 cup ground black pepper	4 tablespoons unsalted butter
2/3 cup chopped sweet onion	2 tablespoons capers, drained and rinsed
24 green olives, pitted	1/2 cup chicken broth
1/2 cup dry white wine	1 teaspoon prepared Dijon mustard
1/2 cup hot sauce	2 cups cooked white rice
1/4 cup fresh chopped parsley	

1. Massage the chicken pieces with salt plus pepper and then brown them in the butter in a large skillet over medium-high heat within 3 minutes on each side. Remove chicken from skillet and place in a greased 4- to 5-quart slow cooker.
2. Sauté the onion in the same skillet for an additional 3–5 minutes. Add onion to slow cooker, along with capers and olives.
3. In a small bowl, whisk the broth, wine, and mustard. Pour over chicken in the slow cooker. Add hot sauce. Cover and cook on high within 3–31/2 hours or low for 51/2–6 hours. When ready to serve,

place the chicken over rice. Spoon sauce and olives over each serving. Garnish with parsley.

Nutrition:
Calories: 703 Fat: 25g Protein: 75g Sodium: 1,373mg Fiber: 2g
Carbohydrates: 34g Sugar: 1.5g

891. Sun-Dried Tomato and Feta Stuffed Chicken

Preparation time: 15 minutes Cooking time: 6 hours Servings: 4

4 (4-ounce) boneless, skinless chicken breasts	1/2 cup chopped oil-packed sun-dried tomatoes
1/3 cup crumbled feta cheese	1/4 cup chopped pitted Kalamata olives
11/2 cups fresh baby spinach leaves	2 tablespoons olive oil
1/2 teaspoon kosher salt	1/2 teaspoon freshly ground black pepper

1. Flatten chicken breasts on a wooden cutting board with a meat mallet's flat side, to 1/2-inch thick. Set chicken breasts aside.
2. In a small bowl, mix the tomatoes, cheese, and olives. Place 3–4 spinach leaves in the middle of each flattened chicken breast. Place 2–3 tablespoons of the tomato filling on top of the spinach leaves.
3. Fold one side of the flattened chicken breast over the filling and continue to roll into a cylinder; secure with 2–3 toothpicks per chicken breast. Place the chicken rolls seam-side down in a greased 4- to 5-quart slow cooker.
4. Drizzle olive oil evenly over the top of the chicken rolls and sprinkle the chicken with salt and pepper. Cook on high within 3 hours or on low for 6 hours.

Nutrition:
Calories: 248 Fat: 12.5g Protein: 27g Sodium: 715mg Fiber: 1g
Carbohydrates: 7g Sugar: 3g

892. Chicken Piccata

Preparation time: 15 minutes Cooking time: 6 hours Servings: 4

2 large (6-ounce) boneless, skinless chicken breasts, cut horizontally into skinny slices	1 cup all-purpose flour
1 tablespoon olive oil	1/4 cup lemon juice
3 tablespoons nonpareil capers	3/4 cup chicken stock
1/4 teaspoon freshly ground black pepper	

1. Dredge both sides of the chicken breast slices in the flour. Discard leftover flour. Heat olive oil in a nonstick pan over medium-high heat. Quickly sear the chicken on both sides to brown, approximately 1 minute per side.
2. Place the chicken, lemon juice, capers, stock, and pepper into a greased 4- to 5-quart slow cooker. Cook on high within 2–3 hours or low for 4–6 hours until the chicken is cooked through and the sauce has thickened.

Nutrition:
Calories: 260 Fat: 6.5g Protein: 22g Sodium: 356mg Fiber: 1g
Carbohydrates: 27g Sugar: 1g

893. Pesto Chicken

Preparation time: 15 minutes Cooking time: 8 hours Servings: 4

2 pounds boneless, skinless chicken thighs	4 medium red potatoes, peeled and diced
1-pint cherry tomatoes	1/2 cup prepared pesto
1/2 teaspoon ground black pepper	1/2 teaspoon kosher salt

1. Place all ingredients in a greased 4- to 5-quart slow cooker. Cook on high for 3–4 hours or on low for 6–8 hours until chicken is tender. Serve.

Nutrition:

Calories: 296 Fat: 5g Protein: 26g Sodium: 407mg Fiber: 4.5g
Carbohydrates: 34g Sugar: 4g

894. Chicken Ragu

Preparation time: 15 minutes Cooking time: 6 hours Servings: 6

1-pound boneless skinless chicken breasts, finely chopped	3 shallots, finely minced
4 cups marinara sauce	2 teaspoons crushed rosemary
2 cloves garlic, minced	1/2 teaspoon freshly ground pepper
1/2 teaspoon oregano	

1. Place all the fixing into a 4- to 5-quart slow cooker. Stir. Cook on low for 4–6 hours. Stir before serving.

Nutrition:
Calories: 247 Fat: 6.5g Protein: 19g Sodium: 771mg Fiber: 5g
Carbohydrates: 27g Sugar: 16g

895. Spiced Chicken with Pancetta

Preparation time: 15 minutes Cooking time: 6 hours Servings: 6

2 ounces pancetta or prosciutto, chopped	6 whole cloves
4 garlic cloves, chopped	3 fresh sage leaves, chopped
1 teaspoon chopped fresh rosemary	4 pounds bone-in chicken breasts, legs, or thighs
salt	1 teaspoon coarsely ground pepper
1/4 cup chicken broth	

1. Spray the insert of a slow cooker using a nonstick cooking spray. Scatter half of the pancetta, 3 of the cloves, and half the garlic, sage, and rosemary in the cooker.
2. Sprinkle the chicken with salt plus pepper to taste. Place it in the slow cooker. Scatter the remaining pancetta, cloves, garlic, sage, and rosemary over the chicken and add the pepper. Pour in the broth. Cover and cook on low within 4 to 6 hours, then serve.

Nutrition:
Calories: 369 Carbs: 4g Fat: 19g Protein: 44g

896. Crunchy Mustard Chicken Diable

Preparation time: 15 minutes Servings: 6

1/4 cup Dijon mustard	2 tablespoons chopped shallots or scallions
1/2 teaspoon dried thyme	1/8 teaspoon cayenne pepper
salt	4 pounds bone-in chicken thighs, skinned
2 tablespoons unsalted butter	3/4 cup fresh bread crumbs, made from French bread, or panko

1. Spray the insert of a slow cooker with nonstick cooking spray. In a small bowl, stir the mustard, shallots, thyme, cayenne, and 1/2 teaspoon salt. Brush the chicken pieces with the mixture, turning to coat all sides. Place the chicken in the cooker. Cover and cook on low within 4 to 6 hours.
2. Meanwhile, melt the butter in a large skillet. Put the bread crumbs and a bit of salt. Cook over medium heat, occasionally stirring, for 5 minutes, or until the crumbs are lightly toasted. Place the chicken pieces on a platter. Sprinkle with the crumb mixture, patting it on so that it adheres. Serve hot or cold.

Nutrition:
Calories: 320 Carbs: 23g Fat: 18g Protein: 15g

897. Spicy Chicken with Green Olives

Preparation: 15 minutes Cooking time: 6 hours & 30 minutes Servings: 6

4 pounds bone-in chicken breasts, legs, or thighs
2 tablespoons olive oil
2 garlic cloves, minced
1 teaspoon ground cumin
¼ teaspoon ground cinnamon
¼ cup chicken broth or vegetable broth
½ cup chopped fresh cilantro or mint

salt and freshly ground pepper

1 medium onion, chopped
2 teaspoons freshly grated ginger
1 teaspoon Spanish smoked paprika
¼ teaspoon ground turmeric
1 cup small pitted green olives, drained

1. Oiled the bottom of a slow cooker with nonstick cooking spray. Flavor the chicken with salt and pepper to taste, then put the pieces in the slow cooker.
2. Warm-up the oil over medium heat in a medium skillet, add the onion and cook within 5 minutes until slightly softened. Add the garlic, ginger, cumin, paprika, cinnamon, turmeric, and broth and bring to a simmer. Cook for 5 minutes more. Pour the mixture over the chicken.
3. Cover and cook on low within 4 to 6 hours. Rinse the olives and drain well. Add the olives to the cooker and cook for 30 minutes more. With a slotted spoon, transfer the chicken and olives to a serving platter. Cover and keep warm.
4. Pour the liquid into a small saucepan. Simmer until slightly reduced. Taste for seasonings. Spoon the sauce over the chicken. Sprinkle with the herbs and serve hot.

Nutrition:
Calories: 239 Carbs: 10g Fat: 10g Protein: 27g

898. Jugged-Chicken

Preparation time: 15 minutes Cooking time: hours Servings: 6

4 pounds bone-in chicken breasts, legs, or thighs
1 cup frozen pearl onions, thawed
4 garlic cloves, chopped
2 cups canned crushed tomatoes
1 tablespoon Dijon mustard

salt and freshly ground pepper

4 ounces prosciutto or pancetta, finely chopped
2 bay leaves
½ cup port wine (tawny or ruby)
chopped fresh flat-leaf parsley

1. Sprinkle the chicken with salt plus pepper to taste. Place the pieces in a large slow cooker. Scatter the onions, prosciutto, garlic, and bay leaves on top. Stir the tomatoes, port, Dijon, ½ teaspoon salt, and pepper to taste. Pour the sauce over the chicken. Cover and cook on low within n 4 to 6 hours. Sprinkle with the parsley. Serve hot with rice.

Nutrition:
Calories: 240 Carbs: 0g Fat: 20g Protein: 15g

899. Balsamic Chicken with Capers

Preparation time: 15 minutes Cooking time: 6 hours Servings: 6

½ cup balsamic vinegar
2 large garlic cloves, finely chopped
2 tablespoons drained capers, chopped
4 pounds bone-in chicken breasts, legs, or thighs

2 tablespoons Dijon mustard
1 tablespoon chopped fresh rosemary
salt and freshly ground pepper

1. Spray the insert of a large slow cooker with nonstick cooking spray. Mix the vinegar, mustard, garlic, rosemary, capers, ½ teaspoon salt, plus pepper to taste in a medium bowl.
2. Soak the chicken pieces into the batter, turning to coat on all sides. Place the chicken in the cooker and pour it on any remaining coating. Cover and cook on low within 4 to 6 hours. Serve hot.

Nutrition:
Calories: 181 Carbs: 13g Fat: 3g Protein: 25g

900. Chicken Tagine

Preparation: 15 minutes Cooking time: 6 hours Servings: 8

3 preserved lemon halves
2 garlic cloves, finely chopped

½ cup chopped fresh cilantro
½ teaspoon ground cumin
2 tablespoons olive oil

4 pounds bone-in chicken breasts, legs, or thighs (legs and thighs skinned if you like)

1 medium onion, finely chopped
1 cup chopped fresh tomatoes or canned tomatoes
1 teaspoon Spanish smoked paprika
½ cup of chicken broth or water
2 pounds Yukon gold potatoes, cut into ¼-inch-thick slices
salt and freshly ground pepper

1. Grease the inside of your slow cooker using a nonstick cooking spray. Rinse the preserved lemon halves and pat dry. Scoop the pulp out of the lemons and chop it finely. Reserve the lemon peel.
2. Place the lemon pulp in a medium bowl with the onion, garlic, tomatoes, ¼ cup of the cilantro, paprika, cumin, broth, and olive oil.
3. Put the potatoes, then add half of the lemon mixture. Toss well. Massage the chicken with salt and pepper to taste. Put the chicken over the potatoes and sprinkle with the remaining lemon mixture.
4. Cover and cook on low within 5 to 6 hours. Transfer the cooked chicken plus potatoes to a platter with a slotted spoon. Keep warm. If there is excess liquid in the cooker, pour it into a saucepan and simmer it until reduced.
5. Put the sauce on the chicken plus potatoes and sprinkle with the reserved lemon peel and the remaining ¼ cup cilantro. Serve hot.

Nutrition:
Calories: 286 Carbs: 19g Fat: 10g Protein: 30g

901. Chicken with Chorizo, Red Wine, and Roasted Peppers

Preparation time: 15 minutes Cooking time: 6 hours Servings: 6

4 pounds bone-in chicken thighs, skinned
8 ounces fully cooked chorizo sausage
2 tablespoons olive oil
1 garlic clove, minced
½ teaspoon chopped fresh thyme

2 tablespoons chopped fresh flat-leaf parsley

salt and freshly ground pepper

1 bay leaf

1 medium onion, chopped
½ cup dry red wine
1 roasted red pepper, thin strips (about 1 cup)

1. Grease the bottom of a slow cooker with nonstick cooking spray. Sprinkle the chicken with salt and pepper. Place the pieces in the cooker, along with the chorizo and bay leaf.
2. In a medium skillet, heat the oil over medium heat. Add the onion, then cook for 10 minutes, or until tender. Stir in the garlic and cook for 1 minute more. Put the red wine and simmer. Stir in the thyme.
3. Scrape the mixture over the chicken and chorizo. Cover and cook on low within 4 to 6 hours. Remove the chorizo and cut into thick slices. Return the chorizo to the slow cooker along with the roasted pepper. Cook on low for 30 minutes more. Discard the bay leaf. Sprinkle with the parsley and serve hot.

Nutrition:
Calories: 158 Carbs: 3g Fat: 14g Protein: 4g

902. Chicken with Feta and Tomatoes

Preparation: 15 minutes Cooking time: 6 hours & 30 minutes Servings: 6

4 pounds bone-in chicken breasts, legs, or thighs
2 garlic cloves, finely chopped
1-pint cherry or grape tomatoes halved
½ cup chopped pitted Kalamata olives

salt and freshly ground pepper
½ teaspoon dried oregano
½ cup chicken broth
½ cup crumbled feta cheese

1. Sprinkle the chicken with salt plus pepper. Place the pieces in the slow cooker, overlapping slightly. Scatter the garlic and oregano over the top. Add the tomatoes and broth.
2. Cover and cook on low within 4 to 6 hours. Add the olives and cheese. Cover and cook on low for 15 to 30 minutes more or until hot. Serve hot.

Nutrition:
Calories: 236 Carbs: 3g Fat: 7g Protein: 36g

903. Chicken Legs with Sausage, Tomatoes, and Black Olives

Preparation: 15 minutes Cooking time: 6 hours Servings: 6

2 tablespoons olive oil	6 sweet Italian sausages (about 1 pound)
1 medium onion, chopped	2 garlic cloves, finely chopped
Pinch of crushed red pepper	½ cup dry red wine
1 28-ounce can crush tomatoes	6 whole chicken legs
salt and freshly ground pepper	1 cup pitted black olives
3 tablespoons chopped fresh flat-leaf parsley	

1. Warm-up oil over medium heat in a large skillet, then put the sausages and brown it within 10 minutes. Transfer the sausages to a large slow cooker. Put the onion in the skillet, and cook, often stirring, until softened. Mix in the garlic plus crushed red pepper. Add the wine and simmer. Cook for 1 minute.
2. Pour the skillet contents into the slow cooker. Add the tomatoes and stir. Massage the chicken pieces with salt plus pepper to taste.
3. Place the chicken in the cooker, spooning the sauce over the top. Cover and cook on low within 4 to 6 hours. Stir in the olives. Taste for seasonings. Serve the chicken, sausages, and sauce hot, sprinkled with the parsley.

Nutrition:
Calories: 212 Carbs: 8g Fat: 10g Protein: 21g

904. Za'atar Roast Chicken and Vegetables

Preparation time: 15 minutes Cooking time: 6 hours Servings: 4

2 medium red onions, sliced	1-pound boiling potatoes, such as Yukon gold, thickly sliced
3 garlic cloves, finely chopped	2 tablespoons za'atar
salt and freshly ground pepper	½ cup chicken broth
1 4-pound chicken	1 cup cherry or grape tomatoes, halved

1. Grease the inside of a slow cooker using a nonstick cooking spray. Scatter the onions, potatoes, and a little of the garlic in the slow cooker. Sprinkle with a bit of the za'atar and salt and pepper to taste. Add the broth.
2. Remove the neck plus giblets from the chicken cavity and reserve them for another use. Trim away any excess fat. Massage and sprinkle the chicken inside and out with the remaining garlic, the remaining za'atar, and salt and pepper to taste.
3. Put the chicken over the vegetables in the cooker. Scatter the tomatoes around the chicken. Cover and cook on low within 5 to 6 hours. Slice the chicken and serve it hot, with the vegetables.

Nutrition:
Calories: 266 Carbs: 11g Fat: 23g Protein: 8g

905. Roast Chicken with Tapenade

Preparation time: 15 minutes Cooking time: 6 hours Servings: 4

2 teaspoons chopped fresh rosemary	3 large garlic cloves
¼ cup store-bought tapenade	2 pounds sliced boiling potatoes, such as Yukon gold
salt and freshly ground pepper	1 4-pound chicken

1. Grease the inside of a slow cooker using a nonstick cooking spray. Chop the rosemary and garlic. Stir half of the mixture into the tapenade. Put the potatoes in the slow cooker and sprinkle them with the remaining garlic and rosemary and salt and pepper to taste. Toss well.
2. Remove the neck plus giblets from the chicken cavity, then set aside for another use. Trim away any excess fat. Flavor the chicken inside and out with salt and pepper. Place about half of the tapenade mixture inside the chicken cavity.
3. Put the rest of the tapenade on the chicken. Place the chicken on the potatoes in the cooker. Cover and cook on low within 5 to 6 hours. Cut the chicken into pieces and serve hot, with the potatoes.

Nutrition:
Calories: 279 Carbs: 4g Fat: 9g Protein: 43g

906. Chicken with Middle Eastern Pesto

Preparation time: 15 minutes Cooking time: 6 hours Servings: 6

1 medium onion, chopped	1 medium zucchini, chopped
½ cup chicken broth	2 preserved lemons or 1 teaspoon grated lemon zest
2 garlic cloves	½ cup chopped fresh cilantro
1 teaspoon ground cumin	1 teaspoon Spanish smoked paprika
½ teaspoon freshly ground pepper	2 tablespoons olive oil
1 4-pound chicken	

1. Grease the large slow cooker with nonstick cooking spray. Scatter the onion and zucchini in the cooker. Add the chicken broth.
2. Rinse the lemons and cut them in half. Scoop out the pulp and discard it. Coarsely chop the lemon skins. Process using a food processor with the garlic, cilantro, cumin, paprika, pepper, and oil. Process until smooth.
3. Remove the neck and giblets, reserve them for another use. Trim away any excess fat. Slide your fingers between the skin and the flesh of the chicken to loosen it. Spread the pesto between the skin and the flesh.
4. Place a little of the pesto inside the chicken. Put the chicken in your slow cooker on top of the vegetables. Cover and cook on low within 4 to 6 hours. Serve hot.

Nutrition:
Calories: 254 Carbs: 12g Fat: 9g Protein: 29g

907. Turkey Breast with Lemon, Capers, and Sage

Preparation time: 15 minutes Cooking time: 3 hours Servings: 6

2 large carrots, peeled and sliced	1 large onion, sliced
1 celery rib, sliced	3 tablespoons unsalted butter, softened
6 sage leaves, chopped	1 teaspoon grated lemon zest
salt and freshly ground pepper	1 boneless turkey breast half
½ cup dry white wine or chicken broth	1 tablespoon cornstarch, blended with 3 tablespoons water
2 tablespoons capers, rinsed, drained, and chopped	1 tablespoon chopped fresh flat-leaf parsley
1–2 tablespoons fresh lemon juice	

1. Grease the inside of a slow cooker using a nonstick cooking spray. Scatter the carrots, onion, and celery in the slow cooker. Blend 2 tablespoons of the butter and the sage, lemon zest, salt, and pepper to taste. Loosen the turkey breast skin, then gently spread the butter mixture inside the skin and meat.
2. Put the turkey breast in your slow cooker. Pour the wine around the turkey. Cover and cook on high within 2 to 3 hours. Remove the turkey from the pot. Cover and keep warm, then drain the cooking liquid into a saucepan. Bring the juices to a boil.
3. Add the cornstarch mixture to the turkey juices and stir well. Cook within 1 minute. Turn off the heat, mix in the remaining 1 tablespoon butter, the capers, parsley, and lemon juice to taste. Carve the turkey and serve it hot, with the sauce.

Nutrition:

Calories: 181 Carbs: 13g Fat: 3g Protein: 25g

908. Turkey Meatloaf with Sun-Dried Tomatoes and Mozzarella

Preparation time: 15 minutes Cooking time: 4 hours Servings: 8

1 cup drained sun-dried tomatoes in oil	2 pounds ground turkey
3 large eggs, beaten	½ cup plain dry bread crumbs
½ cup finely chopped scallions	½ cup freshly grated Parmigiano-Reggiano
¼ cup chopped fresh basil	1½ teaspoons salt
freshly ground pepper	8 ounces mozzarella, cut into ½-inch cubes

1. Place a foil into the insert of a large slow cooker, pressing it against the bottom and up the sides. Spray the foil and the insert with nonstick cooking spray.
2. Rinse the sun-dried tomatoes under warm water. Pat them dry with paper towels. Set aside a few pieces for the top of the meatloaf. Stack the remaining tomatoes and chop them into small pieces.
3. Mix all the fixings except the mozzarella and reserved sun-dried tomatoes in a large bowl. Add the mozzarella. Shape the batter into an oval loaf slightly smaller than the interior of the slow cooker.
4. Carefully place the loaf into the cooker on top of the foil. Press the reserved tomato pieces into the top in a decorative pattern. Cover and cook on high within 3 to 4 hours. Carefully lift the meatloaf out of the slow cooker. Slide the meatloaf onto a serving platter. Cut into slices and serve hot.

Nutrition:
Calories: 388 Carbs: 28g Fat: 18g Protein: 30g

909. Duck Ragu

Preparation time: 15 minutes Cooking time: 5 hours Servings: 8

2 tablespoons olive oil	4 ounces pancetta, chopped
6 whole duck legs and thighs, skinned	salt and freshly ground pepper
4 medium carrots, peeled and chopped	2 celery ribs, chopped
1 large red onion, chopped	2 tablespoons all-purpose flour
1 cup dry red wine	½ cup tomato paste
Pinch of ground cloves	2 cups chicken broth

1. Warm-up, oil over medium heat in a large skillet, then put the pancetta and cook, often stirring, until nicely browned, about 10 minutes. Remove the pancetta to a large slow cooker.
2. Pat the duck legs dry with paper towels. Flavor it all over with salt and pepper. Add the duck legs to the skillet, batches if necessary, and cook until browned on all sides, about 15 minutes in all.
3. Transfer the duck to the cooker. Put the carrots, celery, and onion in the skillet. Cook for 10 minutes, or until the vegetables are tender. Stir in the flour and cook within 1 minute. Add the wine, tomato paste, and cloves and cook, scraping the pan's bottom until the liquid comes to a boil.
4. Scrape the mixture into the slow cooker. Add the broth. Cover and cook on low within 4 to 5 hours, or until the duck is very tender and coming away from the bone.
5. Remove the duck legs, then put it on a cutting board, but leave the cooker on. Cut it into small dice. Discard the bones. Move back the duck meat to the sauce and reheat. Serve hot.

Nutrition:
Calories: 144 Carbs: 4g Fat: 4g Protein: 4g

MEAT

910. Beef Stew with Eggplants

Preparation time: 15 minutes Cooking time: 10 hours Servings: 2

10 oz. of the beef neck, or another tender cut, chopped into bite-sized pieces
2 cups of fire-roasted tomatoes
1 cup of beef broth
2 tbsp. of tomato paste
½ tsp of chili pepper, ground (optional)
Parmesan cheese

1 large eggplant, sliced

½ cup of fresh green peas
4 tbsp. of olive oil
1 tbsp. of Cayenne pepper, ground
½ tsp of salt

1. Grease the bottom of a slow cooker with olive oil. Toss all ingredients in it and add about 1-1 ½ cup of water. Cook within 8-10 hours on low, or until the meat is fork-tender. Sprinkle with Parmesan cheese before serving, but this is optional.

Nutrition:
Calories 195 Proteins 15.3g Carbohydrates 9.6g Fat 11.1g

911. Chopped Veal Kebab

Preparation time: 15 minutes Cooking time: 10 hours Servings: 5

2 lb. boneless veal shoulder, cut into bite-sized pieces
2 tbsp. of all-purpose flour
1 tbsp. of cayenne pepper
1 tbsp. of parsley, finely chopped

3 large tomatoes, roughly chopped

3 tbsp. of butter
1 tsp of salt
1 cup of Greek yogurt (can be replaced with sour cream), for serving

1 pide bread (can be replaced with any bread you have on hand)

1. Oil the bottom of your slow cooker with one tablespoon of butter. Make a layer with veal chops and pour enough water to cover. Season with salt and close the lid. Set to low and simmer within 8-10 hours. Remove, then transfer to a plate.
2. Dissolve the rest of the butter in a small skillet. Add one tablespoon of cayenne pepper, two tablespoons of all-purpose flour, and briefly stir-fry - for about two minutes. Remove from the heat.
3. Chop pide bread and arrange on a serving plate. Place the meat and tomato on top. Drizzle with browned cayenne pepper, top with Greek yogurt, and sprinkle with chopped parsley. Serve immediately.

Nutrition:
Calories 437 Proteins 49.7g Carbohydrates 8.9g Fat 21.8g

912. Garlic Meatballs

Preparation time: 15 minutes Cooking time: 8 hours Servings: 5

1 lb. lean ground beef
2 small onions, peeled and finely chopped
1 egg, beaten
3 tbsp. of extra virgin olive oil

7 oz rice
2 garlic cloves, crushed

1 large potato, peeled and sliced
1 tsp of salt

1. Mix the lean ground beef with rice, finely chopped onions, crushed garlic, one beaten egg, and salt in a large bowl. Shape the batter into 15-20 meatballs.
2. Oiled the bottom of your slow cooker with three tablespoons of olive oil. Make the first layer with sliced potatoes and top with meatballs. Cook low within for 6-8 hours.

Nutrition:
Calories 468 Proteins 33g Carbohydrates 47g Fat 15.3g

913. Meat Pie with Yogurt

Preparation time: 15 minutes Cooking time: 6 hours Servings: 6

2 lb. lean ground beef
1 tsp of salt
1 (16 oz.) pack yufka dough
1 cup of sour cream

5-6 garlic cloves, crushed
½ tsp freshly ground black pepper
½ cup of butter, melted
3 cups of liquid yogurt

1. Mix the ground beef with garlic cloves, salt, and pepper in a large bowl. Mix well until fully incorporated. Lay a sheet of yufka on a work surface and brush with melted butter. Line with the meat mixture and roll-up. Repeat the process until all fixing is used.
2. Gently place in a lightly greased slow cooker and close the lid. Cook for 4-6 hours on low, remove from the cooker, and allow it to cool. Meanwhile, combine sour cream with yogurt. Spread the mixture over the pie and serve cold.

Nutrition:
Calories 503 Proteins 47.4g Carbohydrates 2.6g Fat 32.8g

914. Moussaka

Preparation time: 15 minutes Cooking time: 8 hours Servings: 5

2 lb. large potatoes, peeled and sliced
1 large onion, peeled and finely chopped
½ tsp of black pepper, ground
2 large eggs, beaten
Sour cream or Greek yogurt, for serving

1 lb. lean ground beef

1 tsp of salt

½ cup of milk
Vegetable oil

1. Grease the bottom of your cooker with some vegetable oil. Make one layer with sliced potatoes and brush with some milk. Spread the ground beef and make another layer with potatoes. Brush with the remaining milk, add ½ cup of water and close the lid.
2. Cook within 8 hours on low or 4-6 hours on high. When done, make the final layer with a beaten egg. Cover the cooker and let it stand for about 10 minutes. Top with some sour cream or Greek yogurt and serve!

Nutrition:
Calories 458 Proteins 34.9g Carbohydrates 36g Fat 19.2g

915. Pepper Meat

Preparation time: 15 minutes Cooking time: 10 hours Servings: 6

2 lbs. of beef fillet or another tender cut
3 tbsp. of tomato paste
1 tbsp. of butter, melted
½ tsp of freshly ground black pepper

5 medium-sized onions, peeled and finely chopped
2 tbsp. of oil
2 tbsp. of fresh parsley, finely chopped
1 tsp of salt

1. Oiled the bottom of your slow cooker with some oil. About two tablespoons will be enough. Slice the meat into bite-sized and place them in the cooker.
2. Add finely chopped onions, tomato paste, fresh parsley, salt, and pepper. Mix and put about 2 cups of water. Cook on low for 8-10 hours. Stir in one tablespoon of melted butter and serve warm.

Nutrition:
Calories 382 Proteins 47.3g Carbohydrates 10.3g Fat 16g

916. Roast Lamb

Preparation time: 15 minutes Cooking time: 8 hours Servings: 5

2 lb. lamb leg
2 tsp salt

3 tbsp. extra virgin olive oil

1. Grease the bottom of a slow cooker with three tablespoons of olive oil. Rinse and generously season the meat with salt and place in the cooker. Cook on low within one hour on high and 6-7 hours on low, or until the meat is tender and separates from the bones.

Nutrition:
Calories 473 Proteins 49.7g Carbohydrates 8.9g Fat 21.8g

917. Rosemary Meatballs

Preparation time: 15 minutes Cooking time: 6 hours Servings: 5

1 lb. lean ground beef
¼ cup of all-purpose flour
1 large egg, beaten
3 tbsp. of extra virgin olive oil
2 cups of liquid yogurt
2 tbsp. of fresh parsley

3 garlic cloves, crushed
1 tbsp. of fresh rosemary, crushed
½ tsp of salt
For serving:
1 cup of Greek yogurt
1 garlic clove, crushed

1. Mix the ground beef with crushed garlic, rosemary, one egg, and salt in a large bowl. Lightly dampen hands and shape 1 ½ inch balls transferring into the greased cooker as you work. Slowly add about ½ cup of water.
2. Cook on low for 4-6 hours. Remove from the cooker and cool completely. Meanwhile, combine liquid yogurt with Greek yogurt, parsley, and crushed garlic. Stir well and drizzle over meatballs.

Nutrition:
Calories 477 Proteins 49g Carbohydrates 17.8g Fat 21.4g

918. Spicy White Peas

Preparation time: 15 minutes Cooking time: 9 hours Servings: 4

1 lb. of white peas
1 large onion, finely chopped
2 tbsp. of all-purpose flour
1 tbsp. of cayenne pepper
1 tsp of salt

4 slices of bacon
1 small chili pepper, finely chopped
2 tbsp. of butter
3 bay leaves, dried
½ tsp of freshly ground black pepper

1. Melt two tablespoons of butter in a slow cooker. Add chopped onion and stir well. Now add bacon, peas, finely chopped chili pepper, bay leaves, salt, and pepper.
2. Gently stir in two tablespoons of flour and add three cups of water. Securely close the lid and cook for 8-9 hours on low setting or 5 hours on high.

Nutrition:
Calories 210 Proteins 4g Carbohydrates 24g Fat 12g

919. Stuffed Collard Greens

Preparation time: 15 minutes Cooking time: 4 hours Servings: 5

1 1/2 lb. of collard greens, steamed
2 small onions, peeled and finely chopped
2 tbsp. of olive oil
½ tsp of freshly ground black pepper

1 lb. lean ground beef
½ cup long grain rice

1 tsp of salt
1 tsp of mint leaves, finely chopped

1. Boil a pot of water, then gently put the collard greens. Briefly cook for 2-3 minutes. Drain and gently squeeze the greens and set aside. Mix the ground beef with the chopped onions, rice, salt, pepper, and mint leaves in a large bowl.
2. Oil the slow cooker with some olive oil. Place leaves on your work surface, vein side up. Use one tablespoon of the meat mixture and place it in the bottom center of each leaf.

3. Fold the sides over and roll up tightly. Tuck in the sides and gently transfer to a slow cooker. Cook on low within ten hours, or on high setting for 4 hours.

Nutrition:
Calories 156 Proteins 5.2g Carbohydrates 21g Fat 7g

920. Stuffed Onions

Preparation time: 15 minutes Cooking time: 8 hours Servings: 5

10-12 medium-sized sweet onions, peeled
½ cup of rice
1 tbsp. of dry mint, ground
½ tsp of cumin, ground
½ cup of tomato paste
A handful of fresh parsley, finely chopped

1 lb. of lean ground beef
3 tbsp. of olive oil
1 tsp of Cayenne pepper, ground
1 tsp of salt
½ cup Italian-style bread crumbs

1. Cut a ¼-inch slice from the top of each onion and trim a small amount from the bottom end; this will make the onions stand upright. Place onions in a microwave-safe dish and add about one cup of water. Cover with a tight lid and microwave on HIGH 10 to 12 minutes or until onions are tender.
2. Remove onions from a dish and cool slightly. Now carefully remove inner layers of onions with a paring knife, leaving about a ¼-inch onion shell. Mix the ground beef with rice, olive oil, mint, cayenne pepper, cumin, salt, and bread crumbs in a large bowl. Use one tablespoon of the mixture to fill the onions.
3. Grease the bottom of a slow cooker with some oil and add onions. Put 2 ½ cups of water and cover. Cook within 6-8 hours on a low setting. Sprinkle with chopped parsley or even arugula and serve with sour cream and pide bread.

Nutrition:
Calories 464 Proteins 34g Carbohydrates 48.4g Fat 15.2g

921. Veal Okra

Preparation time: 15 minutes Cooking time: 10 hours Servings: 4

7 oz. veal shoulder, blade chops
3 large Jerusalem artichokes, whole
2-3 fresh cauliflower florets
A handful of fresh broccoli

1 tsp of Himalayan salt

1 lb. okra, rinsed and trimmed
2 medium-sized tomatoes, halved
2 cups of vegetable broth
3 tablespoons of extra virgin olive oil
½ tsp of freshly ground black pepper

1. Grease your slow cooker with three tablespoons of olive oil. Set aside. Cut each okra pod in half lengthwise and place in a slow cooker. Add tomato halves, Jerusalem artichokes, cauliflower florets, a handful of fresh broccoli, and top with meat chops.
2. Season with salt and pepper and add two cups of vegetable broth. Give it a good stir and close the lid. Set the heat to low and cook within 8-10 hours.

Nutrition:
Calories 281 Proteins 19.6g Carbohydrates 17.4g Fat 15.5g

922. Winter Lamb Stew

Preparation time: 15 minutes Cooking time: 10 hours Servings: 4

1 lb. of lamb neck, boneless

2 large carrots, sliced
1 small red bell pepper, chopped
A handful of fresh parsley, finely chopped
¼ cup of lemon juice
½ tsp of black pepper, ground

2 medium-sized potatoes, peeled and chopped into bite-sized pieces
1 medium-sized tomato, diced
1 garlic head, whole
2 tbsp. of extra virgin olive oil

½ tsp of salt

1. Grease the bottom of a slow cooker with olive oil. Place the meat at the bottom of the cooker and season with salt.

2. Now add the other ingredients, tuck in one garlic head in the middle of the pot and add 2 cups of water. Add a handful of fresh parsley and close the lid. Set the heat to low and simmer for 10 hours.

Nutrition:
Calories 379 Proteins 34.6g Carbohydrates 24.2g Fat 15.7g

923.   Beef in Barolo
Preparation time: 15 minutes Cooking time: 6 hours Servings: 6

1/3 cup all-purpose flour	Salt
ground pepper	1 3-pound boneless beef chuck
3 tbsp. olive oil	2 oz. pancetta, chopped
1 onion, chopped	2 garlic cloves, chopped
1 cup dry red wine	2 cups tomatoes, chopped
1 cup Meat Broth	2 medium carrots, sliced
1 medium celery rib, sliced	1 bay leaf
a few grounds clove	

1. Mix the flour with salt plus pepper, put it on wax paper. Roll the meat in the flour mixture. Warm-up oil on medium-high heat in a large skillet, then put the beef and brown within 15 minutes.
2. Put the meat in a slow cooker. Put the pancetta plus onion in the skillet. Reduce the heat to medium and cook within 10 minutes, occasionally stirring, until the onion is tender. Stir in the garlic. Add the wine and simmer.
3. Pour the batter over the beef. Put the tomatoes and broth. Put the carrots, celery, bay leaf, plus ground cloves around the meat. Cover and cook on low within 6 hours, then move the meat to a platter. Discard the bay leaf, then slice the meat and spoon on the sauce.

Nutrition:
Calories: 150 Carbs: 3g Fat: 5g Protein: 19g

924.   Peppery Beef Stew
Preparation time: 15 minutes Cooking time: 8 hours Servings: 6

½ cup all-purpose flour	Salt
3 pounds boneless beef chuck, 2-inch chunks	3 tablespoons olive oil
1 cup dry red wine	2 cups canned tomato puree
2 garlic cloves, chopped, plus 6 whole garlic cloves, peeled	1 tablespoon whole black peppercorns
½ teaspoon freshly ground pepper, or to taste	

1. On a piece of wax paper, stir the flour and salt to taste. Toss the beef with the flour and shake off any excess. Warm-up oil over medium-high heat in a large, heavy skillet, then put the meat in batches, without crowding the pan. Brown the beef well on all sides.
2. Transfer the beef meat to a large slow cooker. Put the wine in the skillet and simmer, scraping the bottom of the pan. Add the tomato puree, garlic, peppercorns, and ground pepper. Cook within 10 minutes.
3. Pour the mixture into the slow cooker. Cook on low within 6 to 8 hours or until the beef is very tender. Taste for seasoning before serving.

Nutrition:
Calories: 187 Carbs: 12g Fat: 5g Protein: 23g

925.   Beef Goulash
Preparation time: 15 minutes Cooking time: 6 hours Servings: 8

3 tablespoons lard, drippings, or vegetable oil	3½ pounds beef chuck, boneless, cut into 2-inch cubes
Salt and freshly ground pepper	4 medium onions, sliced
2 garlic cloves, finely chopped	1 cup dry red wine
2 tablespoons tomato paste	1 bay leaf
¼ cup sweet paprika	1 tablespoon chopped fresh marjoram leaves
1 teaspoon ground cumin	1 2-inch strip lemon zest
Juice of ½ lemon	

1. Heat the lard, drippings in a large skillet over medium-high heat. Pat the meat dry and put in the pan. Cook until browned on all sides. Move the meat to your slow cooker and brown the rest of the meat. Sprinkle the meat with salt and pepper.
2. Adjust the heat to medium, then put the onions in the skillet. Cook, occasionally stirring, until lightly browned. Stir in the garlic. Put the wine plus tomato paste and simmer. Pour the mixture into the slow cooker. Stir in the bay leaf, paprika, marjoram, cumin, and lemon zest.
3. Add enough water to cover the meat barely. Cover and cook on low within 6 hours, or until the beef is very tender when pierced with a fork. Stir in the lemon juice. Remove the bay leaf and lemon zest. Serve hot.

Nutrition:
Calories: 272 Carbs: 25g Fat: 7g Protein: 22g

926.   Braised Beef with Anchovies and Rosemary
Preparation time: 15 minutes Cooking time: 6 hour Servings: 6

2 tablespoons olive oil	4 pounds beef shin or 3 pounds boneless chuck, cut into 2-inch cubes
2 ounces pancetta, chopped	Salt and freshly ground pepper
2 large garlic cloves, finely chopped	6 anchovy fillets
1 cup dry white wine	1 3-inch fresh rosemary sprig

1. Warm-up oil over medium-high heat in a large, heavy skillet. Pat the beef dry. Add only as much of the beef and pancetta to the pan as will fit comfortably without crowding.
2. Cook, then transfer the meat to a large slow cooker and brown the remaining meat. Rub the meat with salt plus pepper to taste. Discard or spoon off the excess fat from the pan and adjust the heat to medium.
3. Put the garlic and anchovies and cook, stirring, within 2 minutes. Put the wine and bring it to a simmer. Pour the liquid into the slow cooker. Add the rosemary. Cover and cook within low for 6 hours. Discard the rosemary and serve hot.

Nutrition:
Calories: 334 Carbs: 0g Fat: 13g Protein: 0g

927.   Braciole in Tomato Sauce
Preparation time: 15 minutes Cooking time: 4 hours Servings: 8

2 ½-inch-thick beef round steaks (each about 1 pound)	Salt and freshly ground pepper
½ cup freshly grated Pecorino Romano	3 tablespoons chopped fresh parsley
4 garlic cloves, finely chopped	2 tablespoons olive oil
1 large onion, chopped	1 28-ounce can tomato puree
6 fresh basil leaves, torn into bits	

1. Put each steak in between two sheets of plastic wrap. Gently pound the steaks with a mallet or the bottom of a small pan to a 1/8-inch thickness. Cut each steak in half.
2. Flavor the meat with salt and pepper to taste, then with the cheese, parsley, and garlic. Roll up each piece of meat. With kitchen twine, tie each roll up like a roast.
3. Warm-up the oil on medium-high heat in a large, heavy skillet. Put the meat rolls and cook until browned on one side. Turn the rolls and scatter the onion around the meat.
4. Cook, then transfer the rolls and onion to a large slow cooker and add the tomato puree and basil. Cover and cook on low within 4 hours, or until the meat is tender. Transfer the meat to a cutting board. Remove the twine, then slice the meat into thick slices. Spoon on the sauce. Serve hot.

Nutrition:
Calories: 220 Carbs: 6g Fat: 15g Protein: 14g

928. Beef Shanks with Red Wine and Tomatoes

Preparation time: 15 minutes Cooking time: 8 hours Servings: 8

About 20 whole garlic cloves (1 large head), peeled	2 cups dry red wine
1 14-ounce can Italian peeled tomatoes with their juice, chopped	1 4-inch fresh rosemary sprig or 1 tablespoon dried
3 pounds bone-in beef shanks, about 2 inches thick, trimmed	Salt and freshly ground pepper
Thick-sliced Italian bread	

1. Scatter the garlic cloves in the slow cooker. Add the wine, tomatoes, and rosemary. Place the beef in the cooker and sprinkle with salt to taste and plenty of pepper.
2. Cover and cook on low within 6 to 8 hours or until the meat is tender and falling off the bone. Skim off the excess fat and taste for seasoning.
3. Toast the bread and place 1 or 2 slices in each serving dish. Crushed the meat up with a spoon and scoop some of the meat, garlic, and pan juices over the bread. Serve with the marrow bones.

Nutrition:
Calories: 479 Carbs: 11g Fat: 17g Protein: 61g

929. Balsamic-Glazed Short Ribs

Preparation time: 15 minutes Cooking time: 8 hours Servings: 6

1 tablespoon olive oil	4 5 pounds bone-in beef short ribs, well-trimmed
Salt and freshly ground pepper	2 large garlic cloves, finely chopped
½ cup dry red wine	1/3 cup balsamic vinegar
1 3-inch fresh rosemary sprig	

1. Warm-up the oil in a large, heavy skillet on medium-high heat. Pat the meat dry and put only as many pieces in the pan as will fit comfortably. Cook, then transfer the meat to a slow cooker. Flavor the ribs with salt plus pepper to taste.
2. Discard all but reserve 1 tablespoon of the fat and adjust the heat to medium. Put the garlic and cook within 1 minute. Add the wine and vinegar and simmer while scraping the bottom of the pan.
3. Put the liquid on the ribs and add the rosemary. Cover and cook on low within 8 hours. Remove the ribs, and discard the rosemary sprig with any loose bones. Skim the fat off the liquid.
4. Pour the rest of all the sauce into a saucepan and cook over medium-high heat until thickened. Put the sauce over the ribs and serve hot.

Nutrition:
Calories: 249 Carbs: 0g Fat: 22g Protein: 11g

930. Roman Oxtail Stew

Preparation time: 15 minutes Cooking time: 6 hours & 30 minutes Servings: 6

¼ cup olive oil	4 pounds oxtails, about 1½ inches thick
1 large onion, chopped	2 garlic cloves, chopped
1 cup dry red wine	1 28-ounce can Italian peeled tomatoes with their juice
¼ teaspoon ground cloves	Salt and freshly ground pepper
6 medium celery ribs, sliced	1 tablespoon chopped bittersweet chocolate
2 tablespoons pine nuts	2 tablespoons raisins

1. Warm-up oil over medium-high heat in a large skillet. Add the oxtails, in batches if necessary, and brown nicely on all sides. Transfer the oxtails to the slow cooker.
2. Put off all but 2 tablespoons of the fat and lower the heat to medium. Add the onion to the skillet and cook until lightly browned, within 10 minutes. Mix in the garlic and cook within 30 seconds.
3. Put the wine and scrape the bottom of the pan. Stir in the tomatoes, cloves, and salt and pepper to taste. Simmer the liquid, then pour over

the oxtails. Cover and cook on low within 6 hours. Boil a large saucepan of water.

4. Add the celery and cook for 1 minute. Drain well. Turn the slow cooker to high. Stir in the chocolate. Add the celery, pine nuts, and raisins. Cook for 30 minutes, or until the flavors blend. Serve hot.

Nutrition:
Calories: 233 Carbs: 19g Fat: 12g Protein: 13g

931. "Big Meatball" Meat Loaf

Preparation time: 15 minutes Cooking time: hours Servings: 8

2 pounds ground beef chuck or round	3 large eggs, beaten
2 garlic cloves, minced	1 cup freshly grated Pecorino Romano
½ cup plain dry bread crumbs	¼ cup chopped fresh parsley
1½ teaspoons salt	Freshly ground pepper
2 cups meatless tomato sauce	

1. Put the foil in a large slow cooker, pressing it against the bottom and up the sides. Mix all the fixing except the tomato sauce in a large bowl. Shape the mixture into a loaf. Carefully place it in the slow cooker on top of the foil.
2. Pour the tomato sauce over the top. Cover and cook on high within 4 hours, or until an instant-read thermometer reads 165° to 170°F. Carefully lift the meatloaf using the ends of the foil as handles. Slide the meatloaf onto a serving platter. Slice and serve.

Nutrition:
Calories: 197 Carbs: 8g Fat: 1g Protein: 20g

932. Springtime Veal Stew

Preparation time: 15 minutes Cooking time: 4 hours & 35 minutes Servings: 6

3 large carrots, cut into ¼-inch-thick slices	2 medium onions, chopped
3 tablespoons olive oil	1 garlic clove, finely chopped
2 teaspoons chopped fresh rosemary	2 pounds veal shoulder or chuck, trimmed and cut into 2-inch pieces
2 cups Chicken Broth	2 tablespoons tomato paste
Salt and freshly ground pepper	4 cups of water
1 cup asparagus, 1-inch pieces	1 cup thawed frozen green peas or baby lima beans

1. Scatter the carrot slices in a large slow cooker. Cook the onions in the oil over medium heat until softened, about 10 minutes in a large skillet. Stir in the garlic and rosemary. Put the veal and cook, occasionally stirring, until the meat is no longer pink. Scrape the veal mixture into the slow cooker.
2. Move back the skillet to the heat and add the broth and tomato paste. Cook until the liquid comes to a simmer, then pour into the slow cooker. Put a pinch of salt plus pepper to taste. Cover and cook on low within 4 hours, or until the veal is tender when pierced with a fork. Boil the water in a medium saucepan.
3. Add the asparagus and salt to taste. Simmer within 3 to 5 minutes, depending on the thickness, until crisp-tender. Drain well. Add the asparagus and the peas or beans to the slow cooker. Cover and cook within 30 minutes more. Serve hot.

Nutrition:
Calories: 280 Carbs: 31g Fat: 4g Protein: 32g

933. Osso Buco with Red

Preparation time: 15 minutes Cooking time: 5 hours Servings: 6

6 1½-inch-thick slices veal shank	¼ cup all-purpose flour
Salt and freshly ground pepper	2 tablespoons unsalted butter
1 tablespoon olive oil	2 medium carrots, chopped
1 medium onion, chopped	1 medium celery rib, chopped
1 cup dry red wine	1 cup peeled, seeded, and chopped fresh tomatoes
1 cup Meat Broth	2 teaspoons chopped fresh thyme or ½ teaspoon dried

1. To help hold the shape of the meat as it cooks, ties a piece of kitchen twine around the circumference of each shank. On a piece of wax paper, stir the flour and salt and pepper to taste. In a large skillet, melt the butter with the oil over medium heat.
2. Dip the cut sides of each piece of meat in the flour mixture and place it in the skillet, in batches if necessary. Cook, turning the meat once until nicely browned, about 10 minutes on each side.
3. Moved the cooked meat to your slow cooker. Add the chopped vegetables to the skillet. Cook, occasionally stirring, until golden brown, about 15 minutes.
4. Put the wine in the skillet, then cook, scraping the bottom of the pan, until the liquid comes to a boil. Stir in the tomatoes, broth, and thyme. Pour the sauce over the veal. Cover and cook on low within 4 to 5 hours. Remove the twine and serve hot.

Nutrition:
Calories: 256 Carbs: 14g Fat: 14g Protein: 19g

934. Milk-Braised Pork Loin

Preparation time: 15 minutes Cooking time: hours Servings: 8

3 pounds boneless pork loin, rolled and tied	Salt and freshly ground pepper
2 tablespoons unsalted butter	1 tablespoon olive oil
2 medium carrots, finely chopped	1 medium onion, finely chopped
1 medium celery rib, finely chopped	2 cups whole milk

1. Pat the meat dry with paper towels. Sprinkle it with salt plus pepper. Dissolve the butter with the oil in a large, heavy skillet over medium-high heat. Cook the meat on one side. Flip it over and put the vegetables around the meat. Cook, then transfer the meat to the slow cooker.
2. Add the milk to the skillet with the vegetables and bring it to a simmer. Pour the contents of the skillet over the meat.
3. Cover and cook on low within 3 to 4 hours. If the sauce is too thin, pour it into a saucepan and reduce it over medium heat. Remove the twine from the meat. Slice the meat, then arrange it on a platter. Spoon the sauce down the center and serve hot.

Nutrition:
Calories: 190 Carbs: 8g Fat: 6g Protein: 25g

935. Pork Chops with Fennel Seeds

Preparation time: 15 minutes Cooking time: 8 hours Servings: 6

6 bone-in pork rib chops (about 3½ pounds total)	Salt and freshly ground pepper
2 tablespoons olive oil	2 large onions, thinly sliced
½ cup dry white wine	1 tablespoon fennel seeds
1 cup Meat Broth	

1. Pat dry the pork chops and sprinkle them on both sides with salt and pepper to taste. Warm-up oil over medium-high heat in a large, heavy skillet. Add as many of the chops as will fit in the pan without touching. Cook, turning the chops occasionally until nicely browned on all sides.
2. Put the cooked chops in your slow cooker. Brown the remaining pork chops. Add the onions to the skillet, reduce the heat to medium, and cook for about 10 minutes. Stir in the wine and fennel seeds and bring it to a simmer.
3. Put the broth, then scrape the bottom of the pan until boiling. Pour the mixture over the chops. Cover and cook on low heat within 6 to 8 hours. Serve hot.

Nutrition:
Calories: 176 Carbs: 313g Fat: 7g Protein: 14g

936. Pork Stew Agrodolce

Preparation time: 15 minutes Cooking time: 6 hours Servings: 8

3 pounds boneless pork shoulder, 2-inch pieces	Salt and freshly ground pepper
3 tablespoons olive oil	3 large onions, chopped
2 large celery ribs, chopped	1 cup dry white wine
3 tablespoons balsamic vinegar	3 large carrots, cut into 1-inch chunks
½ cup golden raisins	

1. Pat the pork dries with paper towels. Sprinkle the meat with salt and pepper. Warm-up oil over medium-high heat in a large, heavy skillet.
2. Put the pork, then brown all sides and move back it to the slow cooker. Reduce the heat to medium. Put the onions plus celery in the skillet and cook until golden.
3. Put the wine and vinegar, then simmer. Transfer the onion batter to the slow cooker. Put the carrots and raisins. Cover and cook on low within 6 hours. Serve hot.

Nutrition:
Calories: 190 Carbs: 0g Fat: 10g Protein: 23g

937. Country-Style Pork Ribs with Tomato and Peppers

Preparation time: 15 minutes Cooking time: hours Servings: 6

4 pounds country-style pork ribs	Salt and freshly ground pepper
2 tablespoons olive oil	2 medium onions, chopped
2 large garlic cloves, chopped	½ cup dry white wine
2 tablespoons tomato paste	1 cup canned tomato puree
1 teaspoon dried oregano	4 medium red bell peppers, ½-inch slices

1. Pat dry the ribs, then flavor them with salt plus pepper. Warm-up oil over medium heat in a large skillet. Put the ribs in the pan without touching. Cook the meat, flipping it occasionally. Put the cooked ribs in the slow cooker and brown the remaining ribs.
2. Put the onions plus garlic in the skillet and cook within 5 minutes. Mix in the wine plus tomato paste and cook until it simmers. Mix in the tomato puree, oregano, plus salt and pepper to taste.
3. Remove, then scatter the peppers over the pork in the slow cooker. Pour on the sauce. Cover and cook on low within 6 hours. Remove any loose bones and skim off the fat. Serve hot.

Nutrition:
Calories: 240 Carbs: 0g Fat: 18g Protein: 18g

VEGETABLES

938. Balsamic Brussels Sprouts

Preparation Time: 10 minutes Cooking Time: 4 hours and 10 minutes
Servings: 6

2 tablespoons brown sugar	½ cup balsamic vinegar
2 lb. Brussels sprouts, trimmed and sliced in half	2 tablespoons olive oil
2 tablespoons butter, cut into cubes	Salt and pepper to taste
¼ cup Parmesan cheese, grated	

1. Put the brown sugar and vinegar in a saucepan over medium heat. Mix and bring to a boil. Reduce heat and simmer for 8 minutes. Let cool and set aside.
2. Mix the brussel sprouts in olive oil plus butter. Season with salt and pepper. Cover the pot. Cook low for 4 hours. Drizzle the balsamic vinegar on top of the Brussels sprouts. Sprinkle the Parmesan cheese on top.

Nutrition:
Calories 193 Fat 10 g Cholesterol 13.2 mg Carbohydrate 21.9 g Fiber 6.2 g Protein 6.9 g Sugars 11.1 g

939. Mediterranean Zucchini & Eggplant

Preparation Time: 15 minutes Cooking Time: 3 hours Servings: 4

1 tablespoon olive oil	1 onion, diced
4 cloves garlic, minced	1 red bell pepper, chopped
4 tomatoes, diced	1 zucchini, chopped
1 lb. eggplant, sliced into cubes	Salt and pepper to taste
2 teaspoons dried basil	4 oz. feta cheese

1. Coat your slow cooker with olive oil. Mix all the fixing except cheese in the pot. Cook on high within 3 hours. Sprinkle feta cheese on top and serve.

Nutrition:
Calories 341 Fat 12 g Cholesterol 25 mg Carbohydrate 51 g Fiber 11 g Protein 13 g Sugars 13 g

940. Roasted Baby Carrots

Preparation Time: 15 minutes Cooking Time: 6 hours Servings: 6

2 lb. baby carrots	¼ cup apricot preserve
6 tablespoons butter	2 tablespoons honey
1 tablespoon sugar	1 teaspoon balsamic vinegar
1 teaspoon garlic powder	Salt and pepper to taste
¼ teaspoon dried thyme	¼ teaspoon ground mustard

1. Combine all the fixing in the slow cooker. Mix well. Cover the pot. Cook on low for 6 hours.

Nutrition:
Calories 218 Fat 11.8g Cholesterol 31mg Sodium 206mg Carbohydrate 29.3g Fiber 4.5g Sugars 20.9g Protein 1.3g

941. Artichokes with Garlic & Cream Sauce

Preparation Time: 15 minutes Cooking Time: 8 hours Servings: 6

Cooking spray	30 oz. canned diced tomatoes
6 cloves garlic, crushed and minced	28 oz. canned artichoke hearts, rinsed, drained, and sliced into quarters
½ cup whipping cream	1 teaspoon dried basil
½ teaspoon dried oregano	Feta cheese

1. Spray the slow cooker with oil. Add the tomatoes with juice, garlic, and artichoke hearts. Season with the basil and oregano. Mix well. Cover the pot. Cook on low for 8 hours. Stir in the cream. Let sit for 5 minutes. Top with the crumbled cheese.

Nutrition:
Calories 403 Fat 5 g Cholesterol 27 mg Carbohydrate 38 g Fiber 5 g Protein 13 g Sugars 17 g

942. Mediterranean Kale & White Kidney Beans

Preparation Time: 30 minutes Cooking Time: 3 hours Servings: 6

1 onion, chopped	4 cloves garlic, crushed
¼ cup celery, chopped	2 carrots, sliced
1 cup farro, rinsed and drained	14 oz. canned roasted tomatoes
4 cups low-sodium vegetable broth	½ teaspoon red pepper, crushed
Salt to taste	3 tablespoons freshly squeezed lemon juice
15-ounce white kidney beans, drained	4 cup kale
½ cup feta cheese, crumbled	Fresh parsley, chopped

1. Put the onion, garlic, celery, carrots, farro, tomatoes, broth, red pepper, and salt in your slow cooker. Seal the pot. Cook on high for 2 hours. Stir in the lemon juice, beans, and kale. Cover and cook for 1 more hour. Sprinkle the cheese and parsley before serving.

Nutrition:
Calories 274 Fat 9 g Cholesterol 11 mg Carbohydrate 46 g Fiber 9 g Protein 14 g Sugars 6 g

943. Creamed Corn

Preparation Time: 10 minutes Cooking Time: 4 hours Servings: 12

16 oz. frozen corn kernels	8 oz. cream cheese
½ cup butter	½ cup milk
1 tablespoon white sugar	Salt and pepper to taste

1. Put all the listed fixing in the slow cooker. Stir well. Cook on high for 4 hours.

Nutrition:
Calories 192 Fat 15 g Cholesterol 42 mg Carbohydrate 13.7 g Fiber 1.3 g Protein 3.4 g - Sugars 3 g

944. Spicy Beans & Veggies

Preparation Time: 20 minutes Cooking Time: 8 hours Servings: 6

15 ounces canned northern beans, drained	15 oz. canned red beans, rinsed and drained
5 teaspoons garlic, minced	1 onion, chopped
1 cup, sliced thinly	½ cup celery, sliced thinly
2 cups green beans, trimmed and sliced	2 red chili peppers, chopped
2 bay leaves	Salt and pepper to taste

1. Mix all the fixing listed above in the slow cooker. Set it on low. Seal and cook for 8 hours. Discard the bay leaves before serving.

Nutrition:
Calories 264 Fat 0.9g Carbohydrate 49g Sugars 3g Protein 17.2g Potassium 1111mg

945. Eggplant Salad

Preparation Time: 10 minutes Cooking Time: 8 hours Servings: 4

1 onion, sliced	1 green bell pepper, sliced
1 red bell pepper, sliced	24 oz. canned tomatoes
1 eggplant, sliced	2 teaspoons cumin
1 tablespoon smoked paprika	1 tablespoon lemon juice
Salt and pepper to taste	

1. Add all the fixings to the slow cooker. Mix well. Cook on low within 8 hours.

Nutrition:
Calories 90 Fat 1.1g Sodium 16mg Carbohydrate 19.7g Fiber 7.9g Sugars 10.9g Protein 3.7g Potassium 826mg

946. Turkish Stuffed Eggplant

Preparation time: 15 minutes Cooking time: 4 hours Servings: 6

½ cup extra-virgin olive oil	3 small eggplants
1 teaspoon of sea salt	½ teaspoon black pepper
1 large yellow onion, finely chopped	4 garlic cloves, minced
one 15-ounce can dice tomatoes, with the juice	¼ cup finely chopped fresh flat-leaf parsley
six 8-inch round pita bread, quartered and toasted	1 cup plain Greek-style yogurt

1. Pour ¼ cup of the olive oil into the slow cooker, and generously coat the interior of the crock. Cut each eggplant in half lengthwise. You can leave the stem on. Score the cut side of each half every ¼ inch.
2. Arrange the eggplant halves, skin-side down, in the slow cooker. Sprinkle with 1 teaspoon salt and ½ teaspoon pepper. In a large skillet, heat the remaining ¼ cup olive oil over medium-high heat. Sauté the onion and garlic for 3 minutes, or until the onion begins to soften.
3. Add the tomatoes and parsley to the skillet. Season with salt and pepper. Sauté for another 5 minutes, until the liquid has almost evaporated. Using a large spoon, spoon the tomato mixture over the eggplants, covering each half with some of the mixtures.
4. Cover and cook on high within 2 hours or on low for 4 hours. Uncover the slow cooker, and let the eggplant rest for 10 minutes. Then transfer the eggplant to a serving dish. If there is any juice in the bottom of the cooker, spoon it over the eggplant. Serve hot with toasted pita wedges and yogurt on the side.

Nutrition:
Calories: 56 Carbs: 10g Fat: 2g Protein: 2g

947. Eggplant Parmigiana

Preparation time: 15 minutes Cooking time: 5 hours Servings: 6

4 mediums to large eggplants, peeled	sea salt for sweating eggplants, plus 1 teaspoon
1/3 cup vegetable stock	2 eggs, lightly beaten
olive oil for frying (about ½ cup)	3 tablespoons all-purpose flour
½ cup grated parmesan cheese, preferably Parmigiano-Reggiano	1/3 cup seasoned bread crumbs
1 yellow onion, chopped	1 tablespoon extra-virgin olive oil
	1 28-ounce can crush tomatoes, with the juice
1 6-ounce can tomato paste	4 tablespoons chopped fresh parsley
2 cloves garlic, minced	1 teaspoon dried oregano
1 teaspoon of sea salt	¼ teaspoon black pepper
½ cup white wine	16 ounces mozzarella cheese, sliced

1. To prepare the eggplant, first, sweat it. Cut the eggplant into ½-inch slices. Put in a large bowl in layers, flavoring each layer with salt. Let it set within 30 minutes to drain excess moisture.
2. Mix the eggs with the stock and flour until smooth in a medium shallow bowl. Soak the eggplant slices in the batter.
3. Warm-up 1 tablespoon of the olive oil for frying in a skillet. Sauté the eggplant in hot olive oil within. Put aside the eggplant on a paper towel-lined plate. Mix the seasoned bread crumbs with the Parmesan cheese in a small bowl. Set aside.

4. Warm-up extra-virgin olive oil in a large skillet over medium heat. Put the onion, then sauté within 3 minutes until the onion begins to soften. Add the crushed tomatoes, tomato paste, parsley, garlic, oregano, 1 teaspoon sea salt, ¼ teaspoon black pepper.
5. Put the fixing in even layers in your slow cooker, in this order: 1/4 of the eggplant slices, 1/4 of the bread crumbs, 1/4 of the tomato mixture, and 1/4 of the mozzarella cheese.
6. Repeat process making three more layers of the eggplant, bread crumbs, tomato mixture, and mozzarella. Cover and cook on low within 4 to 5 hours. Serve hot.

Nutrition:
Calories: 270 Carbs: 26g Fat: 15g Protein: 8g

948. Ratatouille

Preparation time: 15 minutes Cooking time: 9 hours Servings: 6

2 large yellow onions, sliced	1 large eggplant, unpeeled, sliced
4 small zucchinis, sliced	2 garlic cloves, minced
2 green bell peppers, strips	6 large tomatoes, cut into ½-inch wedges
1 teaspoon dried basil	2 teaspoons sea salt
¼ teaspoon black pepper	2 tablespoons chopped fresh flat-leaf parsley
¼ cup olive oil	

1. Layer one-half of each of the vegetables in the slow cooker in the following order: onion, eggplant, zucchini, garlic, bell peppers, and tomatoes. Repeat with the other one-half of the vegetables.
2. Sprinkle with the basil, salt, pepper, and parsley. Drizzle the olive oil over the top. Cover and cook on low within 7 to 9 hours. Serve hot.

Nutrition:
Calories: 189 Carbs: 15g Fat: 12g Protein: 3g

949. Slow Cooker Caponata

Preparation time: 15 minutes Cooking time: 5 hours & 30 minutes Servings: 8

1-pound plum tomatoes, chopped	1 eggplant, not peeled, cut into ½-inch pieces
2 medium zucchinis, cut into ½-inch pieces	1 large yellow onion, finely chopped
3 stalks celery, sliced	½ cup chopped fresh parsley
2 tablespoons red wine vinegar	1 tablespoon brown sugar
¼ cup raisins	¼ cup (4 ounces) tomato paste
1 teaspoon of sea salt	¼ teaspoon black pepper
¼ cup pine nuts	2 tablespoons capers, drained
3 tablespoons oil-cured black olives (optional)	

1. Combine the tomatoes, eggplant, zucchini, onion, celery, and parsley in the slow cooker. Add the vinegar, brown sugar, raisins, and tomato paste. Sprinkle with salt and pepper.
2. Cover and cook on low within 5½ hours, or until thoroughly cooked. Stir in the pine nuts and capers and olives (if using). Serve hot.

Nutrition:
Calories: 68 Carbs: 6g Fat: 4g Protein: 1g

950. Barley-Stuffed Cabbage Rolls with Pine Nuts and Currants

Preparation time: 15 minutes Cooking time: hours Servings: 4

1 large head green cabbage, cored	1 tablespoon olive oil
1 large yellow onion, chopped	3 cups cooked pearl barley
3 ounces feta cheese, crumbled	½ cup dried currants
2 tablespoons pine nuts, toasted	2 tablespoons chopped fresh flat-leaf parsley
½ teaspoon of sea salt	½ teaspoon black pepper
½ cup apple juice	1 tablespoon apple cider vinegar
1 15-ounce can crush tomatoes, with the juice	

1. Steam the cabbage head in a large pot over boiling water for 8 minutes. Remove to a cutting board and let cool slightly. Remove 16 leaves from the cabbage head. Slice off the raised portion of each cabbage leaf (do not cut out the vein).
2. Heat the oil in a large nonstick lidded skillet over medium heat. Add the onion, cover, and cook 6 minutes or until tender. Remove to a large bowl. Stir the barley, feta cheese, currants, pine nuts, and parsley into the onion mixture. Flavor with ¼ teaspoon of the salt and ¼ teaspoon of the pepper.
3. Place cabbage leaves on a work surface. On 1 cabbage leaf, spoon about 1/3 cup of the barley mixture into the center. Fold in the edges of the leaf over the barley mixture and roll the cabbage leaf up. Repeat for the remaining 15 cabbage leaves and filling. Arrange the cabbage rolls in the slow cooker.
4. Combine the remaining ¼ teaspoon salt, ¼ teaspoon pepper, the apple juice, apple cider vinegar, and tomatoes. Pour the apple juice mixture evenly over the cabbage rolls. Cover and cook on high 2 hours or low for 6 to 8 hours. Serve hot.

Nutrition:
Calories: 402 Carbs: 70g Fat: 11g Protein: 11g

951. Balsamic Collard Greens

Preparation time: 15 minutes Cooking time: 4 hours Servings: 5

3 bacon slices	1 cup chopped sweet onion
1-pound fresh collard greens, rinsed, stemmed, and chopped	¼ teaspoon of sea salt
2 garlic cloves, minced	1 bay leaf
2 cups vegetable or chicken stock	3 tablespoons balsamic vinegar
1 tablespoon honey	

1. Cook or brown the bacon in a medium skillet on medium heat until crisp, about 6 minutes. Put the bacon on a paper towel-lined plate to cool. Crumble the bacon. Add the onion to bacon drippings and cook for 5 minutes, or until tender. Add the collard greens and cook 2 to 3 minutes or until the greens begin to wilt, stirring occasionally.
2. Place the collard greens, salt, garlic, bay leaf, and stock in the slow cooker. Cover and cook on low within 3½ to 4 hours. Combine the balsamic vinegar and honey in a small bowl. Stir the vinegar mixture into the collard greens just before serving. Serve hot, sprinkled with the crumbled bacon.

Nutrition:
Calories: 82 Carbs: 0g Fat: 0g Protein: 5g

952. Glazed Brussels Sprouts with Pine Nuts

Preparation time: 15 minutes Cooking time: 3 hours Servings: 6

balsamic glaze	1 cup balsamic vinegar
¼ cup honey	2 pounds brussels sprouts, trimmed and halved
2 cups vegetable or chicken stock	1 teaspoon sea salt & black pepper
2 tablespoons extra-virgin olive oil	¼ cup pine nuts, toasted
¼ cup grated parmesan cheese	

1. Mix the balsamic vinegar plus honey in a small saucepan over medium-high heat. Stir constantly until the sugar has dissolved. Boil, then adjust the heat to low and simmer until the glaze is reduced by half, about 20 minutes. The glaze is finished when it will coat the back of a spoon. Set aside.
2. Combine the Brussels sprouts, stock, and ½ teaspoon salt in the slow cooker. Cover and cook on high within 2 to 3 hours, or until the Brussels sprouts are tender.
3. Drain the Brussels sprouts and transfer to a serving dish. Season with salt and pepper. Drizzle with 2 tablespoons or more of the balsamic glaze and the olive oil, then sprinkle with the pine nuts and Parmesan. Serve hot.

Nutrition:
Calories: 105 Carbs: 4g Fat: 11g Protein: 2g

953. Balsamic Root Vegetables

Preparation time: 15 minutes Cooking time: 5 hours Servings: 8

nonstick cooking oil spray	1-pound parsnips, peeled and cut into 1½-inch cubes
1-pound carrots, peeled and cut into 1½-inch pieces	2 large red onions, coarsely chopped
¾ cup dried apricots or figs	1½ pounds sweet potatoes, 1½-inch cubes
1 tablespoon light brown sugar	3 tbsp. olive oil
2 tbsp. balsamic vinegar	1 tsp sea salt
½ teaspoon black pepper	1/3 cup chopped fresh flat-leaf parsley

1. Coat the interior of the slow cooker crock with nonstick cooking oil spray. Add the parsnips, carrots, onions, and apricots in the prepared slow cooker crock, and layer the sweet potatoes over the top.
2. Whisk the brown sugar, olive oil, balsamic vinegar, salt, and pepper in a small bowl. Pour over vegetable mixture, but do not stir. Cover and cook on high for 4 to 5 hours, or until the vegetables are tender. Toss with parsley just before serving hot.

Nutrition:
Calories: 70 Carbs: 13g Fat: 2g Protein: 1g

954. Sweet Potato Gratin

Preparation time: 15 minutes Cooking time: 4 hours Servings: 12

1 tablespoon butter, at room temperature	1 large sweet onion, thinly sliced
2 pounds sweet potatoes, thinly sliced	1 tablespoon all-purpose flour
1 teaspoon chopped fresh thyme	½ teaspoon of sea salt
½ teaspoon black pepper	2 ounces grated fresh parmesan cheese
nonstick cooking oil spray	½ cup vegetable stock

1. Dissolve the butter in a medium nonstick skillet on medium heat. Add the onion and sauté 5 minutes, or until lightly browned. Remove to a large bowl. Add the sweet potatoes, flour, thyme, salt, pepper, and one-half of the grated Parmesan cheese in the large bowl. Toss gently to coat the sweet potato slices with the flour mixture.
2. Coat the slow cooker with cooking oil spray. Transfer the sweet potato mixture to the slow cooker. Pour the stock over the mixture. Sprinkle with the remaining Parmesan. Cover and cook on low within 4 hours or until the potatoes are tender. Serve hot.

Nutrition:
Calories: 118 Carbs: 26g Fat: 2g Protein: 1g

955. Orange-Glazed Carrots

Preparation time: 15 minutes Cooking time: 6 hours Servings: 8

3 pounds carrots, peeled and cut into ¼-inch slices	1½ cups water, plus extra hot water as needed
1 tablespoon granulated sugar	1 teaspoon of sea salt
½ cup orange marmalade	2 tablespoons unsalted butter, softened
1½ teaspoons fresh sage, minced	
black pepper (optional)	

1. Combine the carrots, 1½ cups water, sugar, and 1 teaspoon salt in the slow cooker. Cover and cook on low within 4 to 6 hours.
2. Drain the carrots, and then return to the slow cooker. Stir in the marmalade, butter, and sage. Season with additional salt and some pepper, if needed. Serve hot.

Nutrition:
Calories: 124 Carbs: 30g Fat: 0g Protein: 2g

956. Lemon-Rosemary Beets

Preparation time: 15 minutes Cooking time: 8 hours Servings: 7

2 pounds beets, slice into wedges
2 tablespoons extra-virgin olive oil
1 tablespoon apple cider vinegar
½ teaspoon black pepper
½ teaspoon lemon zest

2 tablespoons fresh lemon juice
2 tbsp. honey
¾ teaspoon sea salt
2 sprigs fresh rosemary

1. Place the beets in the slow cooker. Whisk the lemon juice, extra-virgin olive oil, honey, apple cider vinegar, salt, and pepper in a small bowl. Pour over the beets.
2. Add the sprigs of rosemary to the slow cooker. Cover and cook on low within 8 hours, or until the beets are tender. Remove and discard the rosemary sprigs. Stir in the lemon zest. Serve hot.

Nutrition:
Calories: 112 Carbs: 18g Fat: 4g Protein: 2g

957. Root Vegetable Tagine

Preparation time: 15 minutes Cooking time: 9 hours Servings: 8

1-pound parsnips, peeled and chopped into bite-size pieces
2 medium yellow onions, chopped into bite-size pieces
6 dried apricots, chopped
1 teaspoon ground turmeric
½ teaspoon ground ginger
¼ teaspoon cayenne pepper
1 tablespoon dried cilantro (or 2 tablespoons chopped fresh cilantro)

1-pound turnips, peeled and chopped into bite-size pieces
1-pound carrots, peeled and chopped into bite-size pieces
6 figs, chopped
1 teaspoon ground cumin
½ teaspoon ground cinnamon
1 tablespoon dried parsley
1¾ cups vegetable stock

1. Combine the parsnips, turnips, onions, carrots, apricots, and figs in the slow cooker. Sprinkle with turmeric, cumin, ginger, cinnamon, cayenne pepper, parsley, and cilantro. Pour in the vegetable stock. Cover and cook within 9 hours on low. Serve hot.

Nutrition:
Calories: 131 Carbs: 31g Fat: 1g Protein: 3g

958. Zucchini Casserole

Preparation time: 15 minutes Cooking time: hours Servings: 4

1 medium red onion, sliced
4 medium zucchinis, sliced

1 teaspoon of sea salt
½ teaspoon basil
¼ cup grated parmesan cheese

1 green bell pepper, thin strips
one 15-ounce can dice tomatoes, with the juice
½ teaspoon black pepper
1 tablespoon extra-virgin olive oil

1. Combine the onion slices, bell pepper strips, zucchini slices, and tomatoes in the slow cooker. Sprinkle with the salt, pepper, and basil.
2. Cover and cook on low within 3 hours. Drizzle the olive oil over the casserole and sprinkle with the Parmesan. Cover and cook on low within for 1½ hours more. Serve hot.

Nutrition:
Calories: 219 Carbs: 3g Fat: 16g Protein: 10g

959. Savory Butternut Squash and Apples

Preparation time: 15 minutes Cooking time: 4 hours Servings: 10

one 3-pound butternut squash, cubed
¾ cup dried currants

1 tablespoon ground cinnamon

4 cooking apples, peeled, cored, and chopped
½ sweet yellow onion such as Vidalia, sliced thin
1½ teaspoons ground nutmeg

Directions:
1. Combine the squash, apples, currants, and onion in the slow cooker. Sprinkle with the cinnamon and nutmeg. Cook on high within 4 hours, or until the squash is tender and cooked through. Stir while cooking, then serve.

Nutrition:
Calories: 300 Carbs: 129g Fat: 2g Protein: 6g

960. Stuffed Acorn Squash

Preparation time: 15 minutes Cooking time: 6 hours Servings: 4

1 acorn squash
1 tablespoon olive oil (not extra-virgin)
¼ cup chopped dried cranberries

1 tablespoon honey
¼ cup chopped pecans or walnuts

sea salt

1. Cut the squash in half. Discard the seeds and pulp from the middle. Cut the halves in half again to make it into quarters.
2. Place the squash quarters cut-side up in the slow cooker. Combine the honey, olive oil, pecans, and cranberries in a small bowl.
3. Spoon the pecan mixture into the center of each squash quarter. Season the squash with salt. Cook on low within 5 to 6 hours, or until the squash is tender. Serve hot.

Nutrition: Calories: 387 Carbs: 42g Fat: 19g Protein: 12g

SOUPS & STEWS

961. Baby - Spinach Soup with Nutmeg

Preparation time: 15 minutes Cooking time: 4 hours Servings: 4

2 tbsp. of olive oil	2 spring onions, sliced
2 garlic cloves, sliced	4 cups of water
1 lb. of baby spinach	Nutmeg, grated
1/4 cup lemon juice	4 tbsp. cream (optional)
Salt	ground black pepper

1. Warm-up oil over medium heat in a large saucepan and sauté onion for 4-5 minutes until soft. Put the onion plus garlic and sauté stirring for another 2 minutes.
2. Add the spinach and stir well; sauté for 2-3 minutes. Transfer the mixture to your Slow Cooker, pour water, lemon juice, and season salt and pepper to taste.
3. Cook on HIGH within 3-4 hours, stirring occasionally. Remove from heat and transfer soup in a blender and blend until smooth. Sprinkle with grated nutmeg. Taste and adjust the lemon juice and salt and pepper. Serve with cream (optional).

Nutrition:
Calories: 272 Carbs: 15g Fat: 20g Protein: 4g

962. Basilico Broccoli Soup

Preparation time: 15 minutes Cooking time: 4 hours Servings: 6

2 tbsp. olive oil	2 green onions finely chopped
2 cloves garlic, chopped	4 lbs. of broccoli, stems peeled and cut into chunks
2 small carrots shredded	2 tbsp. fresh basil finely chopped
1 tsp fresh ginger grated (inner part)	1 cup of water
2 cups of bone broth (preferably homemade)	salt and ground black pepper to taste

1. Place all the fixing in your Slow Cooker and stir well. Cook on LOW within 4 hours. Taste and adjust salt and pepper. Serve.

Nutrition:
Calories: 270 Carbs: 15g Fat: 17g Protein: 16g

963. Light Sour Artichokes

Preparation time: 15 minutes Cooking time: 4 hours Servings: 4

4 large artichoke hearts cleaned	2 tbsp. lard
1/3 cup lemon juice freshly squeezed	Water
Salt and ground black pepper to taste	fresh thyme finely chopped

1. Wash and clean artichokes. With the knife, trim the very bottom of the stem. Grease your Slow Cooker with lard and add artichokes, lemon juice, and season with salt and ground pepper.
2. Pour water enough to cover 3 of the artichokes. Cover the lid and cook on HIGH for 3-4 hours. Sprinkle with fresh thyme and serve.

Nutrition:
Calories: 124 Carbs: 14g Fat: 4g Protein: 10g

964. Cheesy Broccoli Soup

Preparation time: 15 minutes Cooking time: 4 hours Servings: 5

1 of broccoli, cut into medium-size pieces	2 of green onions finely chopped
2 cloves of garlic, chopped	2 cups bone broth (preferably homemade)
2 cups of water	1/4 cup butter melted
1 1/2 cups grated cheese	salt and ground black pepper to taste

1. Add broccoli, green onions, garlic, bone broth, and water in your Slow Cooker. Cover the lid and cook on LOW within 4 hours.
2. Transfer the soup to your high-fast blender, and add melted butter and shredded cheese. Blend until all ingredients combine well, smooth and creamy. Adjust the salt and pepper and serve.

Nutrition:
Calories: 140 Carbs: 13g Fat: 5g Protein: 10g

965. Creamish Chicken Soup with Broccoli

Preparation time: 15 minutes Cooking time: 5 hours Servings: 6

1 tbsp. of chicken fat melted	1 lb. of chicken breasts boneless skinless, cut into cubes
Salt	ground black pepper
4 cups of bone broth	1 green onion, finely chopped
4 tbsp. of almond flour	1 cup of heavy cream
3/4 cup of grated Parmesan	1 1/2 cups of shredded Cheddar
1 large head of broccoli, small florets	

1. Flavor the chicken breasts with salt plus pepper. Pour the chicken fat in your Slow Cooker and add the chicken cubes. Pour the bone broth and green onions. Cover and cook on LOW within 5 hours.
2. Combine the cooking broth, almond flour, cream, Parmesan, and Cheddar. Add broccoli flowerets in a Slow Cooker and pour the broth mixture. Cover and cook on HIGH for 30 to 45 minutes. Serve hot.

Nutrition:
Calories: 178 Carbs: 21g Fat: 4g Protein: 15g

966. Duck Breast Soup

Preparation time: 15 minutes Cooking time: 8 hours & 35 minutes Servings: 6

1 tbsp. of chicken fat	1 lb. of duck breasts boneless cut into pieces
1 carrot sliced	1 bell pepper (chopped)
2 spring onions sliced	1/2 lb. of fresh mushrooms
2 bay leaf	salt and ground black pepper to taste
1 tsp of paprika flakes	3 cups of bone broth or water
2 large eggs	3 tbsp. of sour cream
1/2 cup of parsley, chopped	

1. Add the chicken fat to your Slow Cooker. Flavor the duck meat with salt plus pepper, and place in Slow Cooker. Add carrots, pepper, spring onions, mushrooms, bay leaves, and paprika flakes; season with the salt and pepper and stir well.
2. Pour the bone broth and cover. Cook on LOW heat for 8 hours. Whisk the eggs with sour cream and a pinch of salt and pepper. Pour the mixture into a Slow Cooker. Sprinkle with chopped parsley and stir well. Cook on LOW again within 30 to 45 minutes. Serve hot.

Nutrition:
Calories: 277 Carbs: 23g Fat: 16g Protein: 10g

967. Green Garden Soup

Preparation time: 15 minutes Cooking time: 5 hours - Servings: 6

1 lb. of fresh spinach, rinsed and chopped	2 tbsp. of olive oil
1 large zucchini, sliced	1 carrot, sliced
1 green bell pepper, chopped	3 green onions finely chopped
1/2 tsp of paprika flakes	salt to taste
4 cups of water	

1. Rinse and chop spinach. Pour the oil into a Slow Cooker and add spinach; season with a little salt. Add all remaining ingredients and stir.

Cover and cook on LOW mode for 4 to 5 hours. Taste and adjust salt to taste. Serve.

Nutrition:: Calories: 29 Carbs: 6g Fat: 0g Protein: 2g

968. Meaty Swiss Chard Stew

Preparation time: 15 minutes Cooking time: 4 hours Servings: 4

3 tbsp. of olive oil	2 onions finely diced
Salt and ground pepper to taste	3/4 lbs. ground beef
3/4 lb. of Swiss chard chopped	1/2 cup water
1 tsp garlic powder	1 tsp ground cumin
1 cup of ground or crushed almonds	

1. Warm the oil in a large frying skillet and sauté onions with a pinch of salt. Add the ground meat and sauté for 2 minutes.
2. Add Swiss chard, water, and spices; stir for one minute and pour the mixture into your Slow Cooker. Sprinkle with almonds, stir, and cover. Cook on HIGH mode for 2 hours or on SLOW within 4 to 5 hours. Taste, adjust seasonings, and serve.

Nutrition:
Calories: 238 Carbs: 43g Fat: 1g Protein: 16g

969. Halibut and Shrimp Bisque

Preparation time: 15 minutes Cooking time: 9 hours Servings: 6

1 lb. of halibut fish	2 cups of frozen shrimp
2 cups of potatoes, small cubes	1 onion finely diced
1 cup carrot peeled	1 celery root
6 cloves of garlic	2 tsp half-and-half cream
3 cups of fish broth	Salt
ground black pepper	

1. Cut the fish and place with remaining ingredients (except the cream and the shrimp) into your Slow Cooker.
2. Cover and cook on LOW within 8-10 hours, or until the potatoes are tender. About 30 minutes before cooking time, stir in Slow Cooker a cup of cream and the frozen shrimp. Adjust the salt and pepper. Cook on HIGH within 30 minutes. Serve hot.

Nutrition:
Calories: 190 Carbs: 13g Fat: 10g Protein: 10g

970. Healthy Beef Stew

Preparation time: 15 minutes Cooking time: 8 hours & 45 minutes - Servings: 6

2 tbsp. of olive oil	1 1/2 lbs. beef stewing steak cut into large cubes
1 large tomato grated	2 green chili pepper, finely chopped
2 green onions (green parts only, sliced)	3 cloves garlic finely chopped
1 tbsp. dried oregano	2 tsp ground cumin
1 tsp of red paprika flakes	salt and ground red pepper to taste
1 cup of water	2 to 3 tbsp. breadcrumbs

1. Add all the listed fixing in your Slow Cooker (except breadcrumbs) and stir well. Cover lid and cook on LOW heat 8 hours, or until meat is tender. When ready, open the lid and add in the breadcrumbs; stir well. Cover and cook on LOW again within 30 to 45 minutes. Serve immediately.

Nutrition:
Calories: 170 Carbs: 0g Fat: 7g Protein: 24g

971. Slow Cooked Saffron-Marinated Cod Fillets

Preparation time: 15 minutes Cooking time: 3 hours - Servings: 4

4 Cod fillets without skin	½ cup of olive oil
generous pinch of saffron threads	2 splash of apple cider vinegar
fresh basil finely chopped, to garnish	1/2 tsp sea salt
1/2 tsp black pepper	

1. Combine olive oil, saffron threads, salt, pepper, and vinegar in a deep container. Add the fish fillets and toss well to coat. Sprinkle with a

pinch of ground pepper, cover, and leave to marinate in the fridge for about one hour.

2. Place the cod fillet in your Slow Cooker along with the marinade and cover lid. Cover and cook on LOW within 3 hours. Serve hot with chopped basil.

Nutrition:
Calories: 140 Carbs: 6g Fat: 5g Protein: 17g

972. Julienne Vegetable Soup

Preparation time: 15 minutes Cooking time: 2 hours - Servings: 5

1 carrot cut into julienne strips	1 turnip cut into julienne strips
7 oz. fresh beans cut into julienne strips	2 stalks celery
2 cloves garlic (finely minced)	1 onion finely sliced
2 cups of vegetable broth	2 cups of water
2 bay leaves	1 tsp of fresh thyme finely chopped
1 tsp of fresh basil finely chopped	Salt and ground pepper to taste

1. Cut vegetables into lengthwise julienne strips about 1/4 inch thick. Place all vegetables into Slow Cooker. Pour vegetable broth and water; stir and cover. Season with herbs/spices and with salt and pepper. Cover and cook on HIGH within 2 hours. Remove bay leaves, adjust seasonings, and serve.

Nutrition:
Calories: 70 Carbs: 10g Fat: 3g Protein: 2g

973. Spanish Chorizo and Clams Stew

Preparation time: 15 minutes Cooking time: 40 minutes - Servings: 6

2 tbsp. olive oil	2 onions finely diced
2 cloves of garlic, mashed	12 oz. of Spanish chorizo sausages, finely diced
2 potatoes	5 lbs. clams, rinsed in cold water
2 tbsp. of tomato paste or grated fresh tomato	1 cup of beef broth
1 1 tsp fresh thyme, chopped	2 tsp smoked paprika
Sea salt	ground black pepper

1. Warm olive oil in a frying skillet and sauté the onion and garlic with a pinch of salt. Add sliced chorizo sausages and tomato paste. Cook on medium heat for 5 minutes. Transfer the mixture and all remaining ingredients into your Slow Cooker and add clams; toss to combine well.
2. Pour the beef broth, fresh thyme, and smoked paprika; stir and cover. Season with the salt and pepper; stir. Cook on HIGH for about 30 to 35 minutes or until clams are tender. Serve hot.

Nutrition:
Calories: 166 Carbs: 11g Fat: 6g Protein: 15g

974. Stringing Nettle and Chicken Soup

Preparation time: 15 minutes Cooking time: 4 hours & 45 minutes - Servings: 6

1 tbsp. of chicken fat	2 chicken breasts, cut into pieces
1 carrot sliced	2 onions, sliced
1 bell pepper, chopped	1/2 lb. of nettle cleaned and chopped
1 tbsp. of fresh thyme finely chopped	3 cups of water
salt and ground black pepper to taste	2 eggs from free-range chicken
1 tbsp. of red paprika flakes	

1. Add chicken fat to your Slow Cooker. Add chicken, carrot, onions, bell pepper, nettle, and fresh thyme. Flavor with the salt and pepper, pour water, and stir well. Cover and cook on LOW for 4 hours. Mix the eggs with salt plus paprika flakes, and pour into Slow Cooker. Cover again, and cook on LOW for an additional 30 to 45 minutes. Serve.

Nutrition:: Calories: 121 Carbs: 20g Fat: 3g Protein: 4g

SNACKS

975. Piedmont Fontina Cheese Dip with Truffle Oil Fonduta

Preparation time: 15 minutes Cooking time: 2 hours Servings: 4

4 tsp corn flour (cornstarch)	2/3 cup milk
2 large eggs	1½ cups grated Fontina cheese
2 tbsp. unsalted (sweet) butter, cut into small flakes	Salt and freshly ground black pepper
6 tbsp. single (light) cream	1 tsp truffle oil

1. Whisk the corn flour and milk in a small earthenware pot that will fit in the slow cooker. Whisk in the eggs. Stir in the cheese and add the butter and some salt and pepper. Stand the dish in the crockpot with boiling water to come halfway up the side of the dish.
2. Cover and cook on Low within 2 hours or until thick, stirring well every 30 minutes. Remove from the crockpot and beat well, then beat in the cream. Trickle the truffle oil over and serve straight away with ciabatta bread cut into small chunks for dunking.

Nutrition:
Calories: 120 Carbs: 0g Fat: 12g Protein: 2g

976. Coarse Pork Terrine with Pistachios

Preparation time: 15 minutes Cooking time: 10 hours Servings: 10

12 rashers (slices) of streaky bacon	1 Onion, quartered
2 Garlic cloves, roughly chopped	6 sprigs of fresh parsley
1 lb. belly pork, skinned	4 oz. unsmoked bacon pieces, trimmed of any rind or gristle
12 oz. pig's liver	1 tsp dried herbes de Provence
¼ tsp ground cloves	A good pinch of cayenne
2 tbsp. brandy	¾ cup shelled pistachio nuts
1½ tsp salt	Freshly ground black pepper

1. Line a 6-cup terrine or large loaf tin with some bacon rashers, trimming to fit as necessary. Using a food processor or mincer (grinder), process the onion, garlic, parsley, pork, bacon pieces, and liver but not too finely.
2. Stir in the dried herbs, spices, brandy, pistachios, salt, and a good grinding of pepper. Turn into the prepared terrine and level.
3. Top with the remaining bacon. Cover with greaseproof (waxed) paper, then a lid or foil, twisting and folding it under the rim to secure. Stand the terrine in the crockpot with boiling water to come halfway up of the terrine.
4. Cover and cook on Low within 8-10 hours until firm to the touch and the juices are clear. Remove from the crockpot and remove the cover.
5. Top with some clean greaseproof paper and weigh down with heavy weights or cans of food. Leave until cold, then chill. Serve sliced with crusty bread, mustard, and a side salad.

Nutrition:
Calories: 97 Carbs: 3g Fat: 5g Protein: 9g

977. Chicken Liver Pâté with Button Mushrooms

Preparation time: 15 minutes Cooking time: 8 hours Servings: 10

1 onion, peeled and quartered	2 garlic cloves, peeled and roughly chopped
1 lb. chicken liver, trimmed	2 tbsp. brandy
½ tsp dried mixed herbs 2	1 cup butter, melted
4 tbsp. double (heavy) cream	1 egg, beaten
Salt and freshly ground black pepper	6 oz. button mushrooms, sliced
Mixed salad leaves and lemon	

wedges to garnish

1. Place the onion, garlic, liver, brandy, herbs, three-quarters of butter, cream, and egg in a blender or food processor. Season generously and run the machine to make a smooth paste.
2. Put the remaining melted butter in a saucepan, add the mushrooms, and fry, stirring, for 3 minutes until tender. Turn up the heat, if necessary, to evaporate the liquid. Stir into the pâté mixture.
3. Grease a 6-cup terrine or large loaf tin and line the base with non-stick baking parchment. Spoon the pâté into the tin and level the surface.
4. Cover with greaseproof (waxed) paper, then a lid or foil, twisting and folding under the rim to secure, and place in the slow cooker with enough boiling water to come halfway up the sides of the terrine.
5. Cover and cook on Low within 6-8 hours until firm to the touch. Remove from the crockpot. Remove the lid or foil and re-cover with clean greaseproof paper.
6. Leave to cool, then weigh down with heavy weights or cans of food and chill until firm. Loosen the edge and move it onto a cutting board.
7. Cut into thick slices and arrange on individual plates. Garnish each with a few salad leaves and a lemon wedge and serve with triangles of toast.

Nutrition:
Calories: 200 Carbs: 5g Fat: 17g Protein: 3g

978. Warm Tuscan White Bean Salad

Preparation time: 15 minutes Cooking time: 8 hours Servings: 6

11/3 cup dried haricot (navy) beans, soaked in cold water for several hours or overnight	4¼ cups boiling water
4 slices of Parma (or similar raw) ham, diced 5	1/3 cup black olives
1 red onion, thinly sliced	2 sun-dried tomatoes, chopped
1 red (bell) pepper, chopped	2 tsp chopped fresh rosemary
1 tbsp. chopped fresh basil	1 garlic clove, crushed 6
4 tbsp. olive oil	2 tbsp. white balsamic condiment
Salt and freshly ground black pepper	

1. Drain the beans and boil in a saucepan with water. Return to the boil and boil rapidly for 10 minutes. Tip the beans and liquid into the crockpot, cover, and cook on Low for 6-8 hours until the beans are tender.
2. When ready to serve, drain the beans in a colander and tip into a large salad bowl. Put all the rest of the fixing and season well. Toss well and serve while still warm with ciabatta bread.

Nutrition:
Calories: 321 Carbs: 28g Fat: 20g Protein: 9g

979. Stuffed Garlic Mushrooms with Cream and White Wine

Preparation time: 15 minutes Cooking time: 7 hours Servings: 4

1½ cups soft breadcrumbs	2 spring onions (scallions), finely chopped
2 large garlic cloves, crushed	3 tbsp. chopped fresh parsley
Salt and freshly ground black pepper	1 egg, beaten
2/3 cup dry white wine 8 tiny knobs of butter	2/3 cup double (heavy) cream
4 small sprigs of fresh parsley to garnish	

1. Peel the mushrooms and trim the stalks. Chop the stalks and mix with the breadcrumbs, spring onions, half the garlic, and the parsley. Season well, then mix with the beaten egg.
2. Season the mushroom caps lightly, then press the stuffing mixture onto the gills of each one. Put the wine into the crockpot, add the remaining garlic and a little salt and pepper.

3. Place the mushrooms on top, preferably in a single layer or just overlapping. Top each with a tiny knob of butter.
4. Cover and cook on Low within 5-7 hours until the mushrooms are tender and the stuffing has set. Transfer the mushrooms to small warm plates. Stir the cream into the wine juices, taste, re-season if necessary, and then spoon over. Garnish each plate with a small sprig of parsley and serve with crusty bread.

Nutrition:
Calories: 138 Carbs: 5g Fat: 10g Protein: 4g

980.   Spanish Tortilla with Piquant Tomato Salsa

Preparation time: 15 minutes Cooking time: 6 hours Servings: 4

For the tortilla:	6 tbsp. olive oil
2 onions, thinly sliced	4 large potatoes, thinly sliced
6 eggs	Salt and freshly ground black pepper
For the salsa:	1 tbsp. olive oil
1 small onion, chopped	1 garlic clove, crushed
¼ tsp crushed dried chilies	4 beefsteak tomatoes, skinned and chopped
4 tbsp. apple juice	½ tsp dried oregano
2 tbsp. chopped fresh parsley	

1. To make the tortilla, brush the crockpot with a little of the oil. Warm-up the rest of the oil in a saucepan, add the onions, and fry for 2 minutes, stirring.
2. Add the potatoes and toss well. Cook for within 2 minutes, stirring, then tip the whole lot into the crockpot (keep the pan for making the salsa). Put the mixture as evenly as possible.
3. Cover and cook on Low for 46 hours until the potatoes are tender. Turn the slow cooker to High. Whisk the eggs with salt plus pepper and pour into the pot. Stir well, then cover and cook for 30 minutes until set.
4. Meanwhile, to make the salsa, heat the oil in a saucepan. Put the onion and garlic and cook within 2 minutes until they are softened but not browned. Put all the rest of the fixing except the parsley. Cook rapidly for 5 minutes until pulpy, stirring frequently.
5. Move it to a blender, then blend to a purée. Taste and re-season if necessary, then return to the pan. Reheat when ready to serve. When the tortilla is cooked, remove the crockpot from the base and leave the tortilla cool for 5 minutes. Cut into wedges.
6. Spoon the salsa on to warm plates and place one or two wedges of tortilla on top. Sprinkle with the chopped parsley and serve.

Nutrition:
Calories: 140 Carbs: 18g Fat: 3g Protein: 10g

981. Vine Leaves Stuffed with Rice, Herbs, Pine Nuts, and Raisins

Preparation time: 15 minutes Cooking time: 7 hours Servings: 24

½ cup pine nuts	1/3 cup raisins
½ cup short-grain (pudding) rice	1 garlic clove, crushed
1 small onion, finely chopped	1 tsp dried oregano
1 tsp dried mint	1 tbsp. tomato purée (paste)
½ tsp salt Freshly ground black pepper	½ tsp ground cinnamon
24 vacuum-packed vine leaves, rinsed and dried	5 tbsp. olive oil
Juice of ½ lemon	3 cups boiling vegetable stock

1. Mix the pine nuts with the raisins, uncooked rice, garlic, onion, herbs, tomato purée, salt, lots of pepper, and cinnamon. Put a filling on each vine leaf, fold in the sides, and roll-up. Pack them tightly into the crockpot.
2. Add the oil and lemon juice, then pour over enough of the boiling stock to cover the vine leaves. Cover and cook on Low within 6-7 hours or until the rice is cooked and most of the liquid has been absorbed.
3. Remove the crockpot from the base and leave the vine leaves to cool in the liquid. Transfer the rolls to a serving platter with a draining spoon and serve at room temperature.

Nutrition:
Calories: 170 Carbs: 24g Fat: 2g Protein: 3g

982.   Spanish Mackerel with Roasted Red Peppers

Preparation time: 15 minutes Cooking time: 2 hours Servings: 4

1 large onion, halved and thinly sliced	2 celery sticks, cut into thin matchsticks
2 garlic cloves, finely chopped	2 cloves
2 bay leaves	4 small mackerel, filleted
2/3 cup dry white wine	6 tablespoon of olive oil, plus extra for drizzling
1 tsp light brown sugar	Salt and freshly ground black pepper
4 red (bell) peppers	4 small fresh bay leaves, to garnish

1. Spread out the onion and celery in the crockpot and sprinkle with the garlic. Add the cloves and bay leaves. Cut the mackerel fillets in halves lengthways and lay them on top, preferably in a single layer or, if not, divided by non-stick baking parchment.
2. Heat the wine, oil, and sugar with a little salt and pepper. Bring to the boil and pour over the mackerel. Cover and cook on Low within 2 hours until the mackerel is tender. Remove the pot, and leave to cool but do not chill.
3. Meanwhile, put the peppers under a preheated grill (broiler) and cook, occasionally turning, for about 15 minutes until the skin has blackened. Put the peppers to rub off the skin in a plastic bag. Discard the stalks and seeds, then cut the flesh into thin strips.
4. Lift the mackerel out of the cooking liquid and discard the cloves and bay leaves. Drain the onion and celery and arrange a small pile on each of four small plates.
5. Top each with two mackerel fillets, then a small pile of red pepper strips. Drizzle with olive oil, garnish each with a small bay leaf, and serve with crusty bread.

Nutrition:
Calories: 134 Carbs: 0g Fat: 5g Protein: 20g

DESSERTS

983. Apple Olive Cake

Preparation time: 15 minutes Cooking time: 2 hours Servings: 4

Peeled and chopped Gala apples - 2 large	Ground cinnamon - ½ teaspoon
Whole wheat flour - 3 cups	Orange juice – 2 cups
Baking powder - 1 teaspoon	Ground nutmeg - ½ teaspoon
Sugar - 1 cup	Baking soda - 1 teaspoon
Large eggs - 2	Extra virgin olive oil - 1 cup
Gold raisins, soaked and drained - 2/3 cup	Confectioner's sugar - for dusting purpose

1. In a small bowl, soak the gold raisins in lukewarm water for 15 minutes and drain. Keep aside. Put the chopped apple in a medium bowl and pour orange juice over it. Toss and make sure the apple gets well coated with the orange juice
2. Combine cinnamon, flour, baking powder, nutmeg in a large bowl and keep aside. Add extra virgin olive oil and sugar into the mixture and combine thoroughly.
3. In the large bowl that contains the dry ingredients, make a circular path in the middle part of the flour mixture. Add the olive oil and sugar mixture into this path. Make use of a wooden spoon and stir them well until they blend well with one another. It must be a thick batter.
4. Drain the excess juice from the apples. Add the apples and raisins to the batter and mix it with a spoon to combine. In a six-quart slow cooker, place parchment paper and add the batter over it.
5. Turn the heat setting to low and the timer to two hours or cook until the cake does not have any wet spots over it. Once the cake has cooked well, wait until the cake cools down before cutting them into pieces. Move your cake to a serving dish and sprinkle confectioner's sugar on top.

Nutrition:
Calories: 294 Carbohydrate: 47.7g Protein: 5.3g Sugars: 23.5g Fat: 11g Fiber: 4.3g

984. Strawberry Basil Cobbler

Preparation time: 15 minutes Cooking time: 2 hours & 30 minutes Servings: 5

Divided granulated sugar - 1¼ cups	Divided whole wheat flour - 2½ cups
Ground cinnamon - ½ teaspoon	Baking powder - 2 teaspoons
Skim milk - ½ cup	Eggs - 2
Divided salt - ¼ teaspoon	Canola oil - 4 tablespoons
Rolled oats - ¼ cup	Frozen strawberries - 6 cups
Vanilla frozen yogurt – 3 cups	Chopped fresh basil - ¼ cup
Cooking spray – as required	

1. Mix the sugar, flour, baking powder, salt, plus cinnamon in a large bowl. Add milk, oil, and eggs into the bowl and combine thoroughly. Coat some olive oil in the bottom of the slow cooker. Transfer and spread the mixed batter evenly into the slow cooker.
2. Take another large bowl and combine flour, salt, and sugar. Add basil and strawberries to the bowl and toss it to coat. Put this batter on the top of the batter in the slow cooker. Top up with the rolled oat mixture. Cook on a high heat within 2½ hours. Serve topped with frozen vanilla yogurt and basil.

Nutrition:
Calories: 727 Carbohydrate: 126.8g Sugars: 70.4g Fat: 16.2g Fiber: 5.9g Sodium: 262mg Protein: 19.6g Potassium: 962mg

985. Pumpkin Pecan Bread Pudding

Preparation time: 15 minutes Cooking time: 4 hours Servings: 3

Chopped toasted pecans - ½ cup	Day-old whole-wheat bread cubes - 8 cups
Eggs - 4	Cinnamon chips - ½ cup
Half n half - 1 cup	Canned pumpkin - 1 cup

Melted butter - ½ cup	Brown sugar - ½ cup
Cinnamon - ½ teaspoon	Vanilla - 1 teaspoon
Ground ginger - ¼ teaspoon	Nutmeg - ½ teaspoon
Vanilla ice cream - ¼ cup	Ground cloves – 1/8 teaspoon
Caramel ice cream topping - ¼ cup	

1. Grease a 6-quart crockpot and put the bread cubes, cinnamon, and chopped pecans into it. In a medium bowl, whisk pumpkin, eggs, brown sugar, half-n-half, vanilla, melted butter, nutmeg, cinnamon, cloves, ginger, and pour the mixture over the bread cubes. Stir the mix gently.
2. Cover up the slow cooker and cook for 4 hours. It will be well prepared within 4 hours, which you can check by inserting a toothpick, and if it comes clean, it is ready to serve. Before serving, top up with caramel ice cream and vanilla ice cream.

Nutrition:
Calories: 289 Carbohydrate: 28g Protein: 6g Sugars: 14g Fat: 17g Fiber: 1g Sodium: 216 mg Potassium: 166mg

986. Chocolate Fondue

Preparation time: 15 minutes Cooking time: 2 hours Servings: 3

Chocolate Almonds candy bars	4½ ounces
Butter	1½ tablespoons
Milk	3 tablespoons
Miniature marshmallows	1½ cup
Heavy whipping cream	½ cup

1. Grease a 2-quart slow cooker and put chocolate, butter, milk, marshmallows into it. Close the cooker and cook on low heat setting for 1½ hours. Stir the mix every 30 minutes to melt and mix whipping cream gradually. After adding whipping cream, allow it to settle for 2 hours. Use it as a chocolate dip.

Nutrition:
Calories: 463 Carbohydrate: 3901g Protein: 5.5g Sugars: 29.4g Fat: 31.8g Fiber: 4.5g Sodium: 138mg Potassium: 30mg

987. Chocolate Orange Volcano Pudding

Preparation time: 15 minutes Cooking time: 2 hours Servings: 6

Self-rising flour – ½ pound	Melted butter - 3½ ounces
Sifted cocoa - 2¾ ounces	Caster sugar - 5¼ ounces
Zest and juice of orange - 1	Baking powder - 1 teaspoon
Orange flavored milk chocolate, chopped into chunks - 5¼ ounces	Milk - 1½ cup
Salt – a pinch	Water – 2 cups
For the Sauce:	Cocoa – 1 ounce
Light brown soft sugar - 7½ ounces	**Topping:**
Vanilla ice cream - ¼ cup	Orange wedges – 1 orange
Cream - ¼ cup	

1. Grease the slow cooker with butter. Combine the caster sugar, flour, baking powder, and cocoa, pinch of salt, and orange zest in a large mixing bowl thoroughly. Whisk the eggs, orange juice, milk, and buttermilk in a medium bowl. Put it to the dry fixing and combine to form a smooth mixture.
2. Stir in chocolate pieces and then transfer the mixture into the slow cooker. Prepare the sauce by mixing cocoa and sugar in two cups of boiling water. Pour the sauce over the pudding mixture. Cook on a high heat within two hours. Before serving, top the pudding with vanilla ice cream or cream and orange wedges.

Nutrition: Calories: 733 Carbohydrate: 120.8g Protein: 11.8g Sugars: 79.3g Fat: 25.4g Fiber: 8.3g Cholesterol: 48mg Sodium: 259mg Potassium: 607mg

988. Nutella Fudge

Preparation time: 15 minutes Cooking time: 1 hour & 30 minutes Servings: 5

Vanilla essence - 1 teaspoon	Condensed milk – 14 ounces
70 percent dark chocolate - 7 0unces	Nutella - 1 cup
Chopped toasted hazelnuts - 4 ounces	Icing sugar - 3 ounces

1. In a slow cooker, add vanilla essence, condensed milk, dark chocolate, and Nutella. Cook it for 1½ hours without covering the lid. Make sure to stir the ingredients every ten minutes until they melt completely. Transfer its content into a large-sized mixing bowl
2. Stir in the sieved icing sugar. Take the warm fudge and carefully scrape it flat, and allow it cool. Sprinkle the hazelnuts over the fudge and slightly press them downwards so that they get attached well. Refrigerate this well for 4 hours and then cut them into squares.

Nutrition:
Calories: 191 Carbohydrate: 24.7g Protein: 3.2g Sugars: 22.4g Fat: 9.3gFiber: 1.4g Cholesterol: 5mg Sodium: 25mg

989. Greek Yogurt Chocolate Mousse

Preparation time: 15 minutes Cooking time: 2 hours Servings: 4

Dark chocolate	3½ ounces
Milk	¾ cup
Maple syrup	1 tablespoon
Greek yogurt	2 cups
Vanilla extract	½ teaspoon

1. Pour milk into a glass bowl that can be placed inside the slow cooker. Add the chocolate, either as finely chopped or as a grated one, into the glass bowl. Place the bowl inside the slow cooker. Pour water surrounding the bowl. Cook it within 2 hours on low heat by stirring intermittently.
2. Once the chocolate is combined thoroughly with the milk, turn off the cooker and remove the slow cooker's glass bowl. Put the vanilla extract plus maple syrup in the bowl and stir well. Spoon the Greek yogurt in a large bowl and add the chocolate mixture on top of it. Mix it well before serving. Refrigerate for two hours before serving.

Nutrition:
Calories: 170 Carbohydrate: 20.4g Protein: 3.4g Sugars: 17.9g Fat: 8.3g Fiber: 0.8g Sodium: 42mg Potassium: 130mg

990. Peanut Butter Banana Greek Yogurt Bowl

Preparation time: 15 minutes Cooking time: 2 hours Servings: 4

Sliced bananas	2
Vanilla Greek yogurt	4 cups
Flaxseed meal	¼ cup
Creamy natural peanut butter	¼ cup
Nutmeg	1 teaspoon

1. Divide the yogurt between four different bowls and top it with banana slices. Add peanut butter into a small-sized glass bowl and place it in the slow cooker. Pour water surrounding the glass bowl. Under low heat setting, cook without covering the slow cooker until the peanut butter starts to melt.
2. Once the butter turns to the required thickness, remove the bowl from the slow cooker. Now, scoop one tablespoon of melted peanut butter and serve into the bowl with yogurt and bananas. For each bowl, add about one tablespoon of melted peanut butter. Sprinkle ground nutmeg and flaxseed.

Nutrition:
Calories: 187 Carbohydrate: 19g Protein: 6g Sugars: 9g Fat: 10.7g Fiber: 4.5g Sodium: 77mg Potassium: 375mg

991. Banana Foster

Preparation time: 15 minutes Cooking time: 2 hours Servings: 4

Bananas – 4	Butter, melted – 4 tablespoons
Rum - ¼ cup	Brown sugar – 1 cup
Cinnamon, ground - ½ teaspoon	Vanilla extract – 1 teaspoon
Coconut, shredded - ¼ cup	Walnuts, chopped - ¼ cup

Directions:
1. Peel the bananas, slice, and keep ready to use. Place the sliced bananas in the slow cooker in layers. Mix the brown sugar, vanilla, butter, rum, and cinnamon in a medium bowl thoroughly. Pour the mix over the bananas. Cook on low heat for 2 hours. Sprinkle shredded coconut and walnuts on top before 30 of the end processes.

Nutrition:
Calories: 539 Carbohydrates: 83.7g Cholesterol: 31mg Fiber: 4.7g Protein: 3g Potassium: 567mg Sodium: 101mgSugars: 69g

992. Rice Pudding

Preparation time: 15 minutes Cooking time: 2 hours Servings: 8

Glutinous white rice, uncooked – 1 cup	Evaporated milk – 12 ounces
Cinnamon stick – 1 ounce	White sugar – 1 cup
Nutmeg, ground – 1 teaspoon	Vanilla extract – 1 teaspoon

1. In a 6-quart slow cooker, put all the ingredients. Cover the lid and cook on low heat for 1½ hours. Stir while cooking in progress. Once ready, discard the cinnamon stick and serve.

Nutrition:
Calories: 321 Carbohydrates: 56.4g Cholesterol: 24mg Fiber: 2.6g Protein: 8.2g Sodium: 102mg Potassium: 322mg Sugars: 35g

993. Bittersweet Cocoa Almond Cake

Preparation time: 15 minutes Cooking time: 2 hours & 30 minutes Servings: 8

4 tablespoons (½ stick) unsalted butter, melted and cooled, plus more for the pan	½ cup whole almonds (with skins), lightly toasted
1¼ cups Dutch-process cocoa	1 cup of water
1 teaspoon vanilla extract	¾ cup of sugar
3 large eggs, plus 2 egg whites	Pinch of salt
2 tablespoons sliced almonds (with skins)	Whipped cream

1. Butter a 6-cup soufflé dish. Arrange the bottom of the dish with wax paper, then butter the paper. Place a rack in a large slow cooker. Put the whole almonds in your food processor fitted with the steel blade. Process until finely ground. Remove from the processor.
2. Put the cocoa, water, and vanilla into the processor and process until smooth. Add the 4 tablespoons melted butter and ½ cup of the sugar and mix well for about 30 seconds. While the machine is running, put the whole eggs, one at a time, and process until smooth, about 30 seconds more. Stir in the ground almonds.
3. Whisk the egg whites plus the salt on medium speed until light and fluffy in a large bowl with an electric mixer. Adjust the speed to high and beat in the remaining ¼ cup sugar until soft peaks form about 3 minutes. Mix the cocoa batter into the egg white mixture. Scrape the batter into the prepared dish.
4. Put it on the rack of your slow cooker, then pour hot water about 1 inch. Cook on high within 2½ hours, or until just set. Carefully remove the dish from the cooker. Let cool for 20 minutes.
5. Cover with an inverted bowl and refrigerate for several hours or overnight. Just before serving, sprinkle the cake with the sliced almonds. Slice and serve with whipped cream.

Nutrition:
Calories: 276 Carbs: 20g Fat: 19g Protein: 0g

994. Apricot Almond Cake

Preparation time: 15 minutes Cooking time: 3 hours Servings: 8

4 tablespoons (½ stick) unsalted butter, softened, plus more for the pan	1 cup whole almond (with skins), toasted
1 cup of sugar	½ cup all-purpose flour
¼ teaspoon baking powder	4 large eggs, at room temperature
1 teaspoon vanilla extract	¼ teaspoon almond extract
Apricot Glaze:	1/3 cup apricot jam
2 tablespoons sugar	2–3 tablespoons sliced almonds (with skins), toasted

1. Butter a 7-x-2-inch round cake pan. Put wax paper in the pan and butter the paper. Put a rack in a large slow cooker. Put 2 cups of hot water into the cooker and turn on.
2. Mix the whole almonds and ¼ cup of the sugar in a food processor. Process just until very finely ground, about 1 minute. Put the flour plus baking powder, pulse 2 or 3 times to blend.
3. Whisk the 4 tablespoons butter and the remaining ¾ cup sugar on medium speed until very light and fluffy in a large bowl using an electric mixer. Whisk in the eggs, one at a time, until smooth and well blended. Scrape down the sides of the bowl.
4. Beat in the vanilla and almond extracts. With a rubber spatula, fold in the ground almond mixture. Scrape the batter into the prepared pan. Place the cake pan in the slow cooker. Cook on high within 3 hours. Remove, then let cool for 10 minutes.
5. Make the apricot glaze: Heat the jam and sugar in a small saucepan over medium heat. When the mixture starts to simmer, stir well until melted. Strain the glaze through a fine-mesh sieve into a small bowl, pressing on the solids.
6. Put the glaze over the top of the cake and spread it smooth. Sprinkle the sliced almonds in a border around the top edge of the cake. Let cool before serving.

Nutrition:
Calories: 228 Carbs: 7g Fat: 19g Protein: 8g

995. Walnut Cake with Cinnamon Syrup

Preparation time: 15 minutes Cooking time: 2 hours & 20 minutes Servings: 8

Unsalted butter for the pan	1 cup toasted walnuts
½ cup of sugar	½ cup all-purpose flour
1 teaspoon baking powder	1 teaspoon ground cinnamon
½ teaspoon grated lemon zest	Pinch of salt
2 large eggs, plus 1 egg yolk	½ cup plain Greek-style yogurt
¼ cup olive oil	**Cinnamon Syrup:**
1 cup of sugar	½ cup of water
1 3-inch cinnamon stick	1 2-inch strip lemon zest

1. Butter a 7-x-2-inch round cake pan or a 6-cup soufflé dish. Arrange the bottom of the pan with wax paper plus butter the paper. Put a rack in a large slow cooker. Pour 2 cups hot water into the cooker, and turn on the cooker.
2. Mix the walnuts and ¼ cup of the sugar in a food processor within 1 minute. Add the flour, baking powder, ground cinnamon, lemon zest, and salt. Pulse 2 or 3 times to blend.
3. In another bowl, whisk the whole eggs, the egg yolk, the remaining ¼ cup sugar, the yogurt, and olive oil. Stir in the dry ingredients. Scrape the batter into the prepared pan. Put the cake pan on the rack in the slow cooker. Cook on high within 2¼ hours. Let it cool.
4. For the cinnamon syrup, mix all the syrup ingredients in a small saucepan. Simmer within 10 minutes, or until slightly thickened. Let cool.
5. Slide the cake onto a serving dish. Remove the cinnamon stick and the lemon zest from the syrup. Pour the syrup over the cake. Let it stand within 1 hour before serving so that the cake can absorb some of the syrup.

Nutrition:
Calories: 260 Carbs: 32g Fat: 13g Protein: 3g

996. Sunny Orange Cake with Orange Syrup

Preparation time: 15 minutes Cooking time: 2 hours & 30 minutes Servings: 8

4 tablespoons (½ stick) unsalted butter, softened, plus more for the pan	½ cup all-purpose flour
½ cup fine semolina or farina	1 teaspoon baking powder
½ cup of sugar	2 large eggs, separated
1 teaspoon vanilla extract	½ teaspoon grated orange zest
½ cup whole milk	Pinch of salt
Orange Syrup:	¾ cup of sugar
¾ cup of orange juice	½ teaspoon grated orange zest
Fresh orange slices and mint leaves	

1. Put a rack in a large slow cooker. Butter a round cake pan. Line the bottom of the pan with wax paper and butter the paper. Stir the flour, semolina, and baking powder. Whisk the 4 tablespoons butter and the sugar in a large bowl using an electric mixer on medium speed within 2 minutes.
2. Put the egg yolks, then beat until light, about 3 minutes. Beat in the vanilla and orange zest. Put the flour batter in 3 additions, alternating with the milk and beginning and ending with the flour.
3. Beat the egg whites and the salt in a medium bowl on medium speed until soft peaks form. Fold the egg whites with the semolina mixture. Scrape the mixture into the prepared pan. Place the pan on in the slow cooker. Put the hot water around the cake pan to a depth of 1 inch. Cook on high within 2 to 2½ hours.
4. For the orange syrup, combine the sugar and orange juice in a small saucepan. Simmer the mixture within 5 minutes. Stir in the orange zest. Remove from the heat and let cool.
5. Slowly put the orange syrup on the cake. Let it set within 1 hour so that the cake can absorb some of the syrup. Serve with the orange slices and mint leaves.

Nutrition:
Calories: 300 Carbs: 36g Fat: 15g Protein: 7g

997. Two-Berry Clafouti

Preparation time: 15 minutes Cooking time: 2 hours Servings: 6

2 cups fresh blueberries	1 cup fresh raspberry
1 3-ounce package cream cheese, softened	½ cup of sugar
3 large eggs	½ cup milk
½ teaspoon grated lemon or orange zest	¼ cup all-purpose flour
Confectioners' sugar for sprinkling	

1. Oiled the insert of a large slow cooker with nonstick cooking spray. Scatter the berries in the slow cooker. Mix the cream cheese and sugar in a blender. Add the eggs, milk, and zest and blend well. Put the flour and blend within 1 minute. Pour the mixture over the berries.
2. Cook on high within 1½ to 2 hours, or until the clafouti is slightly puffed and the center jiggles slightly when the sides are tapped. Allow cooling to room temperature. Scoop onto serving plates and serve, sprinkled with confectioners' sugar.

Nutrition:
Calories: 200 Carbs: 6g Fat: 0g Protein: 0g

998. Cannoli Cheesecake

Preparation time: 15 minutes Cooking time: 2 hours & 30 minutes Servings: 8

Unsalted butter for the pan	1 15- to 16-ounce container whole-milk ricotta
6 ounces cream cheese, softened	2/3 cup confectioners' sugar
½ teaspoon ground cinnamon	1 teaspoon vanilla extract
2 large eggs	½ cup miniature semisweet chocolate chips
2 tablespoons chopped candied orange peel or 1 teaspoon grated orange zest	½ cup coarsely chopped unsalted pistachios

1. Put a rack in a large slow cooker. Butter a 7-inch pan. Put the pan in the center of an aluminum foil and wrap the foil around the sides so that water cannot enter.
2. Whisk the ricotta and cream cheese with the confectioners' sugar, cinnamon, and vanilla until very smooth, about 5 minutes in a food processor. Add the eggs and process until blended, about 2 minutes.
3. With a spoon, lightly stir in the chocolate chips and candied orange peel. Pour the mixture into the prepared pan. Put hot water around the pan. Cook on high within 2½ hours. Press the pistachios onto the sides of the cake. Cut into wedges and serve.

Nutrition:
Calories: 358 Carbs: 36g Fat: 20g Protein: 12

999.   Chocolate Hazelnut Cheesecake

Preparation time: 15 minutes Cooking time: hours Servings: 8

3 tbsp. dissolved unsalted butter, plus more for the pan	2/3 cup chocolate wafer, cookie crumbs
1 15- to 16-ounce container whole-milk ricotta	2/3 cup Nutella or other chocolate hazelnut spread
¼ cup of sugar	2 large eggs

1. Put a rack in a slow cooker. Butter a 7-inch pan. Put the pan in the center of a large sheet of aluminum foil and wrap it around the sides so that water cannot enter. Mix the cookie crumbs, and the 3 tablespoons melted butter in a small bowl. Put the mixture firmly into the base of the prepared pan. Place the pan in the refrigerator.
2. Beat the ricotta and Nutella with the sugar until very smooth, about 2 minutes in a food processor. Put the eggs, one at a time, and process until blended. Pour the mixture into the pan. Put the pan on the rack of your slow cooker. Put hot water to a depth of about 1 inch around the pan. Cook on high within 2½ hours. Cut into wedges and serve.

Nutrition:
Calories: 210 Carbs: 22g Fat: 13g Protein: 1g

1000.   Coffee Caramel Flan

Preparation time: 15 minutes Cooking time: 2 hours & 30 minutes Servings: 8

1 cup of sugar	¼ cup of water
1 12-ounce can evaporate milk	1 14-ounce can sweeten condensed milk
2 large eggs, plus 2 egg yolks	2 tbsp. espresso powder melted in 1 tablespoon hot water

1. Put a rack in your large slow cooker. Mix the sugar plus water in a small saucepan. Cook over medium heat within 5 minutes. Simmer the mixture within 10 minutes.
2. Put the hot syrup into a 6-cup soufflé dish, then let it cool. Whisk the evaporated milk and condensed milk in a medium bowl. Beat in the eggs, yolks, and espresso until blended. Pour the mixture into the soufflé dish.
3. Put the dish on the rack in your slow cooker. Put hot water to a depth of 1 inch around. Cook on high within 2 to 2½ hours. Let it cool, and refrigerate within several hours or overnight. Carefully remove the dish. Cut into wedges and serve.

Nutrition:
Calories: 130 Carbs: 25g Fat: 3g Protein: 3g

1001.   Coconut Flan

Preparation time: 15 minutes Cooking time: 3 hours & 30 minutes Servings: 8

½ cup of sugar	¼ cup of water
1 12-ounce can evaporate milk	1 15-ounce can cream of coconut
4 large eggs	1 tablespoon brandy or rum or 1 teaspoon vanilla extract

1. Put a rack in a large slow cooker. Mix the sugar plus water in a saucepan. Cook on medium heat within 5 minutes. Simmer within 10 minutes, then put the hot syrup into a 6-cup soufflé dish.
2. In a medium bowl, whisk the evaporated milk and cream of coconut. Beat in the eggs and brandy until blended. Pour the mixture into the soufflé dish.
3. Put it on the rack in the slow cooker. Pour hot water of 1 inch around it. Cover and cook on high within 3 to 3½ hours. Carefully remove the dish, then slice into wedges and serve.

Nutrition:
Calories: 290 Carbs: 46g Fat: 9g Protein: 7g

1002.   Lemon Cheese Flan

Preparation time: 15 minutes Cooking time: 2 hours & 30 minutes Servings: 8

1½ cups sugar	¼ cup of water
1 8-ounce package cream cheese, softened	1 12-ounce can evaporate milk
3 large eggs	1 teaspoon grated lemon zest
1 teaspoon vanilla extract	

1. Put a rack in the slow cooker. Mix one cup of the sugar and the water in a small saucepan. Cook on medium heat within 5 minutes. Simmer within 10 minutes. Put the hot syrup into a 6-cup soufflé dish, let it cool until the caramel is just set.
2. Mix the remaining ½ cup sugar, the cream cheese, evaporated milk, eggs, lemon zest, and vanilla until blended in a large bowl. Pour the mixture into the soufflé dish, then in your slow cooker. Put hot water to a depth of 1 inch around the soufflé dish.
3. Cover and cook on high within 2 to 2½ hours. Remove, then let it cool until chilled in the fridge, several hours or overnight. Serve.

Nutrition:
Calories: 359 Carbs: 31g Fat: 24g Protein: 13g

1003.   Apple Raisin Soufflé Pudding

Preparation time: 15 minutes Cooking time: 2 hours Servings: 8

6 large sweet apples, such as Golden Delicious, peeled and thinly sliced	1 cup golden raisins
¼ cup of sugar	2 tablespoons unsalted butter, melted
1 teaspoon grated lemon zest	2 tablespoons all-purpose flour
2 tablespoons cognac or rum	Topping:
8 tablespoons (1 stick) unsalted butter, softened	½ cup of sugar
3 large eggs, separated	1 cup milk
2 tablespoons cognac or rum (optional)	½ cup all-purpose flour
Pinch of salt	

1. Grease the insert of your large slow cooker with nonstick cooking spray. Add the apples, raisins, sugar, butter, lemon zest, flour, and cognac and toss well. Cover and cook on high within 1½ to 2 hours, or until the apples are softened but not quite tender.
2. Make the topping: When the apples are almost ready, beat the butter with the sugar using an electric mixer in a bowl within 3 minutes. Add the egg yolks and blend well. In a small bowl, stir the milk and cognac, if using. Gently stir the milk mixture into the sugar mixture in 3 additions, alternating with the flour in 2 additions.
3. Whisk the egg whites plus salt on medium speed until foamy in a large bowl with clean beaters. Continue beating until soft peaks form. Mix the egg whites into the yolk batter. Stir the apples. Scrape the topping over the apples.
4. Cover and cook on high within 1 hour. Uncover and remove the insert from the cooker. Let cool slightly. Scoop the pudding onto serving plates and serve warm or at room temperature.

Nutrition:
Calories: 300 Carbs: 47g Fat: 9g Protein: 9g

1004.   Pistachio and Golden Raisin Bread Pudding

Preparation time: 15 minutes Cooking time: 3 hours Servings: 8

8 ounces French bread, torn into bite-size pieces and lightly toasted (about 6 cups)	½ cup golden raisins
½ cup unsalted pistachios	6 large eggs
½ cup of sugar	1 teaspoon ground cinnamon
¼ cup honey	1 tablespoon grated orange zest
3 cups of milk	1½ teaspoons vanilla extract

1. Oiled the insert of a large slow cooker with nonstick cooking spray. Scatter the bread, raisins, and pistachios in the cooker. Mix the eggs

until frothy in a large bowl. Beat in the sugar, cinnamon, honey, and orange zest. Stir in the milk and vanilla.

2. Put the liquid over the bread mixture and stir. Cook on high within 2½ to 3 hours, or until the center is just barely set and slightly puffed. Uncover and remove the insert from the cooker. Let cool slightly. Scoop the pudding into bowls and serve warm.

Nutrition:
Calories: 120 Carbs: 27g Fat: 0g Protein: 3g

1005. White Chocolate Bread Pudding with Rasp Berried Strawberries
Preparation time: 15 minutes Cooking time: 2 hours & 30 minutes
Servings: 8

1 cup chopped white chocolate (10 ounces)	2 cups milk, heated until hot
2/3 cup sugar	1 cup heavy cream
4 large eggs, beaten	2 teaspoons vanilla extract
8 ounces brioche or challah bread, cut into 1-inch cubes and lightly toasted (about 6 cups)	1-pint strawberries, sliced
2–3 tablespoons seedless raspberry jam	

1. Oiled the insert of a large slow cooker with nonstick cooking spray. Place the white chocolate in a large, heatproof bowl. Add the hot milk and sugar and let stand for 5 minutes. Stir until the white chocolate is melted and the sugar is dissolved.
2. Whisk the cream, eggs, and vanilla and stir the mixture into the white chocolate mixture. Scatter the bread cubes in the slow cooker. Pour the white chocolate mixture over the bread. Cover and cook on high for 1 hour. Adjust the heat to low and cook within 1½ hours, or until the pudding is softly set in the center.
3. Uncover and remove the insert from the cooker. Let cool slightly. Meanwhile, toss the berries with the jam and let stand for 30 minutes, until juicy. Scoop the pudding into bowls. Top with the marinated strawberries and serve.

Nutrition:
Calories: 372 Carbs: 31g Fat: 25g Protein: 5g

1006. Rice Pudding Brûlée
Preparation time: 15 minutes Cooking time: 3 hours Servings: 8

4 cups of milk	1 cup heavy cream
¾ cup Arborio rice or another short-grain white rice	2 2-inch strips of orange zest
1 3-inch cinnamon stick	Pinch of salt
2 tablespoons brandy	¾ cup of sugar
Pinch of ground cinnamon	

1. Oiled the insert of a large slow cooker with nonstick cooking spray. Put the milk and cream into the slow cooker. Stir in the rice, orange zest, cinnamon stick, and salt.
2. Cover and cook on high within 2½ to 3 hours, stirring 2 or 3 times so that the rice doesn't stick to the bottom until the rice is tender. Stir in the brandy and ½ cup of the sugar.
3. Cover and cook for 20 minutes more, or until the sugar dissolves. Remove the cinnamon stick and orange zest. Spread the pudding in a shallow, flameproof baking dish and smooth the top.
4. Put a piece of plastic wrap on the pudding and chill within 2 hours or overnight. Just before serving, position an oven rack about 3 inches from the broiler. Turn the broiler to high. Remove the plastic wrap and place the dish on a baking sheet.
5. Stir the remaining ¼ cup sugar and the ground cinnamon. Put the mixture over the surface of the pudding. Place under the broiler for 2 to 3 minutes, or until the sugar is browned and bubbling. Remove the baking dish and let cool for 5 minutes before serving.

Nutrition:
Calories: 70 Carbs: 12g Fat: 2g Protein: 2g

1007. Blushing Pomegranate Pears
Preparation time: 15 minutes Cooking time: 3 hours & 5 minutes
Servings: 8

2/3 cup sugar	2 cups pomegranate juice
2 3-inch strips of orange zest	10 whole black peppercorns
8 firm-ripe pears, such as Bosc or Anjou, peeled	2 tablespoons chopped unsalted pistachios or sliced almonds

1. In a large slow cooker, stir the sugar and juice. Add the orange zest and peppercorns. Put the pears upright in the cooker and put some of the liquid over them. Cook on high within 3 hours, or until the pears are tender when pierced with a knife. Move the pears to a serving dish.
2. Drain the juices through a fine-mesh sieve into a small saucepan. Simmer the juices within 5 minutes. Pour the syrup over the pears. Chill until serving time. Just before serving, sprinkle the pears with the nuts.

Nutrition:
Calories: 210 Carbs: 30g Fat: 8g Protein: 4g

1008. Tea-Spiced Pears
Preparation time: 15 minutes Cooking time: 4 hours Servings: 8

2 Earl Grey tea bags	1 cup boiling water
1 cup dry white wine	¾ cup of sugar
1 2-inch strip orange zest	4 whole cloves
2 whole star anise	8 Bosc, Bartlett, or Anjou pears
Crème fraîche or whipped cream	

1. Let the tea bags stand in boiling water within 3 minutes. Remove, then pour the tea into a large slow cooker. Add the wine, sugar, orange zest, cloves, and star anise and stir well. Wash the pears and place them standing upright in the slow cooker.
2. Cook on low within 4 hours, or until the pears are tender when pierced with a knife. Remove the pears from the syrup. Strain the syrup over the pears. Let cool slightly, then cover and refrigerate. Serve chilled with a dollop of crème fraîche.

Nutrition:
Calories: 200 Carbs: 51g Fat: 0g Protein: 1g

1009. Honeyed Pears with Goat Cheese and Thyme Pears
Preparation time: 15 minutes Cooking time: 4 hours Servings: 8

8 Bosc, Bartlett, or Anjou pears	1 lemon
½ cup of water	½ cup honey
4 ounces fresh goat cheese, sliced	Fresh thyme sprigs

1. Wash the pears and place them standing upright in a large slow cooker. Peel off a 2-inch strip of lemon zest. Squeeze the lemon to get 2 tablespoons juice. In a measuring cup, combine the water, honey, and lemon juice and stir well. Pour the liquid over the pears. Add the zest. Cover and cook on low within 4 hours or on high for 2 hours.
2. Carefully remove the pears from the cooker and pour the juices overall. Cover and chill until serving time. Place a pear on each serving plate. Add a slice or two of goat cheese and garnish with a few thyme sprigs.

Nutrition:
Calories: 165 Carbs: 4g Fat: 13g Protein: 9g

1010. Lemon Pots de Crème Smooth

Preparation time: 15 minutes Cooking time: 2 hours Servings: 4

1/3 cup fresh lemon juice	½ teaspoon grated lemon zest
½ cup of sugar	4 large egg yolks
1 cup heavy cream	

1. Stir the lemon juice, zest, and sugar until the sugar is dissolved. Whisk the egg yolks plus cream until blended in a large bowl. Stir in the lemon juice mixture. Scrape the mixture into four ½-cup custard cups or ramekins. Put a rack in the insert of a large slow cooker. Put the cups on the rack.
2. Put within 1 inch of hot water into the cooker. Cook on high within 2 hours, or until the creams are softly set and slightly jiggly in the center. Uncover and let stand for 10 minutes. Carefully remove the cups from the cooker. Refrigerate within 2 hours, or up to 3 days, before serving.

Nutrition:
Calories: 192 Carbs: 20g Fat: 11g Protein: 4g

1011. Bittersweet Chocolate Creams

Preparation time: 15 minutes Cooking time: 1 hour & 30 minutes Servings: 8

2 tablespoons sugar	3 large eggs
2 cups heavy cream	¼ cup espresso or strong coffee
8 ounces bittersweet (not unsweetened) chocolate, broken into small pieces	1 teaspoon vanilla extract
Chocolate-covered coffee beans (optional)	Whipped cream (optional)

1. Beat the sugar, eggs, cream, and espresso in a heatproof bowl that will fit in the slow cooker until blended and the sugar is dissolved. Add the chocolate and stir well. Place a rack in the insert of a large slow cooker. Place the bowl on the rack. Pour hot water around the bowl to a depth of 1 inch.
2. Cover and cook on high for 1½ hours, or until the chocolate is melted and the surface appears foamy. Carefully remove the bowl from the cooker. Whisk the mixture until blended. Add the vanilla. Spoon the mixture into eight ramekins or demitasse cups. Refrigerate until chilled and serve plain or garnished with the coffee beans and whipped cream.

Nutrition:
Calories: 170 Carbs: 16g Fat: 13g Protein: 3g

1012. Bistro Crème Caramel

Preparation time: 15 minutes Cooking time: hours Servings: 8

1 cup of sugar	¼ cup of water
1 12-ounce can evaporate whole milk	1 14-ounce can sweeten condensed milk
4 large eggs	1 teaspoon vanilla extract

1. Mix the sugar plus water in a saucepan. Cook on medium heat, swirling the pan until the sugar is dissolved. Simmer, then gently swirl the pan until the syrup is evenly caramelized. Protect your hand with an oven mitt and put the hot syrup into a 6-cup soufflé dish.
2. Let it cool until the caramel is just set. Whisk the evaporated and condensed milk in a large bowl. Mix in the eggs plus vanilla until blended. Pour the mixture into the soufflé dish.
3. Put a rack inside a large slow cooker, then arrange the dish on the rack. Put hot water around the dish to a depth of 1 inch. Cover and cook on high within 2 to 2½ hours, then remove. Let it cool in the fridge within several hours or overnight. Cut into wedges and serve.

Nutrition:
Calories: 136 Carbs: 24g Fat: 3g Protein: 4g

2-WEEK MEAL PLAN

Day	Breakfast	Lunch	Snack	Dinner	Dessert
1	Egg & Vegetable Breakfast Casserole	Butcher Style Cabbage Rolls- Pork & Beef Version	Piedmont Fontina Cheese Dip with Truffle Oil Fonduta	Greek Style Lamb Shanks	Apple Olive Cake
2	Breakfast Stuffed Peppers	One-Pot Oriental Lamb	Coarse Pork Terrine with Pistachios	Homemade Meatballs & Spaghetti Squash	Strawberry Basil Cobbler
3	Slow Cooker Frittata	Zucchini Lasagna with Minced Pork	Chicken Liver Pâté with Button Mushrooms	Beef & Cabbage Roast	Pumpkin Pecan Bread Pudding
4	Cranberry Apple Oatmeal	Stuffed Bell Peppers Dolma Style	Warm Tuscan White Bean Salad	Simple Chicken Chili	Chocolate Fondue
5	Blueberry Banana Steel Cut Oats	Slow BBQ Ribs	Stuffed Garlic Mushrooms with Cream and White Wine	Beef Shoulder in BBQ Sauce	Chocolate Orange Volcano Pudding
6	Berry Breakfast Quinoa	Steak & Salsa	Spanish Tortilla with Piquant Tomato Salsa	Moist & Spicy Pulled Chicken Breast	Nutella Fudge
7	Mediterranean Crockpot Breakfast	Beef Pot Roast with Turnips	Vine Leaves Stuffed with Rice, Herbs, Pine Nuts and Raisins	Whole Roasted Chicken	Greek Yogurt Chocolate Mousse
8	Slow Cooker Mediterranean Potatoes	Chili Beef Stew	Spanish Mackerel with Roasted Red Peppers	Pot Roast Beef Brisket	Peanut Butter Banana Greek Yogurt Bowl
9	Mediterranean Crockpot Quiche	Pork Shoulder Roast	Piedmont Fontina Cheese Dip with Truffle Oil Fonduta	Seriously Delicious Lamb Roast	Banana Foster
10	Slow Cooker Meatloaf	Easy & Delicious Chicken Stew	Coarse Pork Terrine with Pistachios	Dress Pork Leg Roast	Rice Pudding
11	Crockpot Chicken Noodle Soup	Chili Con Steak	Chicken Liver Pâté with Button Mushrooms	Rabbit & Mushroom Stew	Bittersweet Cocoa Almond Cake
12	Hash Brown & Cheddar Breakfast	One-Pot Chicken and Green Beans	Warm Tuscan White Bean Salad	Italian Spicy Sausage & Bell Peppers	Walnut Cake with Cinnamon Syrup
13	Slow Cooker Fava Beans	Two-Meat Chili	Stuffed Garlic Mushrooms with Cream and White Wine	Chicken in Salsa Verde	Sunny Orange Cake with Orange Syrup
14	Pork Sausage Breakfast	Slightly Addictive Pork Curry	Spanish Tortilla with Piquant Tomato Salsa	Salmon Poached in White Wine & Lemon	Two-Berry Clafouti

CONCLUSION

The Mediterranean is a prominent place. Dozens of different cultures and languages and cuisines blend together, but this and its lush climate are part of the reason it's such a culinary powerhouse today. It's a bounty for both the soul and the body, fit for a peasant or an emperor. Hopefully, this carried you to wherever you wanted to be – whether that was health, performance, or simple curiosity.

This cookbook was not intended to be the be-all-end-all publication on Mediterranean food, but it was structured to serve as a knowledge basis – to give you a complete idea of the most basics of where to look when it comes to making choices for yourself. Just the essentials and then enough to get you started, with enough to carry you in confidence. We also tried to give you a reliable, calorie-precise guide to what you'll be eating, not so you can obsessively track every calorie, but so you can start thinking about the food choices you make every day in hopes that it will encourage you to find your way to a healthy lifestyle.

Changing your diet isn't a simple thing, but hopefully, we'll provided enough examples to inspire you on a culinary journey. Cooking and eating is a fundamental part of existence, and it is also one of the most rewarding for the body and spirit.

We emphasize how the Mediterranean diet and slow cookers can be a beautiful combination if you want to try a healthier version of the food you eat. Slow cooking can be a radical change to those that have lived their entire lives hectically and impatiently. However, once you get used to the genuine taste that great food can deliver through a slow cooker, you will quickly adjust your schedule.

Quicker and faster is not always better, especially when it comes to instant food or fast foods, which is unhealthy, as we have seen in an overweight society and harnesses several ailments. This was designed to learn the basics and assets that slow cooking can bring to your life with a little twist of Mediterranean cuisine. You will find that there is no extra burden of time placed upon your schedule but a simple rearrangement of habit.

Once you have this new form of cooking blended into your routine, several cookbooks are designed for specific weight-loss diets, diabetic slow cooking, or even going Vegetarian. A slow cooker is one of the best and fabulous appliances that you can own. Follow the 2-week plan for putting menus in place and discover that you have more time than you did by opening a box and preparing the contents. You will find yourself switching to healthier foods, saving on groceries, and using less energy.

The slow cooker can be an essential part of your life when you realize the multiple advantages it provides in cooking healthy meals. Keep this cookbook handy and learn why slow cooker cooking is making such a famous comeback. You will discover that the slow cooker has always been a valuable tool, but perhaps, a little ahead of its time, for being noticed and appreciated.

At the very least, we have enriched your life in the smallest way. Enjoy your Mediterranean meals with your friends and family to the best effect. Whatever you've gleaned from this cookbook, the one thing we must say is Bon appétit!

CPSIA information can be obtained
at www.ICGtesting.com
Printed in the USA
LVHW051509191122
733599LV00004B/69